Inside you'll find easy-to-read entries such as . . .

Zantac 75
Pronounced ZAN-tack
Generic name: Ranitidine hydrochloride

What this drug is used for

Zantac 75 relieves heartburn, acid indigestion, and sour stomach. It is part of a family of acid-blocking prescription drugs recently released in over-the-counter formulations. Other members of the family are Axid AR, Mylanta AR, Pepcid AC, and Tagamet HB.

How should you take this medication?

Swallow 1 tablet with water. Do not chew. Take no more than 2 tablets a day.

■ STORAGE
Store at room temperature. Protect from high heat or humidity.

Do not take this medication if . . .

Not for children under 12, unless your doctor approves.

Special warnings about this medication

Do not take 2 tablets of Zantac 75 every day for more than 2 weeks without your doctor's approval. If you have trouble swallowing, or you have stomach pain that does not go away, see your doctor right away. You may have a serious condition that needs treatment.

Possible food and drug interactions when taking this medication

Alcohol, blood-thinning drugs, diabetes medications

THE PDR®
FAMILY GUIDE
TO OVER-THE-COUNTER DRUGS™

BALLANTINE BOOKS • NEW YORK

A Ballantine Book
Published by The Ballantine Publishing Group
Copyright © 1997 by Medical Economics Company, Inc.

All rights reserved under International and Pan-American Copyright Conventions. Published in the United States by The Ballantine Publishing Group, a division of Random House, Inc., New York, and simultaneously in Canada by Random House of Canada Limited, Toronto.

None of the content of this publication may be reproduced or transmitted in any form or by any means, electronic or mechanical, including photocopying, recording, or by any information storage and retrieval system, without permission in writing from Medical Economics Company, Inc., Five Paragon Drive, Montvale, NJ 07645.

http://www.randomhouse.com

Library of Congress Catalog Card Number: 97-97165

ISBN 0-345-41716-X

Manufactured in the United States of America

First Edition: February 1998

10 9 8 7 6 5 4

PHYSICIANS' DESK REFERENCE®, PDR®, PHYSICIANS' DESK REFERENCE for Nonprescription Drugs®, PDR for Nonprescription Drugs®, and The PDR® Family Guide to Prescription Drugs® are registered trademarks used herein under license. PDR® Family Guides™, The PDR® Family Guide to Over-The-Counter Drugs™, The PDR® Family Guide to Women's Health and Prescription Drugs™, The PDR® Family Guide to Nutrition and Health™, and PDR Guide to Interactions, Side Effects, Indications, Contraindications™ are trademarks used herein under license.

Contents

Publisher's Note

The drug information contained in this book is based on product labeling published in the 1997 editions of *Physicians' Desk Reference®* and *Physicians' Desk Reference for Nonprescription Drugs®,* supplemented with facts from other sources the publisher believes reliable. While diligent efforts have been made to assure the accuracy of this information, the book does not list every possible action, adverse reaction, interaction, and precaution; and all information is presented without guarantees by the authors, consultants, and publisher, who disclaim all liability in connection with its use.

This book is intended only as an aid in the rational selection and use of nonprescription health products. It is not a subsitiute for a doctor's professional judgement on matters of health. All readers are urged to consult with a physician whenever a question arises about the safety or efficacy of any medication, be it available over-the-counter or by prescription only.

Brand names listed in this book are intended to represent only the more commonly used products. Inclusion of a brand name does not signify endorsement of the product; absense of a name does not imply a criticism or rejection of the product. The publisher is not advocating the use of any product described in this book, does not warrant or guarantee any of these products, and has not performed any independent analysis in connection with the product information contained herein.

The PDR® Family Guide
to Over-the-Counter Drugs™

Editor-in-Chief: David W. Sifton
Director of Professional Services: Mukesh Mehta, R.Ph.
Art Director: Robert Hartman

Assistant Editors: Paula Benus; Gwynned L. Kelly, Ann Marevis

Writers: Lynn H. Buechler; Deborah Epstein, Gregory A. Freeman; Kris Hallam; Jayne Jacobson; Lisa A. Maher; James Morelli, R.Ph.; Kavitha Pareddy, R.Ph., M.S.; Theresa Waldron

Editorial Production: *Vice President of Production:* David Pitler; *Director of Print Purchasing:* Marjorie A. Duffy; *Director of Production:* Carrie Williams; *Manager of Production:* Kimberly Hiller-Vivas; *Electronic Publishing Coordinator:* Joanne M. Pearson; *Electronic Publishing Designer:* Robert K. Grossman; *Senior Digital Imaging Coordinator:* Shawn W. Cahill; *Digital Imaging Coordinator:* Frank J. McElroy, III

Medical Economics Company

**Executive Vice President
and Chief Operating Officer:** Rick Noble

Vice President of Directory Services: Stephen B. Greenberg

Product Manager: Mark A. Friedman

Director of Trade and Direct Marketing Sales: Robin B. Bartlett; **National Sales Manager:** Bill Gaffney

Getting the Most out of Over-the-Counter Medications

If you feel confused when you go to buy an over-the-counter drug, you're far from alone. Available everywhere without a prescription, these remarkable household remedies promise relief from an ever-growing number of troubling ailments. But as more and more reach the market, the blizzard of claims and counterclaims is becoming almost impossible to sort out.

That's the dilemma the first section of this book sets out to solve. To help you zero in on the best products to consider, the Product Selection Tables in Part 1 allow you to make the kind of point-by-point comparisons you never have time for in the store. The Product Profiles in Part 2 follow up with detailed information on when, how, and why to take each product, who should avoid it, and what to watch out for while using it.

If you're taking any prescription medications, you also need to worry about possible interactions; so Part 3 provides you with detailed lists of the conflicts you could encounter. And because even over-the-counter drugs sometimes cause unpleasant side effects, Part 4 lists the products responsible for each type of reaction. Together, these four references can help you quickly find the product that best fits your own unique needs.

The selection process is really quite simple. Here, step by step, is what you need to do.

1. Decide on the problem
Many over-the-counter drugs attack a variety of symptoms; and the more symptoms they cover, the more ingredients they're likely to have. With each extra ingredient, the chance of a conflict with other medical conditions increases, as do the chances of side effects and interactions with other medications.

It's wise, therefore, to look for products that target only the symptoms that trouble you. If you have a cough, use a simple cough remedy with few, if any, side effects instead of a multi-symptom cold product that could cause drowsiness, dizziness, and more. Likewise, if your main problem is a stuffy nose, stick with a nasal decongestant rather than a general hay fever remedy—most decongestants won't cause drowsiness, many allergy products will.

The tables in Part 1 are organized by the symptom or group of symptoms that each product fights. Look through the list of headings at the beginning of the section and find the one that best describes your problem. Then consider only the products under that heading. This automatically limits the number of products you need to evaluate and assures that you'll be getting a medicine specifically designed to relieve your main problems, and those problems alone.

2. Check active ingredients

In the Part 1 comparison tables, each product's active ingredients appear right next to the brand name. Checking these ingredients can save you a lot of frustration. You'll quickly find that many brands contain the same basic medicine—and if one of these brands doesn't work for you, you can be relatively certain that the others won't either.

For example, if Afrin 12 Hour Nasal Spray doesn't clear up your stuffy nose, there's little reason to try 4-Way 12 Hour Nasal Spray, which contains exactly the same medicine. Instead, you might want to try brands such as Privine or Sudafed, which contain completely different active ingredients.

The ingredient listings also allow you to quickly identify products that contain a medicine you need to avoid. If, for instance, you have an ulcer and can't take aspirin, the comparison tables will show you at a glance which products contain that ingredient.

3. Compare dosing instructions

Some people like short-acting medications that can be taken only as needed. Others want a long-acting product they can take once and forget for the rest of the day. To help you find the type you prefer, the comparison tables include each product's recommended frequency of dosing.

4. Look for medical conflicts

The comparison tables also list the chronic medical conditions—such as asthma, high blood pressure, or diabetes—that a product may aggravate. This allows you to quickly identify the brands you may need to avoid. (Check with your doctor to make certain.)

If you have kidney problems, for example, you'll find that certain antacids—such as Di-Gel and Maalox—should be avoided, while others—Tums, Rolaids, Pepcid AC—are okay to take.

If you're taking any prescription medicines, you'll also want to check the table in Part 3, which lists possible interactions with each over-the-counter remedy.

5. Check for unwanted extras

In addition to their active ingredients, many over-the-counter products contain small amounts of alcohol, sugar, lactose, or sodium. If you need to watch your intake of one of these substances, the comparison tables will quickly alert you to the products that contain it. If you find that a brand you're considering *does* include the offending ingredient, you can almost always find a comparable product doesn't.

6. Read up on your choices

Once you've narrowed the field down to two or three promising candidates, you can get additional information on all of them in Part 2, where each brand is profiled in full. There you'll find the following:

■ WHAT THIS DRUG IS USED FOR: Presents a detailed summary of the symptoms the product relieves, plus information on available forms, strengths, and related products.

■ HOW YOU SHOULD TAKE THIS MEDICATION: Provides complete instructions for use, plus the usual dosage for each age group and the manufacturer's storage recommendations.

■ DO NOT TAKE THIS MEDICATION IF: Gives the circumstances in which you should completely avoid the product, and those in which you should get a doctor's approval before beginning its use.

■ SPECIAL WARNINGS ABOUT THIS MEDICATION: Lists the signs that mean you need professional care. Gives possible side effects and what to do if they occur.

■ POSSIBLE FOOD AND DRUG INTERACTIONS: Summarizes the harmful combinations to avoid.

■ OVERDOSAGE: Lists specific symptoms that should alert you to danger. ·

Choosing a vitamin supplement

Multivitamin products—many with over two dozen ingredients—pose an especially difficult challenge for consumers. It's just about impossible to compare so many ingredients in the scores of products competing for attention, so most people tend to throw in the towel, read only the big type, and select on the basis of catchwords like "antioxidant," "complete," or "therapeutic."

To get you past this problem, Section II of this book includes Product Selection Tables that line up the exact amounts of each government-recommended vitamin and mineral found in the most common vitamin/mineral supplements. If you're especially concerned about your intake of Vitamin E, for example, all you need do is glance down the appropriate column to instantly find the products with the largest amounts. And if you're wondering just how much of a vitamin you really need—and how much you're already getting—you can turn to the Vitamin/Mineral Profiles in Section II for at least an approximate answer.

These profiles are designed to quickly give you the essential facts about each of the most common nutrients, answering questions such as:

■ WHAT IT IS: Gives a brief overview of the substance's role in your diet.

■ WHAT IT DOES: Describes the nutrient's action inside the body; tells which systems and functions it affects the most.

■ WHY YOU NEED IT: Summarizes the nutrient's impact on your health; gives the symptoms of a deficiency.

■ CAN YOU TAKE TOO MUCH: Many vitamins and minerals can be extremely toxic when taken in massive amounts. In this section, you'll find the symptoms of long-term overdosage.

■ RECOMMENDED DAILY ALLOWANCES: Gives official or commonly accepted daily requirements; tells which groups need more, and who may need to avoid extra amounts.

■ BEST DIETARY SOURCES: Lists foods with the highest content of the nutrient.

Making a savvy purchase

Whether you're simply deciding on a new vitamin supplement or need to find an over-the-counter remedy that precisely fits your needs, the Product Selection Tables, the detailed Product Profiles, and the Interaction Tables, you have just about all the information you need to make an effective, economical purchase.

When choosing a medication, always focus on these two key concerns:

■ YOUR SPECIFIC SYMPTOMS
■ THE PRODUCT'S INGREDIENTS

Many cold products, for instance, rely on the same limited set of active ingredients, mixed and matched a dozen different ways. If one brand works well for you, chances are there's another that contains the same mixture—possibly at a lower price. Using the tables in Part 1, it's easy to find these comparable brands. And when you do, you can usually substitute the thriftier choice.

Don't, however, let special deals or sales enter into your decision unless the products are completely comparable. And don't pay attention to marketing hype. You'll find, for instance, that many products are labeled "extra strength" or "maximum strength" even though the brand comes in no other strength at all. When that's the case, you can usually ignore the verbiage and buy strictly on the basis of ingredients that work well for you.

On the other hand, don't let your natural doubts and skepticism stand between you and an important new remedy. The drug industry is bringing more medical breakthroughs to market each year—most recently the acid blockers that keep heartburn from ever happening, several potent new pain relievers, and yeast-infection cures that formerly required a doctor's prescription.

These products can make a real difference in your health and well-being. Never hesitate to give them a try. Medical science is making more progress now than ever before, and you owe it to yourself to take full advantage of its benefits.

Using Over-the-Counter Medicines Safely

Compared with many of the potent medications prescribed by doctors, medicines available without a prescription pose relatively little risk. Still, it's important to remember that they are drugs. Misused or overused, they can cause unpleasant—even dangerous—side effects. Here are some precautions to remember whenever you take an over-the-counter drug.

■ When pregnant, check with your doctor before using any drug.

Most over-the-counter medicines have never been implicated in a case of harm or damage to an unborn child. On the other hand, few drugs have ever been conclusively *proven* safe through scientific tests on pregnant women. Therefore, if you're pregnant—or even think you may be—your most prudent course is to ask your doctor about any medication you plan to take.

A few over-the-counter products, including aspirin, are definitely known to pose some degree of risk and should be avoided almost without question. When that's the situation, you'll see it noted in the drug's profile in Part 2 of this book.

■ After an overdose, always seek medical assistance

Even if you see no ill effects, call your doctor or go to an emergency room immediately. Massive overdoses of over-the-counter products can be dangerous, and the toxic effects sometimes take several hours to develop. If you wait for symptoms to appear, you'll have wasted crucial hours that could have been used for emergency treatment.

Don't be lulled into a false sense of safety by a relatively minor reaction, either. An overdose of some over-the-counter drugs may cause little more than a stomach upset at first, yet wreak hidden damage as the days go by. Early treatment of such an overdose can make the difference between complete recovery and lasting injury.

■ Never exceed the recommended dose.

It's tempting to assume that if a little is good, a lot will be better; but drugs don't work that way. Higher-than-called-for doses usually yield no extra benefit and sometimes make symptoms worse. Excessive doses also dramatically increase the odds of side effects that rarely if ever appear at recommended dosage levels. With drugs it's especially easy to get too much of a good thing.

■ Never take a drug more often than recommended.

Taking a drug too often is the same as taking too much. Doses are timed to keep an effective level of medicine in your body. Speeding up that timetable can lead to a buildup of the drug, ending in the same toxic effects you would get from an overdose. (With some drugs, it takes months for this to happen; but happen it will.)

■ Don't use a drug after its expiration date.

Expiration dates are like the last-sale date on meat, poultry, and seafood—after that date, you can assume the product's gone bad. An expired drug may not make you as sick as rancid fish, but it probably won't help you either.

■ Keep all drugs away from children.

Over-the-counter drugs are no exception to this rule. Indeed, an over-the-counter overdose is likely to pose more of a danger to the very young. For safety's sake, follow these six simple guidelines:

1. Keep all medications—including "harmless" pain relievers and laxatives—in a locked cabinet or in a spot well out of the reach of children.

2. When buying over-the-counter remedies, look for childproof caps.

3. Avoid mixups—make sure you're fully awake and alert when giving a child medication.

4. Make sure that children know any medication can be dangerous if misused.

5. Keep antidotes such as Syrup of Ipecac on hand, in case your doctor recommends one.

6. Always have the numbers of your local emergency medical service and poison control center close at hand.

■ Be cautious when mixing over-the-counter remedies and prescription drugs.

Most over-the-counter medicines can—and will—interfere with certain prescription drugs, either reducing their benefits or aggravating their side effects. Here's how to avoid potential conflicts:

1. Make sure your doctor is aware of all medications you are taking—including over-the-counter remedies.

2. When your doctor gives you a new prescription, ask if there are any drugs you should avoid combining with it.

3. When buying an over-the-counter drug, check the interactions listings in Part 3 of this book. If any of your prescriptions are on the list, check with your doctor before you buy.

4. If an over-the-counter drug gives you a reaction, let your doctor know. It could mean you need to avoid a whole class of similar drugs and could even signal an unsuspected medical condition.

■ Make sure you know what you're taking.

Keep all medicines—both prescription and over-the-counter—in their original bottles. Don't mix pills together in a single bottle; it's too easy to forget what the different pills are. And always check the label before taking a drug. Taking pills in the dark could be dangerous if you grab the wrong ones.

I. Over-the-Counter Remedies

1. Product Selection Tables

This section provides you with the key facts you need to find a sensible choice among the host of over-the-counter remedies competing for your dollars. To locate the leading medicines for any particular problem, simply skim through the *Medication Finder* on the next page and turn to the heading that best describes your symptoms. There, you'll find each product listed with its active ingredients and manufacturer, its recommended frequency of administration, a list of medical conditions that could make the product an unwise choice, and a handy checklist of the product's alcohol, sugar, lactose, and sodium content. When available, products formulated specifically for children are listed separately.

The tables will quickly show you which brands contain the same active ingredients, which conflict with any chronic problems you may have, and which are free of a substance you may need to avoid. Because most of this information involves a product's effects *within* your system, coverage is limited primarily to oral medications. The ingredients in creams, salves, and ointments sometimes get into the system in trace amounts, but usually pose little, if any, problem. Such products have therefore been left out.

The information in these tables is extracted from the manufacturer's own package labeling as published in *PDR for Nonprescription Drugs*, the physician's professional guide to over-the-counter medications. The tables include only brands listed by PDR; store brands and generics do not appear.

Medication Finder

ACID STOMACH, ADULTS

BRAND	ACTIVE INGREDIENTS (MANUFACTURER)	HOW OFTEN TO TAKE	GET MD APPROVAL IF YOU HAVE:	ALCOHOL-FREE	SUGAR-FREE	LACTOSE-FREE	SODIUM-FREE
Alka-Mints	Calcium carbonate (Bayer)	Every 2 hours	—	Yes	No	Yes	No
Alka-Seltzer Gold	Citric acid, Potassium bicarbonate, Sodium bicarbonate (Bayer)	Every 4 hours	—	Yes	Yes	Yes	No
ALternaGEL	Aluminum hydroxide, Sodium (J & J Merck)	Between meals and at bedtime	Kidney disease	Yes	Yes	Yes	No
Amphojel	Aluminum hydroxide, Sodium (Wyeth-Ayerst)	5 to 6 times a day	Kidney disease	Yes	Yes	Yes	No
Axid AR	Nizatidine (Whitehall-Robins)	1 or 2 times a day	Persistent abdominal pain, difficulty swallowing	Yes	Yes	Yes	Yes
Basaljel	Aluminum carbonate (Wyeth-Ayerst)	Every 2 hours	Kidney disease	Yes	Yes	Yes	Yes

Di-Gel Tablets	Calcium carbonate, Magnesium hydroxide, Simethicone (*Schering-Plough*)	Every 2 hours	Kidney disease	Yes	No	No	Yes
Di-Gel Liquid	Aluminum hydroxide, Magnesium hydroxide, Simethicone (*Schering-Plough*)	Every 2 hours	Kidney disease	Yes	Yes	Yes	Yes
Gaviscon	Aluminum hydroxide, Magnesium (*SmithKline Beecham*)	4 times a day	Kidney disease (liquid only)	Tablets only	Liquid only	Liquid only	No
Maalox	Aluminum hydroxide, Magnesium (*Novartis*)	4 times a day	Kidney disease	Yes	Yes	Yes	Yes
Maalox Antacid/ Anti-Gas	Aluminum hydroxide, Magnesium hydroxide, Simethicone (*Novartis*)	4 times a day	Kidney disease	Yes	Liquid only	Liquid only	No
Mylanta AR	Famotidine (*J&J Merck*)	1 or 2 times a day	Persistent abdominal pain, difficulty swallowing	Yes	Yes	Yes	Yes

BRAND	ACTIVE INGREDIENTS (MANUFACTURER)	HOW OFTEN TO TAKE	GET MD APPROVAL IF YOU HAVE:	ALCOHOL-FREE	SUGAR-FREE	LACTOSE-FREE	SODIUM-FREE
Mylanta Liquid	Aluminum hydroxide, Magnesium hydroxide, Simethicone (J&J Merck)	Between meals and at bedtime	Kidney disease	Yes	Yes	Yes	No
Mylanta Tablets and Gelcaps	Calcium carbonate, Magnesium hydroxide (J&J Merck)	Gelcaps: as needed; Tablets: between meals and at bedtime	Kidney disease	Tablets only	Gelcaps only	Gelcaps Yes	No
Mylanta Soothing Lozenges	Calcium carbonate (J&J Merck)	Every 2 hours	—	Yes	No	Yes	Yes
Nephrox	Aluminum hydroxide, Mineral oil (Fleming)	At bedtime	Pregnancy, nursing	Yes	Yes	Yes	No
Pepcid AC	Famotidine (J&J Merck)	1 or 2 times a day	Persistent abdominal pain, difficulty swallowing	Yes	Yes	Yes	Yes

Product	Ingredients (Manufacturer)	Dosage	Warning				
Phillips' Milk of Magnesia	Magnesium hydroxide (*Bayer*)	4 times a day	Kidney disease	Yes	Orig. and Mint only	Yes	Orig. only
Rolaids	Calcium carbonate, Magnesium hydroxide (*Warner-Lambert*)	Every hour	—	Yes	No	Yes	Yes
Tagamet HB	Cimetidine (*SmithKline Beecham*)	1 or 2 times a day	Persistent abdominal pain, difficulty swallowing	Yes	Yes	Yes	No
Titralac	Calcium carbonate (*3M*)	Every 2 to 3 hours	—	Yes	Yes	Yes	No
Titralac Plus	Calcium carbonate, Simethicone (*3M*)	Tablets: Every 2 to 3 hours; Liquid: between meals and at bedtime	—	Tablets only	Yes	Yes	No

BRAND	ACTIVE INGREDIENTS (MANUFACTURER)	HOW OFTEN TO TAKE	GET MD APPROVAL IF YOU HAVE:	ALCOHOL-FREE	SUGAR-FREE	LACTOSE-FREE	SODIUM-FREE
Tums (Regular, E-X, Ultra)	Calcium carbonate (*SmithKline Beecham*)	Hourly	—	Yes	Sugar-free varieties only	Yes	Reg. and sugar-free only
Tums Antigas/Antacid Formula	Calcium carbonate, Simethicone (*SmithKline Beecham*)	Hourly	—	Yes	No	Yes	Yes
Zantac 75	Ranitidine (*Warner-Lambert*)	1 or 2 times a day	Persistent abdominal pain, difficulty swallowing	Yes	Yes	Yes	Yes

ACID STOMACH, CHILDREN

BRAND	ACTIVE INGREDIENTS (MANUFACTURER)	HOW OFTEN TO TAKE	GET MD APPROVAL IF YOU HAVE:	ALCOHOL-FREE	SUGAR-FREE	LACTOSE-FREE	SODIUM-FREE
Children's Mylanta	Calcium carbonate (*J&J Merck*)	Up to 3 times a day	—	Yes	Liquid only	Yes	Tablets only

APPETITE SUPPRESSION

Acutrim (*Novartis*)	Phenylpropanolamine	Once a day	High blood pressure, depression, eating disorder, heart disease, diabetes, thyroid disease, enlarged prostate gland	Steady Control and Maximum Strength only	Yes	Yes	Yes
Dexatrim (*Thompson Medical*)	Phenylpropanolamine	Once a day	High blood pressure, depression, eating disorder, heart disease, diabetes, thyroid disease	Yes	Yes	Yes	Vit. C form has sodium

ARTHRITIS PAIN, MINOR

Actron (*Bayer*)	Ketoprofen	Every 4 to 6 hours	Redness or swelling in painful area, an allergy to pain relievers, last 3 months of pregnancy	Yes	Yes	No	No
Advil (*Whitehall-Robins*)	Ibuprofen	Every 4 to 6 hours	An allergy to aspirin, problems with other pain relievers, last 3 months of pregnancy	Yes	Gel caplets only	Yes	No

BRAND	ACTIVE INGREDIENTS (MANUFACTURER)	HOW OFTEN TO TAKE	GET MD APPROVAL IF YOU HAVE:	ALCOHOL-FREE	SUGAR-FREE	LACTOSE-FREE	SODIUM-FREE
Aleve	Naproxen sodium (Procter & Gamble)	Every 8 to 12 hours (adults over 65: Every 12 hours)	An allergy to pain relievers, last 3 months of pregnancy	Yes	Yes	Yes	Yes
Ascriptin	Alumina-magnesia, Aspirin, Calcium carbonate (Novartis)	Every 4 hours; Maximum Strength: Every 6 hours	Asthma, heartburn, upset stomach, stomach pain, ulcers, bleeding problems, an allergy to aspirin, last 3 months of pregnancy	Yes	Yes	Yes	Yes
Ascriptin Enteric	Aspirin (Novartis)	Every 4 hours	Asthma, heartburn, upset stomach, stomach pain, ulcers, bleeding problems, an allergy to aspirin, last 3 months of pregnancy	Yes	Yes	Yes	No
Bayer Aspirin Regimen	Aspirin (Bayer)	Every 4 to 6 hours	Asthma, heartburn, upset stomach, stomach pain, ulcers, bleeding problems, an allergy to aspirin, last 3 months of pregnancy	Yes	Yes	325-mg caplet only	325-mg caplet only

Product	Ingredients	Dosage	Warnings				
Bayer (Genuine, Extra Strength, Extended-Release, Arthritis Pain)	Aspirin (*Bayer*)	Every 4 hours; Arthritis Pain: Every 6 hours; Extended-Release: Every 8 hours	Asthma, heartburn, upset stomach, stomach pain, ulcers, bleeding problems, an allergy to aspirin, last 3 months of pregnancy	Yes	Yes	Yes	Yes
BC Powder	Aspirin, Caffeine, Salicylamide (*Block Drug*)	Every 3 to 4 hours	An allergy to aspirin, last 3 months of pregnancy	NA	NA	NA	NA
Bufferin (Regular, Extra, and Arthritis Strengths)	Aspirin, Calcium carbonate, Magnesium carbonate, Magnesium oxide (*Bristol-Myers*)	Every 4 hours; Extra and Arthritis Strengths: Every 6 hours	Asthma, heartburn, upset stomach, stomach pain, ulcers, bleeding problems, an allergy to aspirin, last 3 months of pregnancy	Yes	Yes	Yes	No

BRAND	ACTIVE INGREDIENTS (MANUFACTURER)	HOW OFTEN TO TAKE	GET MD APPROVAL IF YOU HAVE:	ALCOHOL-FREE	SUGAR-FREE	LACTOSE-FREE	SODIUM-FREE
Ecotrin	Aspirin (SmithKline Beecham)	Every 4 to 6 hours	Asthma, heartburn, upset stomach, stomach pain, ulcers, bleeding problems, an allergy to aspirin, last 3 months of pregnancy	Yes	Yes	Yes	81-mg tablet only
Excedrin	Acetaminophen, Aspirin, Caffeine (Bristol-Myers)	Every 6 hours	Asthma, heartburn, upset stomach, stomach pain, ulcers, bleeding problems, an allergy to aspirin, last 3 months of pregnancy	Yes	Yes	Yes	No
Excedrin, Aspirin Free	Acetaminophen, Caffeine (Bristol-Myers)	Every 6 hours	—	Yes	Yes	Yes	No
Goody's	Acetaminophen, Aspirin, Caffeine (Block Drug)	Every 4 to 6 hours	An allergy to aspirin, last 3 months of pregnancy	Yes	Yes	Tablets only	Yes
Motrin IB	Ibuprofen (Pharmacia & Upjohn)	Every 4 to 6 hours	An allergy to aspirin, problems with other pain relievers, last 3 months of pregnancy	Caplets and tablets only	Yes	Yes	Caplets and tablets only

Nuprin	Ibuprofen (*Bristol-Myers*)	Every 4 to 6 hours	An allergy to aspirin, problems with other pain relievers, last 3 months of pregnancy	Yes	Yes	Yes	Yes
Orudis KT	Ketoprofen (*Whitehall-Robins*)	Every 4 to 6 hours	Redness or swelling in painful area, an allergy to pain relievers, last 3 months of pregnancy	Yes	No	Yes	No
Panadol	Acetaminophen (*SmithKline Beecham*)	Every 4 hours	—	Yes	Yes	Yes	Yes
Tylenol	Acetaminophen (*McNeil*)	Every 4 to 6 hours; Extended Relief: Every 8 hours	—	Caplets and tablets only	Tablets, caplets, gelcaps, and geltabs only	Yes	No
Vanquish	Acetaminophen, Aluminum hydroxide, Aspirin, Caffeine, Magnesium hydroxide (*Bayer*)	Every 4 hours	Asthma, heartburn, upset stomach, stomach pain, ulcers, bleeding problems, an allergy to aspirin, last 3 months of pregnancy	Yes	Yes	Yes	Yes

BACKACHE

BRAND	ACTIVE INGREDIENTS (MANUFACTURER)	HOW OFTEN TO TAKE	GET MD APPROVAL IF YOU HAVE:	ALCOHOL-FREE	SUGAR-FREE	LACTOSE-FREE	SODIUM-FREE
Actron	Ketoprofen (Bayer)	Every 4 to 6 hours	Redness or swelling in painful area, an allergy to pain relievers, last 3 months of pregnancy	Yes	Yes	No	No
Advil	Ibuprofen (Whitehall-Robins)	Every 4 to 6 hours	Side effects from pain relievers, a serious medical condition, last 3 months of pregnancy	Yes	Gel caplets only	Yes	No
Aleve	Naproxen sodium (Procter & Gamble)	Every 8 to 12 hours; Adults over 65: Every 12 hours	An allergy to pain relievers, last 3 months of pregnancy	Yes	Yes	Yes	Yes
Backache Caplets	Magnesium salicylate tetrahydrate (Bristol-Myers)	Every 6 hours	Asthma, heartburn, upset stomach, stomach pain, ulcers, bleeding problems, an allergy to salicylates (aspirin)	Yes	Yes	Yes	Yes

Product	Active Ingredient (Maker)	Dosage	Do Not Use If You Have					
Bayer 8-Hour Extended-Release	Aspirin (*Bayer*)	Every 8 hours	Asthma, heartburn, upset stomach, stomach pain, ulcers, bleeding problems, an allergy to aspirin, last 3 months of pregnancy	Yes	Yes	Yes	Yes	Yes
Doan's	Magnesium salicylate tetrahydrate (*Novartis*)	Every 4 hours; Extra Strength: Every 6 hours	Heartburn, upset stomach, stomach pain, ulcers, bleeding problems, an allergy to salicylates (aspirin)	Yes	Yes	Yes	Yes	Yes
Doan's P.M.	Diphenhydramine, Magnesium salicylate tetrahydrate (*Novartis*)	At bedtime	Breathing problems, glaucoma, prostate enlargement, stomach problems, ulcers, bleeding problems, an allergy to salicylates (aspirin)	Yes	Yes	Yes	Yes	No
Goody's	Acetaminophen, Aspirin, Caffeine (*Block Drug*)	Every 4 to 6 hours	An allergy to aspirin, last 3 months of pregnancy	Yes	Yes	Yes	Tablets only	Yes
Midol Menstrual Formula	Acetaminophen, Caffeine, Pyrilamine (*Bayer*)	Every 4 hours	Breathing problems, glaucoma	Yes	Yes	Yes	Yes	No

BRAND	ACTIVE INGREDIENTS (MANUFACTURER)	HOW OFTEN TO TAKE	GET MD APPROVAL IF YOU HAVE:	ALCOHOL-FREE	SUGAR-FREE	LACTOSE-FREE	SODIUM-FREE
Midol PMS Formula	Acetaminophen, Pamabrom, Pyrilamine (*Bayer*)	Every 4 hours	Breathing problems, glaucoma	Yes	Yes	Yes	No
Midol Teen Menstrual Formula	Acetaminophen, Pamabrom (*Bayer*)	Every 4 hours	—	Yes	Yes	Yes	No
Motrin IB	Ibuprofen (*Pharmacia & Upjohn*)	Every 4 to 6 hours	An allergy to aspirin, problems with other pain relievers, last 3 months of pregnancy	Caplets and tablets only	Yes	Yes	Caplets and tablets only
Nuprin	Ibuprofen (*Bristol-Myers*)	Every 4 to 6 hours	An allergy to aspirin, problems with other pain relievers, last 3 months of pregnancy	Yes	Yes	Yes	Yes
Orudis KT	Ketoprofen (*Whitehall-Robins*)	Every 4 to 6 hours	Redness or swelling in painful area, an allergy to pain relievers, last 3 months of pregnancy	Yes	No	Yes	No

Product	Ingredients (Manufacturer)	Dosage	Don't use if you have				
Pamprin Maximum Pain Relief	Acetaminophen, Magnesium salicylate, Pamabrom (*Chattem*)	Every 4 to 6 hours	An allergy to salicylates (aspirin), last 3 months of pregnancy	Yes	Yes	Yes	No
Pamprin Multi-Symptom	Acetaminophen, Pamabrom, Pyrilamine (*Chattem*)	Every 4 to 6 hours	Breathing problems, glaucoma	Yes	Yes	Yes	No
Panadol	Acetaminophen (*SmithKline Beecham*)	Every 4 hours	—	Yes	Yes	Yes	Yes
St. Joseph	Aspirin (*Schering-Plough*)	Every 4 hours	Asthma, heartburn, upset stomach, stomach pain, ulcers, bleeding problems, an allergy to aspirin, last 3 months of pregnancy	Yes	Yes	Yes	Yes
Tylenol (Regular, Extra Strength, Extended Relief)	Acetaminophen (*McNeil*)	Every 4 to 6 hours; Extended Relief: Every 8 hours	—	Caplets and tablets only	Tablets, caplets, gelcaps, and geltabs only	Yes	No

BRAND	ACTIVE INGREDIENTS (MANUFACTURER)	HOW OFTEN TO TAKE	GET MD APPROVAL IF YOU HAVE:	ALCOHOL-FREE	SUGAR-FREE	LACTOSE-FREE	SODIUM-FREE
Vanquish	Acetaminophen, Aluminum hydroxide, Aspirin, Caffeine, Magnesium hydroxide (*Bayer*)	Every 4 hours	Asthma, heartburn, upset stomach, stomach pain, ulcers, bleeding problems, an allergy to aspirin, last 3 months of pregnancy	Yes	Yes	Yes	Yes

BRONCHIAL ASTHMA

BRAND	ACTIVE INGREDIENTS (MANUFACTURER)	HOW OFTEN TO TAKE	GET MD APPROVAL IF YOU HAVE:	ALCOHOL-FREE	SUGAR-FREE	LACTOSE-FREE	SODIUM-FREE
Primatene Mist	Epinephrine (*Whitehall-Robins*)	Every 3 hours	Heart disease, high blood pressure, thyroid disease, diabetes, enlarged prostate gland	No	Yes	Yes	Yes
Primatene Tablets	Ephedrine, Guaifenesin (*Whitehall-Robins*)	Every 4 hours	Heart disease, high blood pressure, thyroid disease, diabetes, enlarged prostate gland, chronic cough, cough with excessive phlegm, been hospitalized for asthma	Yes	Yes	Yes	Yes

CHEST CONGESTION, ADULTS

Product	Ingredients	Dosage	Don't take if you have					
Novahistine DMX	Dextromethorphan, Guaifenesin, Pseudoephedrine (SmithKline Beecham)	Every 4 hours	Heart disease, clogged coronary arteries, high blood pressure, thyroid disease, diabetes, enlarged prostate gland, chronic cough, cough with excessive phlegm, an allergy to any ingredient, a nursing baby	No	No	No	Yes	No
Primatene Tablets	Ephedrine, Guaifenesin (Whitehall-Robins)	Every 4 hours	Heart disease, high blood pressure, thyroid disease, diabetes, enlarged prostate gland, chronic cough, cough with excessive phlegm, been hospitalized for asthma	Yes	Yes	Yes	Yes	Yes
Robitussin	Guaifenesin (Whitehall-Robins)	Every 4 hours	Chronic cough, cough with excessive phlegm, allergy to any ingredient	Yes	No	No	Yes	No
Robitussin-DM	Dextromethorphan, Guaifenesin (Whitehall-Robins)	Every 4 hours	Chronic cough, cough with excessive phlegm, allergy to any ingredient	Yes	No	No	Yes	No
Robitussin-PE	Guaifenesin, Pseudoephedrine (Whitehall-Robins)	Every 4 hours	Chronic cough, cough with excessive phlegm, heart disease, high blood pressure, thyroid disease, diabetes, enlarged prostate gland	Yes	No	No	Yes	No

BRAND	ACTIVE INGREDIENTS (MANUFACTURER)	HOW OFTEN TO TAKE	GET MD APPROVAL IF YOU HAVE:	ALCOHOL-FREE	SUGAR-FREE	LACTOSE-FREE	SODIUM-FREE
Robitussin Severe Congestion Liqui-Gels	Guaifenesin, Pseudoephedrine (Whitehall-Robins)	Every 4 hours	Chronic cough, cough with excessive phlegm, heart disease, high blood pressure, thyroid disease, diabetes, enlarged prostate gland	Yes	Yes	Yes	Yes
Sinutab	Guaifenesin, Pseudoephedrine (Warner-Lambert)	Every 4 hours	Chronic cough, cough with excessive phlegm, heart disease, high blood pressure, thyroid disease, diabetes, enlarged prostate gland	Yes	Yes	Yes	Yes
Sudafed Non-Drying Sinus	Guaifenesin, Pseudoephedrine (Warner-Lambert)	Every 4 hours	Chronic cough, cough with excessive phlegm, heart disease, high blood pressure, thyroid disease, diabetes, enlarged prostate gland	Yes	Yes	Yes	Yes
Triaminic Expectorant	Guaifenesin, Phenylpropanolamine (Novartis)	Every 4 hours	Chronic cough, cough with excessive phlegm, heart disease, high blood pressure, thyroid disease, diabetes, enlarged prostate gland	Yes	No	Yes	Yes
Vicks 44E	Dextromethorphan, Guaifenesin (Procter & Gamble)	Every 4 hours	Chronic cough, cough with excessive phlegm	No	No	Yes	No

CHEST CONGESTION, CHILDREN

Product	Ingredients (Manufacturer)	Dosage	Cautions				
Vicks 44E, Pediatric	Dextromethorphan, Guaifenesin (*Procter & Gamble*)	Every 4 hours	Chronic cough, cough with excessive phlegm	Yes	No	Yes	No

COMMON COLD (MULTI-SYMPTOM), ADULTS

Product	Ingredients (Manufacturer)	Dosage	Cautions				
Actifed Cold & Allergy	Pseudoephedrine, Triprolidine (*Warner-Lambert*)	Every 4 to 6 hours	Heart disease, high blood pressure, thyroid disease, diabetes, glaucoma, enlarged prostate gland, breathing problems	Yes	No	No	Yes
Actifed Cold & Sinus	Acetaminophen, Pseudoephedrine, Triprolidine (*Warner-Lambert*)	Every 6 hours	Heart disease, high blood pressure, thyroid disease, diabetes, glaucoma, enlarged prostate gland, breathing problems	Yes	Yes	Yes	Yes
Advil Cold and Sinus	Ibuprofen, Pseudoephedrine (*Whitehall-Robins*)	Every 4 to 6 hours	Heart disease, high blood pressure, thyroid disease, diabetes, enlarged prostate gland, an allergy to aspirin, last 3 months of pregnancy	Yes	No	Yes	No
Alka-Seltzer Plus Cold Medicine Liqui-Gels	Acetaminophen, Chlorpheniramine, Pseudoephedrine (*Bayer*)	Every 4 hours	Heart disease, high blood pressure, thyroid disease, diabetes, glaucoma, enlarged prostate gland, breathing problems	Yes	Yes	Yes	Yes

BRAND	ACTIVE INGREDIENTS (MANUFACTURER)	HOW OFTEN TO TAKE	GET MD APPROVAL IF YOU HAVE:	ALCOHOL-FREE	SUGAR-FREE	LACTOSE-FREE	SODIUM-FREE
Alka-Seltzer Plus Cold Medicine Tablets	Aspirin, Chlorpheniramine, Phenylpropanolamine (*Bayer*)	Every 4 hours	Heart disease, high blood pressure, thyroid disease, diabetes, glaucoma, enlarged prostate gland, breathing problems, bleeding problems, an allergy to aspirin, last 3 months of pregnancy	Yes	Yes	Yes	No
Alka-Seltzer Plus Cold & Cough Medicine Liqui-Gels	Acetaminophen, Chlorpheniramine, Dextromethorphan, Pseudoephedrine (*Bayer*)	Every 4 hours	Chronic cough, cough with excessive phlegm, heart disease, high blood pressure, thyroid disease, diabetes, glaucoma, enlarged prostate gland, breathing problems	Yes	Yes	Yes	Yes
Alka-Seltzer Plus Cold & Cough Medicine Tablets	Aspirin, Chlorpheniramine, Dextromethorphan, Phenylpropanolamine (*Bayer*)	Every 4 hours	Chronic cough, cough with excessive phlegm, heart disease, high blood pressure, thyroid disease, diabetes, glaucoma, enlarged prostate gland, breathing problems, bleeding problems, an allergy to aspirin, last 3 months of pregnancy	Yes	Yes	Yes	No

Alka-Seltzer Plus Flu & Body Aches Liqui-Gels	Acetaminophen, Dextromethorphan, Pseudoephedrine (*Bayer*)	Every 4 hours	Chronic cough, cough with excessive phlegm, heart disease, high blood pressure, thyroid disease, diabetes, enlarged prostate gland	Yes	Yes	Yes	Yes
Alka-Seltzer Plus Flu & Body Aches Tablets	Acetaminophen, Chlorpheniramine, Dextromethorphan, Phenylpropanolamine (*Bayer*)	Every 4 hours	Chronic cough, cough with excessive phlegm, heart disease, high blood pressure, thyroid disease, diabetes, glaucoma, enlarged prostate gland, breathing problems	Yes	Yes	Yes	No
Alka-Seltzer Plus Night-Time Cold Medicine Liqui-Gels	Acetaminophen, Dextromethorphan, Doxylamine, Pseudoephedrine (*Bayer*)	Once a day	Chronic cough, cough with excessive phlegm, heart disease, high blood pressure, thyroid disease, diabetes, glaucoma, enlarged prostate gland, breathing problems	Yes	Yes	Yes	Yes
Alka-Seltzer Plus Night-Time Cold Medicine Tablets	Aspirin, Dextromethorphan, Doxylamine, Phenylpropanolamine (*Bayer*)	Every 4 hours	Chronic cough, cough with excessive phlegm, heart disease, high blood pressure, thyroid disease, diabetes, glaucoma, enlarged prostate gland, breathing problems, bleeding problems, an allergy to aspirin, last 3 months of pregnancy	Yes	Yes	Yes	No

BRAND	ACTIVE INGREDIENTS (MANUFACTURER)	HOW OFTEN TO TAKE	GET MD APPROVAL IF YOU HAVE:	ALCOHOL-FREE	SUGAR-FREE	LACTOSE-FREE	SODIUM-FREE
BC Allergy Sinus Cold Powder	Aspirin, Chlorpheniramine, Phenylpropanolamine (Block Drug)	Every 3 to 4 hours	Heart disease, high blood pressure, thyroid disease, diabetes, glaucoma, enlarged prostate gland, breathing problems, an allergy to aspirin, last 3 months of pregnancy	NA	NA	NA	NA
BC Sinus Cold Powder	Aspirin, Phenylpropanolamine (Block Drug)	Every 3 to 4 hours	Heart disease, high blood pressure, thyroid disease, diabetes, glaucoma, enlarged prostate gland, breathing problems, an allergy to aspirin, last 3 months of pregnancy	NA	NA	NA	NA
Benadryl Allergy Capsules and Tablets	Diphenhydramine (Warner-Lambert)	Every 4 to 6 hours	Breathing problems, glaucoma, enlarged prostate gland	Yes	Yes	Tablets only	Yes
Benadryl Allergy Chewables	Diphenhydramine (Warner-Lambert)	Every 4 to 6 hours	Breathing problems, glaucoma, enlarged prostate gland	Yes	Yes	Yes	Yes
Benadryl Allergy Liquid	Diphenhydramine (Warner-Lambert)	Every 4 to 6 hours	Breathing problems, glaucoma, enlarged prostate gland	Yes	No	Yes	No

Product	Ingredients	Dosage	Do Not Use If You Have				
Benadryl Allergy/Cold Tablets	Acetaminophen, Diphenhydramine, Pseudoephedrine (*Warner-Lambert*)	Every 6 hours	Heart disease, high blood pressure, thyroid disease, diabetes, glaucoma, enlarged prostate gland, breathing problems	Yes	Yes	Yes	No
Benadryl Allergy Decongestant Liquid and Tablets	Diphenhydramine, Pseudoephedrine (*Warner-Lambert*)	Every 4 to 6 hours	Heart disease, high blood pressure, thyroid disease, diabetes, glaucoma, enlarged prostate gland, breathing problems	Yes	Yes	Yes	No
Cheracol Plus	Chlorpheniramine, Dextromethorphan, Phenylpropanolamine (*Roberts*)	Every 4 hours	Chronic cough, cough with excessive phlegm, heart disease, high blood pressure, thyroid disease, diabetes, glaucoma, enlarged prostate gland, breathing problems	No	Yes	Yes	No
Comtrex Cold & Flu Reliever Tablets and Caplets	Acetaminophen, Chlorpheniramine, Dextromethorphan, Pseudoephedrine (*Bristol-Myers*)	Every 6 hours	Chronic cough, cough with excessive phlegm, heart disease, high blood pressure, thyroid disease, diabetes, glaucoma, enlarged prostate gland, breathing problems	Yes	Yes	Yes	Yes

BRAND	ACTIVE INGREDIENTS (MANUFACTURER)	HOW OFTEN TO TAKE	GET MD APPROVAL IF YOU HAVE:	ALCOHOL-FREE	SUGAR-FREE	LACTOSE-FREE	SODIUM-FREE
Comtrex Cold & Flu Reliever Liquid	Acetaminophen, Chlorpheniramine, Dextromethorphan, Pseudoephedrine (*Bristol-Myers*)	Every 6 hours	Chronic cough, cough with excessive phlegm, heart disease, high blood pressure, thyroid disease, diabetes, glaucoma, enlarged prostate gland, breathing problems	No	No	Yes	No
Comtrex Cold & Flu Reliever Liqui-Gels	Acetaminophen, Chlorpheniramine, Dextromethorphan, Phenylpropanolamine (*Bristol-Myers*)	Every 6 hours	Chronic cough, cough with excessive phlegm, heart disease, high blood pressure, thyroid disease, diabetes, glaucoma, enlarged prostate gland, breathing problems	Yes	Yes	Yes	Yes
Comtrex Deep Chest Cold	Acetaminophen, Dextromethorphan, Guaifenesin, Phenylpropanolamine (*Bristol-Myers*)	Every 4 hours	Chronic cough, cough with excessive phlegm, heart disease, high blood pressure, thyroid disease, diabetes, enlarged prostate gland	Yes	Yes	Yes	Yes
Comtrex Non-Drowsy Caplets	Acetaminophen, Dextromethorphan, Pseudoephedrine (*Bristol-Myers*)	Every 6 hours	Chronic cough, cough with excessive phlegm, heart disease, high blood pressure, thyroid disease, diabetes, enlarged prostate gland	Yes	Yes	Yes	Yes

Product	Ingredients	Dosage	Don't take if you have				
Comtrex Non-Drowsy Liqui-Gels	Acetaminophen, Dextromethorphan, Phenylpropanolamine (*Bristol-Myers*)	Every 6 hours	Chronic cough, cough with excessive phlegm, heart disease, high blood pressure, thyroid disease, diabetes, enlarged prostate gland	Yes	Yes	Yes	Yes
Contac (Regular Strength)	Chlorpheniramine, Phenylpropanolamine (*SmithKline Beecham*)	Every 12 hours	Heart disease, high blood pressure, thyroid disease, diabetes, glaucoma, enlarged prostate gland, breathing problems	No	No	Yes	No
Contac (Maximum Strength)	Chlorpheniramine, Phenylpropanolamine (*SmithKline Beecham*)	Every 12 hours	Heart disease, high blood pressure, thyroid disease, diabetes, glaucoma, enlarged prostate gland, breathing problems	Yes	Yes	No	Yes
Contac Day & Night Cold/Flu	Day Caplets: Acetaminophen, Dextromethorphan, Pseudoephedrine; Night Caplets: Acetaminophen, Diphenhydramine, Pseudoephedrine (*SmithKline Beecham*)	Every 6 hours	Chronic cough, cough with excessive phlegm, heart disease, high blood pressure, thyroid disease, diabetes, glaucoma, enlarged prostate gland, breathing problems	Yes	Yes	Yes	Yes

BRAND	ACTIVE INGREDIENTS (MANUFACTURER)	HOW OFTEN TO TAKE	GET MD APPROVAL IF YOU HAVE:	ALCOHOL-FREE	SUGAR-FREE	LACTOSE-FREE	SODIUM-FREE
Contac Severe Cold and Flu	Acetaminophen, Chlorpheniramine, Dextromethorphan, Phenylpropanolamine (SmithKline Beecham)	Every 6 hours	Chronic cough, cough with excessive phlegm, heart disease, high blood pressure, thyroid disease, diabetes, glaucoma, enlarged prostate gland, breathing problems	Yes	Yes	Yes	No
Contac Severe Cold and Flu Non-Drowsy	Acetaminophen, Dextromethorphan, Pseudoephedrine (SmithKline Beecham)	Every 6 hours	Chronic cough, cough with excessive phlegm, heart disease, high blood pressure, thyroid disease, diabetes, enlarged prostate gland	Yes	Yes	Yes	Yes
Coricidin Cold & Flu Tablets	Acetaminophen, Chlorpheniramine (Schering-Plough)	Every 4 to 6 hours	Breathing problems, glaucoma, enlarged prostate gland	Yes	No	No	Yes
Coricidin Cough & Cold Tablets	Chlorpheniramine, Dextromethorphan (Schering-Plough)	Every 6 hours	Chronic cough, cough with excessive phlegm, breathing problems, glaucoma, enlarged prostate gland	Yes	No	No	No
Coricidin 'D'	Acetaminophen, Chlorpheniramine, Phenylpropanolamine (Schering-Plough)	Every 4 hours	Heart disease, high blood pressure, thyroid disease, diabetes, glaucoma, enlarged prostate gland, breathing problems	Yes	No	Yes	Yes

Product	Ingredients (Manufacturer)	Dosage	Don't use if you have				
Coricidin Nighttime Cold & Cough Liquid	Acetaminophen, Diphenhydramine (*Schering-Plough*)	Every 4 hours	Chronic cough, cough with excessive phlegm, breathing problems, glaucoma, enlarged prostate gland	Yes	No	Yes	No
Dimetapp Elixir	Brompheniramine, Phenylpropanolamine (*Whitehall-Robins*)	Every 4 hours	Heart disease, high blood pressure, thyroid disease, diabetes, glaucoma, enlarged prostate gland, breathing problems	Yes	Yes	Yes	No
Dimetapp Extentabs	Brompheniramine, Phenylpropanolamine (*Whitehall-Robins*)	Every 12 hours	Heart disease, high blood pressure, thyroid disease, diabetes, glaucoma, enlarged prostate gland, breathing problems	No	No	Yes	Yes
Dimetapp Tablets and Liqui-Gels	Brompheniramine, Phenylpropanolamine (*Whitehall-Robins*)	Every 4 hours	Heart disease, high blood pressure, thyroid disease, diabetes, glaucoma, enlarged prostate gland, breathing problems	Yes	Yes	Yes	Yes
Dimetapp Allergy Sinus	Acetaminophen, Brompheniramine, Phenylpropanolamine (*Whitehall-Robins*)	Every 6 hours	Heart disease, high blood pressure, thyroid disease, diabetes, glaucoma, enlarged prostate gland, breathing problems	Yes	Yes	Yes	Yes

BRAND	ACTIVE INGREDIENTS (MANUFACTURER)	HOW OFTEN TO TAKE	GET MD APPROVAL IF YOU HAVE:	ALCOHOL-FREE	SUGAR-FREE	LACTOSE-FREE	SODIUM-FREE
Dimetapp Cold & Cough Liqui-Gels	Brompheniramine, Dextromethorphan, Phenylpropanolamine (*Whitehall-Robins*)	Every 4 hours	Chronic cough, cough with excessive phlegm, heart disease, high blood pressure, thyroid disease, diabetes, glaucoma, enlarged prostate gland, breathing problems	Yes	Yes	Yes	Yes
Dimetapp DM Elixir	Brompheniramine, Dextromethorphan, Phenylpropanolamine (*Whitehall-Robins*)	Every 4 hours	Chronic cough, cough with excessive phlegm, heart disease, high blood pressure, thyroid disease, diabetes, glaucoma, enlarged prostate gland, breathing problems	Yes	Yes	Yes	No
Drixoral Allergy/Sinus	Acetaminophen, Dexbrompheniramine, Pseudoephedrine (*Schering-Plough*)	Every 12 hours	Heart disease, high blood pressure, thyroid disease, diabetes, glaucoma, enlarged prostate gland, breathing problems	Yes	Yes	Yes	Yes
Drixoral Cold & Allergy	Dexbrompheniramine, Pseudoephedrine (*Schering-Plough*)	Every 12 hours	Heart disease, high blood pressure, thyroid disease, diabetes, glaucoma, enlarged prostate gland, breathing problems	Yes	No	No	Yes

Product	Ingredients (Manufacturer)	Dosage	Warnings				
Drixoral Cold & Flu	Acetaminophen, Dexbrompheniramine, Pseudoephedrine (Schering-Plough)	Every 12 hours	Heart disease, high blood pressure, thyroid disease, diabetes, glaucoma, enlarged prostate gland, breathing problems	Yes	Yes	Yes	Yes
Novahistine	Chlorpheniramine, Phenylephrine (SmithKline Beecham)	Every 4 hours	Heart disease, high blood pressure, thyroid disease, diabetes, glaucoma, enlarged prostate gland, breathing problems, ulcers, a nursing baby, an allergy to any ingredient	No	Yes	Yes	No
Robitussin Cold & Cough	Dextromethorphan, Guaifenesin, Pseudoephedrine (Whitehall-Robins)	Every 4 hours	Chronic cough, cough with excessive phlegm, heart disease, high blood pressure, thyroid disease, diabetes, enlarged prostate gland	Yes	Yes	Yes	Yes
Robitussin Cold, Cough & Flu	Acetaminophen, Dextromethorphan, Guaifenesin, Pseudoephedrine (Whitehall-Robins)	Every 4 hours	Chronic cough, cough with excessive phlegm, heart disease, high blood pressure, thyroid disease, diabetes, enlarged prostate gland	Yes	Yes	Yes	Yes
Robitussin Night-Time Cold Formula	Acetaminophen, Dextromethorphan, Doxylamine, Pseudoephedrine (Whitehall-Robins)	Every 6 hours	Chronic cough, cough with excessive phlegm, heart disease, high blood pressure, thyroid disease, diabetes, enlarged prostate gland	Yes	Yes	Yes	No

BRAND	ACTIVE INGREDIENTS (MANUFACTURER)	HOW OFTEN TO TAKE	GET MD APPROVAL IF YOU HAVE:	ALCOHOL-FREE	SUGAR-FREE	LACTOSE-FREE	SODIUM-FREE
Ryna Liquid	Chlorpheniramine, Pseudoephedrine (Wallace)	Every 4 to 6 hours	Heart disease, high blood pressure, thyroid disease, diabetes, glaucoma, enlarged prostate gland, breathing problems	Yes	Yes	Yes	No
Ryna-C Liquid	Chlorpheniramine, Codeine, Pseudoephedrine (Wallace)	Every 4 to 6 hours	Chronic cough, cough with excessive phlegm, heart disease, high blood pressure, thyroid disease, diabetes, glaucoma, enlarged prostate gland, breathing problems	Yes	Yes	Yes	No
Ryna-CX Liquid	Codeine, Guaifenesin, Pseudoephedrine (Wallace)	Every 4 to 6 hours	Chronic cough, cough with excessive phlegm, heart disease, high blood pressure, thyroid disease, diabetes, glaucoma, enlarged prostate gland, breathing problems	Yes	Yes	Yes	No
Sine-Off	Acetaminophen, Diphenhydramine, Pseudoephedrine (Hogil)	Every 6 hours	Heart disease, high blood pressure, thyroid disease, diabetes, glaucoma, enlarged prostate gland, breathing problems	Yes	Yes	Yes	No

Singlet	Acetaminophen, Chlorpheniramine, Pseudoephedrine (*SmithKline Beecham*)	Every 4 to 6 hours	Heart disease, high blood pressure, thyroid disease, diabetes, glaucoma, enlarged prostate gland, breathing problems	Yes	No	Yes	No
Sinulin	Acetaminophen, Chlorpheniramine, Phenylpropanolamine (*Carnrick*)	Every 4 to 6 hours	Heart disease, high blood pressure, thyroid disease, diabetes, glaucoma, enlarged prostate gland, breathing problems	Yes	NA	NA	NA
Sudafed Cold & Allergy	Chlorpheniramine, Pseudoephedrine (*Warner-Lambert*)	Every 4 to 6 hours	Heart disease, high blood pressure, thyroid disease, diabetes, glaucoma, enlarged prostate gland, breathing problems	Yes	Yes	No	Yes
Sudafed Cold & Cough	Acetaminophen, Dextromethorphan, Guaifenesin, Pseudoephedrine (*Warner-Lambert*)	Every 4 hours	Chronic cough, cough with excessive phlegm, heart disease, high blood pressure, thyroid disease, diabetes, enlarged prostate gland	Yes	Yes	Yes	Yes
Sudafed Cold & Sinus	Acetaminophen, Pseudoephedrine (*Warner-Lambert*)	Every 4 to 6 hours	Heart disease, high blood pressure, thyroid disease, diabetes, enlarged prostate gland	Yes	Yes	Yes	No

BRAND	ACTIVE INGREDIENTS (MANUFACTURER)	HOW OFTEN TO TAKE	GET MD APPROVAL IF YOU HAVE:	ALCOHOL-FREE	SUGAR-FREE	LACTOSE-FREE	SODIUM-FREE
Sudafed Severe Cold Formula	Acetaminophen, Dextromethorphan, Pseudoephedrine (Warner-Lambert)	Every 6 hours	Chronic cough, cough with excessive phlegm, heart disease, high blood pressure, thyroid disease, diabetes, enlarged prostate gland	Yes	Yes	Yes	Yes
Sudafed Sinus	Acetaminophen, Pseudoephedrine (Warner-Lambert)	Every 6 hours	Heart disease, high blood pressure, thyroid disease, diabetes, enlarged prostate gland	Yes	Yes	Yes	Yes
Theraflu Flu and Cold Medicine	Acetaminophen, Chlorpheniramine, Pseudoephedrine (Novartis)	Every 4 to 6 hours	Heart disease, high blood pressure, thyroid disease, diabetes, glaucoma, enlarged prostate gland, breathing problems	Yes	No	Yes	No
Theraflu Flu, Cold & Cough (Regular and Nighttime)	Acetaminophen, Chlorpheniramine, Dextromethorphan, Pseudoephedrine (Novartis)	Every 6 hours	Chronic cough, cough with excessive phlegm, heart disease, high blood pressure, thyroid disease, diabetes, glaucoma, enlarged prostate gland, breathing problems	Yes	No	Hot liquid only	No

Theraflu Flu, Cold & Cough (Non-Drowsy)	Acetaminophen, Dextromethorphan, Pseudoephedrine (*Novartis*)	Every 6 hours	Chronic cough, cough with excessive phlegm, heart disease, high blood pressure, thyroid disease, diabetes, enlarged prostate gland	Yes	No	Hot liquid only	No
Triaminic	Chlorpheniramine, Phenylpropanolamine (*Novartis*)	Every 4 to 6 hours	Heart disease, high blood pressure, thyroid disease, diabetes, glaucoma, enlarged prostate gland, breathing problems	Yes	No	Yes	No
Triaminic Night Time	Chlorpheniramine, Dextromethorphan, Pseudoephedrine (*Novartis*)	Every 6 hours	Chronic cough, cough with excessive phlegm, heart disease, high blood pressure, thyroid disease, diabetes, glaucoma, enlarged prostate gland, breathing problems	Yes	No	Yes	No
Triaminic Sore Throat Formula	Acetaminophen, Dextromethorphan, Pseudoephedrine (*Novartis*)	Every 6 hours	Chronic cough, cough with excessive phlegm, heart disease, high blood pressure, thyroid disease, diabetes, enlarged prostate gland	Yes	No	Yes	No
Triaminicol	Chlorpheniramine, Dextromethorphan, Phenylpropanolamine (*Novartis*)	Every 4 to 6 hours	Chronic cough, cough with excessive phlegm, heart disease, high blood pressure, thyroid disease, diabetes, glaucoma, enlarged prostate gland, breathing problems	Yes	No	Yes	No

BRAND	ACTIVE INGREDIENTS (MANUFACTURER)	HOW OFTEN TO TAKE	GET MD APPROVAL IF YOU HAVE:	ALCOHOL-FREE	SUGAR-FREE	LACTOSE-FREE	SODIUM-FREE
Triaminicin	Acetaminophen, Chlorpheniramine, Phenylpropanolamine (Novartis)	Every 4 to 6 hours	Heart disease, high blood pressure, thyroid disease, diabetes, glaucoma, enlarged prostate gland, breathing problems	Yes	Yes	No	No
Tylenol Cold Medication (Tablets and Caplets)	Acetaminophen, Chlorpheniramine, Dextromethorphan, Pseudoephedrine (McNeil)	Every 6 hours	Chronic cough, cough with excessive phlegm, heart disease, high blood pressure, thyroid disease, diabetes, glaucoma, enlarged prostate gland, breathing problems	Yes	Yes	Yes	No
Tylenol Cold Medication Packets	Acetaminophen, Chlorpheniramine, Dextromethorphan, Pseudoephedrine (McNeil)	Every 6 hours	Chronic cough, cough with excessive phlegm, heart disease, high blood pressure, thyroid disease, diabetes, glaucoma, enlarged prostate gland, breathing problems	Yes	No	Yes	No
Tylenol Cold (No Drowsiness Caplets and Gelcaps)	Acetaminophen, Dextromethorphan, Pseudoephedrine (McNeil)	Every 6 hours	Chronic cough, cough with excessive phlegm, heart disease, high blood pressure, thyroid disease, diabetes, enlarged prostate gland	Caplets only	Yes	Yes	No

Product	Ingredients	Dosage	Precautions				
Tylenol Cold Severe Congestion	Acetaminophen, Dextromethorphan, Guaifenesin, Pseudoephedrine (*McNeil*)	Every 6 to 8 hours	Chronic cough, cough with excessive phlegm, heart disease, high blood pressure, thyroid disease, diabetes, enlarged prostate gland	Yes	Yes	Yes	No
Tylenol Flu NightTime (Gelcaps)	Acetaminophen, Diphenhydramine, Pseudoephedrine (*McNeil*)	Every 6 hours	Heart disease, high blood pressure, thyroid disease, diabetes, glaucoma, enlarged prostate gland, breathing problems	No	Yes	Yes	No
Tylenol Flu NightTime (Hot Medication Packets)	Acetaminophen, Diphenhydramine, Pseudoephedrine (*McNeil*)	Every 6 hours	Heart disease, high blood pressure, thyroid disease, diabetes, glaucoma, enlarged prostate gland, breathing problems	Yes	No	Yes	No
Tylenol Flu No Drowsiness Formula	Acetaminophen, Dextromethorphan, Pseudoephedrine (*McNeil*)	Every 6 hours	Chronic cough, cough with excessive phlegm, heart disease, high blood pressure, thyroid disease, diabetes, enlarged prostate gland	No	Yes	Yes	No

BRAND	ACTIVE INGREDIENTS (MANUFACTURER)	HOW OFTEN TO TAKE	GET MD APPROVAL IF YOU HAVE:	ALCOHOL-FREE	SUGAR-FREE	LACTOSE-FREE	SODIUM-FREE
Vicks 44M	Acetaminophen, Chlorpheniramine, Dextromethorphan, Pseudoephedrine (Procter & Gamble)	Every 6 hours	Chronic cough, cough with excessive phlegm, heart disease, high blood pressure, thyroid disease, diabetes, glaucoma, enlarged prostate gland, breathing problems	No	No	Yes	No
Vicks DayQuil	Acetaminophen, Dextromethorphan, Pseudoephedrine (Procter & Gamble)	Every 4 hours	Chronic cough, cough with excessive phlegm, heart disease, high blood pressure, thyroid disease, diabetes, enlarged prostate gland, breathing problems	Yes	Softgels only	Yes	Softgels only
Vicks DayQuil Allergy	Brompheniramine, Phenylpropanolamine (Procter & Gamble)	Every 12 hours	Heart disease, high blood pressure, thyroid disease, diabetes, glaucoma, enlarged prostate gland, breathing problems	Yes	Yes	No	Yes
Vicks DayQuil Sinus Pressure & Pain Relief	Ibuprofen, Pseudoephedrine (Procter & Gamble)	Every 4 to 6 hours	Heart disease, high blood pressure, thyroid disease, diabetes, enlarged prostate gland, an allergy to aspirin, last 3 months of pregnancy	Yes	No	Yes	No

Vicks NyQuil Liquicaps	Acetaminophen, Dextromethorphan, Doxylamine, Pseudoephedrine (*Procter & Gamble*)	Every 4 hours	Chronic cough, cough with excessive phlegm, heart disease, high blood pressure, thyroid disease, diabetes, glaucoma, enlarged prostate gland, breathing problems	Yes	Yes	Yes	Yes
Vicks NyQuil Liquid	Acetaminophen, Dextromethorphan, Doxylamine, Pseudoephedrine (*Procter & Gamble*)	Every 6 hours	Chronic cough, cough with excessive phlegm, heart disease, high blood pressure, thyroid disease, diabetes, glaucoma, enlarged prostate gland, breathing problems	No	No	Yes	No
Vicks NyQuil Hot Therapy	Acetaminophen, Dextromethorphan, Doxylamine, Pseudoephedrine (*Procter & Gamble*)	Every 6 hours	Chronic cough, cough with excessive phlegm, heart disease, high blood pressure, thyroid disease, diabetes, glaucoma, enlarged prostate gland, breathing problems	Yes	No	Yes	Yes

COMMON COLD (MULTI-SYMPTOM), CHILDREN

BRAND	ACTIVE INGREDIENTS (MANUFACTURER)	HOW OFTEN TO TAKE	GET MD APPROVAL IF YOU HAVE:	ALCOHOL-FREE	SUGAR-FREE	LACTOSE-FREE	SODIUM-FREE
Dimetapp Cold & Allergy (Chewable and Quick-Dissolving Tablets)	Brompheniramine, Phenylpropanolamine (Whitehall-Robins)	Every 4 hours	Heart disease, high blood pressure, thyroid disease, diabetes, glaucoma, breathing problems	Yes	Yes	Yes	Yes
Dimetapp Cold and Fever Suspension	Acetaminophen, Brompheniramine, Pseudoephedrine (Whitehall-Robins)	Every 4 hours	Heart disease, high blood pressure, thyroid disease, diabetes, glaucoma, breathing problems	Yes	No	Yes	No
PediaCare Cough-Cold (Liquid and Chewable Tablets)	Chlorpheniramine, Dextromethorphan, Pseudoephedrine (McNeil)	Every 4 to 6 hours	Chronic cough, cough with excessive phlegm, heart disease, high blood pressure, thyroid disease, diabetes, glaucoma, breathing problems	Yes	Tablets only	Tablets Yes	Tablets only

COMMON COLD, CHILDREN/**51**

Product	Ingredients	Dosage	Warnings				
PediaCare Cough-Cold (NightRest Liquid) (*McNeil*)	Chlorpheniramine, Dextromethorphan, Pseudoephedrine	Every 6 to 8 hours	Chronic cough, cough with excessive phlegm, heart disease, high blood pressure, thyroid disease, diabetes, glaucoma, breathing problems	Yes	No	Yes	No
Tylenol Children's Cold (*McNeil*)	Acetaminophen, Chlorpheniramine, Pseudoephedrine	Every 4 to 6 hours	Heart disease, high blood pressure, thyroid disease, diabetes, glaucoma, breathing problems	Yes	Tablets only	Yes	Tablets only
Tylenol Children's Cold Plus Cough (*McNeil*)	Acetaminophen, Chlorpheniramine, Dextromethorphan, Pseudoephedrine	Every 4 to 6 hours	Chronic cough, cough with excessive phlegm, heart disease, high blood pressure, thyroid disease, diabetes, glaucoma, breathing problems	Yes	Tablets only	Yes	Tablets only
Tylenol Children's Flu Liquid (*McNeil*)	Acetaminophen, Chlorpheniramine, Dextromethorphan, Pseudoephedrine	Every 6 to 8 hours	Chronic cough, cough with excessive phlegm, heart disease, high blood pressure, thyroid disease, diabetes, glaucoma, breathing problems	Yes	No	Yes	No
Tylenol Infants' Cold Drops (*McNeil*)	Acetaminophen, Pseudoephedrine	Every 4 to 6 hours	Heart disease, high blood pressure, thyroid disease, diabetes	Yes	No	Yes	No

BRAND	ACTIVE INGREDIENTS (MANUFACTURER)	HOW OFTEN TO TAKE	GET MD APPROVAL IF YOU HAVE:	ALCOHOL-FREE	SUGAR-FREE	LACTOSE-FREE	SODIUM-FREE
Vicks Children's NyQuil	Chlorpheniramine, Dextromethorphan, Pseudoephedrine (*Procter & Gamble*)	Every 6 hours	Chronic cough, cough with excessive phlegm, heart disease, high blood pressure, thyroid disease, diabetes, glaucoma, breathing problems	Yes	No	Yes	No
Vicks Pediatric 44M	Chlorpheniramine, Dextromethorphan, Pseudoephedrine (*Procter & Gamble*)	Every 6 hours	Chronic cough, cough with excessive phlegm, heart disease, high blood pressure, thyroid disease, diabetes, glaucoma, breathing problems	Yes	No	Yes	No

CONSTIPATION, CHRONIC, ADULTS

BRAND	ACTIVE INGREDIENTS (MANUFACTURER)	HOW OFTEN TO TAKE	GET MD APPROVAL IF YOU HAVE:	ALCOHOL-FREE	SUGAR-FREE	LACTOSE-FREE	SODIUM-FREE
Citrucel	Methylcellulose (*SmithKline Beecham*)	Up to 3 times a day (adults); once a day (children)	Abdominal pain, nausea, vomiting, sudden change in bowel habits lasting 2 weeks	Yes	Sugar-free variety only	Yes	Sugar-free variety only

Konsyl Fiber Tablets	Calcium polycarbophil (*Konsyl*)	1 to 4 times a day (adults); 1 to 3 times a day (children)	Difficulty swallowing, bowel obstruction, fecal impaction	Yes	Yes	Yes	Yes
Konsyl Powder	Psyllium (*Konsyl*)	1 to 3 times a day	Difficulty swallowing, bowel obstruction, fecal impaction	Yes	Yes	Yes	No
Metamucil	Psyllium (*Procter & Gamble*)	1 to 3 times a day	Difficulty swallowing, bowel obstruction, fecal impaction, rectal bleeding, abdominal pain, nausea, vomiting, sudden change in bowel habits lasting 2 weeks	Yes	Sugar-free varieties and powder only	Yes	No
Peri-Colace	Casanthranol, Docusate sodium (*Roberts*)	1 or 2 times a day (adults), once a day (children)	Abdominal pain, nausea, vomiting	Caps only	Caps only	Yes	Caps only
Senokot	Senna (*Purdue Frederick*)	Once a day	Abdominal pain, nausea, vomiting, sudden change in bowel habits lasting 2 weeks	Yes	Yes	Yes	Yes

BRAND	ACTIVE INGREDIENTS (MANUFACTURER)	HOW OFTEN TO TAKE	GET MD APPROVAL IF YOU HAVE:	ALCOHOL-FREE	SUGAR-FREE	LACTOSE-FREE	SODIUM-FREE
Senokot-S	Docusate sodium, Senna (*Purdue Frederick*)	Once a day	Abdominal pain, nausea, vomiting, sudden change in bowel habits lasting 2 weeks	Yes	Yes	Yes	No

CONSTIPATION, CHRONIC, CHILDREN

BRAND	ACTIVE INGREDIENTS (MANUFACTURER)	HOW OFTEN TO TAKE	GET MD APPROVAL IF YOU HAVE:	ALCOHOL-FREE	SUGAR-FREE	LACTOSE-FREE	SODIUM-FREE
Senokot Children's Syrup	Senna (*Purdue Frederick*)	Once a day	Abdominal pain, nausea, vomiting, sudden change in bowel habits lasting 2 weeks	Yes	No	Yes	Yes

CONSTIPATION, TEMPORARY, ADULTS

BRAND	ACTIVE INGREDIENTS (MANUFACTURER)	HOW OFTEN TO TAKE	GET MD APPROVAL IF YOU HAVE:	ALCOHOL-FREE	SUGAR-FREE	LACTOSE-FREE	SODIUM-FREE
Citrucel	Methylcellulose (*SmithKline Beecham*)	Up to 3 times a day (adults); once a day (children)	Abdominal pain, nausea, vomiting, sudden change in bowel habits lasting 2 weeks	Yes	Sugar-free variety only	Yes	Sugar-free variety only
Colace	Docusate sodium (*Roberts*)	Once a day	—	Caps and liquid only	Caps and liquid only	Yes	No

Product	Ingredient (Manufacturer)	Dosage	Warning					
Correctol	Bisacodyl (*Schering-Plough*)	Once a day	Difficulty swallowing, abdominal pain, nausea, vomiting, sudden change in bowel habits lasting 2 weeks	Yes	No	No	No	Yes
Correctol Herbal Tea	Senna (*Schering-Plough*)	1 to 3 times a day	Abdominal pain, nausea, vomiting, sudden change in bowel habits lasting 2 weeks	Yes	Yes	Yes	Yes	Yes
Correctol Stool Softener	Docusate sodium (*Schering-Plough*)	1 to 3 times a day (adults); once a day (children)	Abdominal pain, nausea, vomiting, sudden change in bowel habits lasting 2 weeks	Yes	Yes	Yes	Yes	No
Dialose	Docusate sodium (*J&J Merck*)	1 to 3 times a day (adults); once a day (children)	Abdominal pain, nausea, vomiting	Yes	No	No	Yes	No
Dialose Plus	Docusate sodium, Yellow phenolphthalein (*J&J Merck*)	Once a day	Abdominal pain, nausea, vomiting	Yes	No	No	Yes	No
Dulcolax	Bisacodyl (*Novartis*)	Once a day	Abdominal pain, nausea, vomiting	Yes	Supp. only	Supp. only	Supp. only	Yes

BRAND	ACTIVE INGREDIENTS (MANUFACTURER)	HOW OFTEN TO TAKE	GET MD APPROVAL IF YOU HAVE:	ALCOHOL-FREE	SUGAR-FREE	LACTOSE-FREE	SODIUM-FREE
Ex-Lax Regular-Strength Laxative Pills	Sennosides (Novartis)	1 or 2 times a day	Abdominal pain, nausea, vomiting	Yes	No	Yes	Yes
Ex-Lax Chocolated Laxative	Sennosides (Novartis)	1 or 2 times a day	Abdominal pain, nausea, vomiting	Yes	No	No	Yes
Ex-Lax Maximum-Strength Laxative Pills	Sennosides (Novartis)	1 or 2 times a day	Abdominal pain, nausea, vomiting	Yes	No	Yes	Yes
Ex-Lax Gentle Nature Pills	Senna (Novartis)	Once a day	Abdominal pain, nausea, vomiting	Yes	Yes	Yes	Yes
Ex-Lax Stool Softener Caplets	Docusate sodium (Novartis)	1 to 3 times a day (adults); once a day (children)	Abdominal pain, nausea, vomiting, sudden change in bowel habits lasting 2 weeks	Yes	No	Yes	No

Product	Ingredient (Manufacturer)	Dosage	Warnings				
Fibercon	Calcium polycarbophil (*Lederle*)	1 to 4 times a day	Difficulty swallowing, abdominal pain, nausea, vomiting, sudden change in bowel habits lasting 2 weeks	Yes	No	Yes	No
Fleet Sof-Lax	Docusate sodium (*Fleet*)	Once a day	Abdominal pain, nausea, vomiting, sudden change in bowel habits lasting 2 weeks	NA	NA	NA	NA
Fleet Sof-Lax Overnight	Casanthranol, Docusate sodium (*Fleet*)	Once a day	Abdominal pain, nausea, vomiting, sudden change in bowel habits lasting 2 weeks	NA	NA	NA	NA
Kondremul	Mineral oil (*Novartis*)	2 to 5 times a day	Difficulty swallowing, abdominal pain, nausea, vomiting, sudden change in bowel habits lasting 2 weeks, pregnancy, bed confinement	Yes	Yes	Yes	Yes
Maltsupex	Malt soup extract (*Wallace*)	2 times a day (liquid and powder); 4 times a day (tablets)	Abdominal pain, nausea, vomiting, sudden change in bowel habits lasting 2 weeks	Yes	Yes	Yes	No
Perdiem	Psyllium, Sennosides (*Novartis*)	1 to 2 times a day	Difficulty swallowing, abdominal pain, nausea, vomiting, sudden change in bowel habits lasting 2 weeks	Yes	No	Yes	Yes

BRAND	ACTIVE INGREDIENTS (MANUFACTURER)	HOW OFTEN TO TAKE	GET MD APPROVAL IF YOU HAVE:	ALCOHOL-FREE	SUGAR-FREE	LACTOSE-FREE	SODIUM-FREE
Perdiem Fiber	Psyllium (Novartis)	1 to 2 times a day	Difficulty swallowing, abdominal pain, nausea, vomiting, sudden change in bowel habits lasting 2 weeks	Yes	No	Yes	No
Peri-Colace	Casanthranol, Docusate sodium (Roberts)	1 or 2 times a day (adults), once a day (children)	Abdominal pain, nausea, vomiting	Caps only	Caps only	Yes	Caps only
Phillips' Gelcaps	Docusate sodium, Phenolphthalein (Bayer)	1 to 2 times a day	Abdominal pain, nausea, vomiting, sudden change in bowel habits lasting 2 weeks	Yes	Yes	Yes	No
Phillips' Milk of Magnesia	Magnesium hydroxide (Bayer)	Once a day	Kidney disease	Yes	No	Yes	No
Senokot	Senna (Purdue Frederick)	Once a day	Abdominal pain, nausea, vomiting, sudden change in bowel habits lasting 2 weeks	Yes	Yes	Yes	Yes

CONSTIPATION, TEMPORARY, CHILDREN

Product		Dosage	Symptoms				
Fletcher's Castoria	Senna concentrate (Mentholatum Co.)	1 to 2 times a day	Abdominal pain, nausea, vomiting, sudden change in bowel habits lasting 2 weeks	Yes	No	Yes	No
Senokot Children's Syrup	Senna (Purdue Frederick Co.)	Once a day	Abdominal pain, nausea, vomiting, sudden change in bowel habits lasting 2 weeks	Yes	No	Yes	Yes

COUGH, ADULTS

Product		Dosage	Symptoms				
Benylin Adult Formula Cough Suppressant	Dextromethorphan (Warner-Lambert)	Every 6 to 8 hours	Chronic cough, cough with excessive phlegm	Yes	Yes	Yes	No
Benylin Cough Suppressant Expectorant	Dextromethorphan, Guaifenesin (Warner-Lambert)	Every 4 hours	Chronic cough, cough with excessive phlegm	Yes	Yes	Yes	No

BRAND	ACTIVE INGREDIENTS (MANUFACTURER)	HOW OFTEN TO TAKE	GET MD APPROVAL IF YOU HAVE:	ALCOHOL-FREE	SUGAR-FREE	LACTOSE-FREE	SODIUM-FREE
Cheracol D	Dextromethorphan, Guaifenesin (Roberts)	Every 4 hours	Chronic cough, cough with excessive phlegm	No	No	Yes	No
Delsym Cough Formula	Dextromethorphan (Medeva)	Every 12 hours	Chronic cough, cough with excessive phlegm	Yes	No	Yes	Yes
Halls Cough Drops	Menthol (Warner-Lambert)	Every hour as needed	Chronic cough, cough with excessive phlegm	Yes	Sugar-Free Drops only	Yes	Yes
N'Ice Sore Throat and Cough Lozenges	Menthol (SmithKline Beecham)	Every hour as needed	Chronic cough, cough with excessive phlegm	Yes	Yes	Yes	Not all flavors
Pertussin DM	Dextromethorphan (Blairex)	Every 6 to 8 hours	Chronic cough, cough with excessive phlegm	No	No	Yes	No
Robitussin	Guaifenesin (Whitehall-Robins)	Every 4 hours	Chronic cough, cough with excessive phlegm, allergy to any ingredient	Yes	No	Yes	No

Product	Ingredients (Manufacturer)	Dosage	Don't use if you have				
Robitussin-DM	Dextromethorphan, Guaifenesin (Whitehall-Robins)	Every 4 hours	Chronic cough, cough with excessive phlegm. allergy to any ingredient	Yes	No	Yes	No
Robitussin Cough Suppressant	Dextromethorphan (Whitehall-Robins)	Every 6 to 8 hours	Chronic cough, cough with excessive phlegm	No	No	Yes	No
Sucrets 4 Hour Cough Suppressant	Dextromethorphan (SmithKline Beecham)	Every 4 hours (Age 6 to 12: Every 6 hours)	Chronic cough, cough with excessive phlegm	Yes	No	Yes	Yes
Tylenol Cough Medication	Acetaminophen, Dextromethorphan (McNeil)	Every 6 to 8 hours	Chronic cough, cough with excessive phlegm	No	No	Yes	No
Vicks 44 Cough Relief (Procter & Gamble)	Dextromethorphan	Every 6 to 8 hours	Chronic cough, cough with excessive phlegm	No	No	Yes	No
Vicks 44E	Dextromethorphan, Guaifenesin (Procter & Gamble)	Every 4 hours	Chronic cough, cough with excessive phlegm	No	No	Yes	No

BRAND	ACTIVE INGREDIENTS (MANUFACTURER)	HOW OFTEN TO TAKE	GET MD APPROVAL IF YOU HAVE:	ALCOHOL- FREE	SUGAR- FREE	LACTOSE- FREE	SODIUM- FREE
Vicks Chloraseptic Cough & Throat Drops	Menthol (Procter & Gamble)	Every hour as needed	Chronic cough, cough with excessive phlegm	Yes	No	Yes	Yes
Vicks Cough Drops (Oval)	Menthol (Procter & Gamble)	Every hour as needed	Chronic cough, cough with excessive phlegm	Cherry Flavor only	No	Yes	Yes
Vicks Cough Drops (Triangular)	Menthol (Procter & Gamble)	Every hour as needed	Chronic cough, cough with excessive phlegm	Yes	No	Yes	Yes

COUGH, CHILDREN

BRAND	ACTIVE INGREDIENTS (MANUFACTURER)	HOW OFTEN TO TAKE	GET MD APPROVAL IF YOU HAVE:	ALCOHOL- FREE	SUGAR- FREE	LACTOSE- FREE	SODIUM- FREE
Benylin Pediatric Cough Suppressant	Dextromethorphan (Warner-Lambert)	Every 6 to 8 hours	Chronic cough, cough with excessive phlegm	Yes	Yes	Yes	No
Halls Juniors	Menthol (Warner-Lambert)	Every hour as needed	Chronic cough, cough with excessive phlegm	Yes	Yes	Yes	Yes

Pertussin CS	Dextromethorphan (Blairex)	Every 4 hours	Chronic cough, cough with excessive phlegm	Yes	No	Yes	Yes
Robitussin Pediatric Cough Suppressant	Dextromethorphan (Whitehall-Robins)	Every 6 to 8 hours	Chronic cough, cough with excessive phlegm, allergy to any ingredient	Yes	Yes	Yes	No
Vicks 44E, Pediatric	Dextromethorphan, Guaifenesin (Procter & Gamble)	Every 4 hours	Chronic cough, cough with excessive phlegm	Yes	No	Yes	No

COUGH WITH HEAD CONGESTION, ADULTS

Benylin Multi-Symptom	Dextromethorphan, Guaifenesin, Pseudoephedrine (Warner-Lambert)	Every 4 hours	Chronic cough, cough with excessive phlegm, heart disease, high blood pressure, thyroid disease, diabetes, enlarged prostate gland	Yes	Yes	Yes	No
Cerose DM	Chlorpheniramine, Dextromethorphan, Phenylephrine (Wyeth-Ayerst)	Every 4 hours	Chronic cough, cough with excessive phlegm, heart disease, high blood pressure, thyroid disease, diabetes, glaucoma, enlarged prostate gland, breathing problems	No	Yes	Yes	No

BRAND	ACTIVE INGREDIENTS (MANUFACTURER)	HOW OFTEN TO TAKE	GET MD APPROVAL IF YOU HAVE:	ALCOHOL-FREE	SUGAR-FREE	LACTOSE-FREE	SODIUM-FREE
Novahistine DMX	Dextromethorphan, Guaifenesin, Pseudoephedrine (SmithKline Beecham)	Every 4 hours	Heart disease, clogged coronary arteries, high blood pressure, thyroid disease, diabetes, enlarged prostate gland, chronic cough, cough with excessive phlegm, an allergy to any ingredient, a nursing baby	No	No	Yes	No
Robitussin-CF	Dextromethorphan, Guaifenesin, Phenylpropanolamine (Whitehall-Robins)	Every 4 hours	Chronic cough, cough with excessive phlegm, heart disease, high blood pressure, thyroid disease, diabetes, enlarged prostate gland	Yes	Yes	Yes	No
Robitussin Cough & Cold	Dextromethorphan, Pseudoephedrine (Whitehall-Robins)	Every 6 hours	Chronic cough, cough with excessive phlegm, heart disease, high blood pressure, thyroid disease, diabetes, enlarged prostate gland	No	No	Yes	No
Robitussin-PE	Guaifenesin, Pseudoephedrine (Whitehall-Robins)	Every 4 hours	Chronic cough, cough with excessive phlegm, heart disease, high blood pressure, thyroid disease, diabetes, enlarged prostate gland	Yes	No	Yes	No

Product	Ingredients	Dose	Don't use if you have				
Robitussin Severe Congestion Liqui-Gels	Guaifenesin, Pseudoephedrine (*Whitehall-Robins*)	Every 4 hours	Chronic cough, cough with excessive phlegm, heart disease, high blood pressure, thyroid disease, diabetes, enlarged prostate gland	Yes	Yes	Yes	Yes
Sinutab	Guaifenesin, Pseudoephedrine (*Warner-Lambert*)	Every 4 hours	Chronic cough, cough with excessive phlegm, heart disease, high blood pressure, thyroid disease, diabetes, enlarged prostate gland	Yes	Yes	Yes	Yes
Sudafed Non-Drying Sinus	Guaifenesin, Pseudoephedrine (*Warner-Lambert*)	Every 4 hours	Chronic cough, cough with excessive phlegm, heart disease, high blood pressure, thyroid disease, diabetes, enlarged prostate gland	Yes	Yes	Yes	Yes
Triaminic AM Cough and Decongestant Formula	Dextromethorphan, Pseudoephedrine (*Novartis*)	Every 6 hours	Chronic cough, cough with excessive phlegm, heart disease, high blood pressure, thyroid disease, diabetes, enlarged prostate gland	Yes	No	Yes	No
Triaminic DM	Dextromethorphan, Phenylpropanolamine (*Novartis*)	Every 4 hours	Chronic cough, cough with excessive phlegm, heart disease, high blood pressure, thyroid disease, diabetes, enlarged prostate gland	Yes	No	Yes	No

BRAND	ACTIVE INGREDIENTS (MANUFACTURER)	HOW OFTEN TO TAKE	GET MD APPROVAL IF YOU HAVE:	ALCOHOL-FREE	SUGAR-FREE	LACTOSE-FREE	SODIUM-FREE
Tylenol Cough Medication with Decongestant	Acetaminophen, Dextromethorphan, Pseudoephedrine (McNeil)	Every 6 to 8 hours	Chronic cough, cough with excessive phlegm, heart disease, high blood pressure, thyroid disease, diabetes, enlarged prostate gland	No	No	Yes	No
Vicks 44D	Dextromethorphan, Pseudoephedrine (Procter & Gamble)	Every 6 hours	Chronic cough, cough with excessive phlegm, heart disease, high blood pressure, thyroid disease, diabetes, enlarged prostate gland, breathing problems	No	No	Yes	No

COUGH WITH HEAD CONGESTION, CHILDREN

BRAND	ACTIVE INGREDIENTS (MANUFACTURER)	HOW OFTEN TO TAKE	GET MD APPROVAL IF YOU HAVE:	ALCOHOL-FREE	SUGAR-FREE	LACTOSE-FREE	SODIUM-FREE
Pediacare Infant's Drops Decongestant Plus Cough	Dextromethorphan, Pseudoephedrine (McNeil)	Every 4 to 6 hours	Chronic cough, cough with excessive phlegm, heart disease, high blood pressure, thyroid disease, diabetes	Yes	Yes	Yes	No

Robitussin Pediatric Cough & Cold Formula	Dextromethorphan, Pseudoephedrine (*Whitehall-Robins*)	Every 6 hours	Chronic cough, cough with excessive phlegm, heart disease, high blood pressure, thyroid disease, diabetes	Yes	Yes	Yes	No
Robitussin Pediatric Drops	Dextromethorphan, Guaifenesin, Pseudoephedrine (*Whitehall-Robins*)	Every 4 hours	Chronic cough, cough with excessive phlegm, heart disease, high blood pressure, thyroid disease, diabetes	Yes	No	Yes	No

CRAMPS, ABDOMINAL

Donnagel	Attapulgite (*Wyeth-Ayerst*)	1 to 7 times a day	Fever	Tablets only	Yes	Yes	No
Gas-X	Simethicone (*Novartis*)	After meals and at bedtime	—	Yes	Soft-gels only	Yes	Yes

DEHYDRATION, ADULTS

Kao Lectrolyte	Dextrose, Potassium chloride, Sodium chloride, Sodium citrate (*Pharmacia & Upjohn*)	As needed	—	Yes	No	Yes	No

BRAND	ACTIVE INGREDIENTS (MANUFACTURER)	HOW OFTEN TO TAKE	GET MD APPROVAL IF YOU HAVE:	ALCOHOL-FREE	SUGAR-FREE	LACTOSE-FREE	SODIUM-FREE
Rehydralyte	Dextrose, Potassium citrate, Sodium chloride, Sodium citrate (Ross)	As needed	—	Yes	No	Yes	No

DEHYDRATION, CHILDREN

BRAND	ACTIVE INGREDIENTS (MANUFACTURER)	HOW OFTEN TO TAKE	GET MD APPROVAL IF YOU HAVE:	ALCOHOL-FREE	SUGAR-FREE	LACTOSE-FREE	SODIUM-FREE
Pedialyte	Dextrose, Potassium citrate, Sodium chloride, Sodium citrate (Ross)	As needed	—	Yes	No	Yes	No

DIARRHEA

BRAND	ACTIVE INGREDIENTS (MANUFACTURER)	HOW OFTEN TO TAKE	GET MD APPROVAL IF YOU HAVE:	ALCOHOL-FREE	SUGAR-FREE	LACTOSE-FREE	SODIUM-FREE
Donnagel	Attapulgite (Wyeth-Ayerst)	1 to 7 times a day	Fever	Tablets only	Yes	Yes	No

Product	(Ingredient / Maker)	Dose	Do not use if you have...				
Imodium A-D	Loperamide (*McNeil*)	1 to 3 times a day (Children 9 to 11: 1 to 5 times a day)	Fever of 101 degrees+, blood or mucus in the stool, liver disease	Caplets only	Caplets only	Caplets only	Caplets only
Pepto Diarrhea Control	Loperamide (*Procter & Gamble*)	1 to 3 times a day (Children 9 to 11: 1 to 5 times a day)	Fever of 101 degrees+, blood or mucus in the stool, liver disease	Yes	Yes	No	Yes
Pepto-Bismol	Bismuth subsalicylate (*Procter & Gamble*)	8 times a day (Maximum Strength: 4 times a day)	High fever, aspirin allergy, chickenpox or flu (in children)	Yes	Yes	Yes	No
Rheaban	Attapulgite (*Pfizer*)	1 to 6 times a day	Fever	Yes	No	Yes	No

FEVER, ADULTS

BRAND	ACTIVE INGREDIENTS (MANUFACTURER)	HOW OFTEN TO TAKE	GET MD APPROVAL IF YOU HAVE:	ALCOHOL-FREE	SUGAR-FREE	LACTOSE-FREE	SODIUM-FREE
Actron	Ketoprofen (Bayer)	Every 4 to 6 hours	Redness or swelling in painful area, an allergy to pain relievers, last 3 months of pregnancy	Yes	Yes	No	No
Advil	Ibuprofen (Whitehall-Robins)	Every 4 to 6 hours	An allergy to aspirin, problems with other pain relievers, last 3 months of pregnancy	Yes	Gel caplets only	Yes	No
Aleve	Naproxen sodium (Procter & Gamble)	Every 8 to 12 hours (Adults over 65: Every 12 hours)	An allergy to pain relievers, last 3 months of pregnancy	Yes	Yes	Yes	Yes
Bayer (Genuine, Extra Strength, and Extended-Release)	Aspirin (Bayer)	Every 4 hours; Extended-Release: Every 8 hours	Asthma, heartburn, upset stomach, stomach pain, ulcers, bleeding problems, an allergy to aspirin, last 3 months of pregnancy	Yes	Yes	Yes	Yes

BC Powder	Aspirin, Caffeine, Salicylamide (*Block Drug*)	Every 3 to 4 hours	An allergy to aspirin, last 3 months of pregnancy	NA	NA	NA	NA
BC Sinus Cold Powder	Aspirin, Phenylpropanolamine, Chlorpheniramine (Allergy Sinus only) (*Block Drug*)	Every 3 to 4 hours	Heart disease, high blood pressure, thyroid disease, diabetes, glaucoma, enlarged prostate, breathing problems, an allergy to aspirin, last 3 months of pregnancy	NA	NA	NA	NA
Bufferin (Regular and Extra Strengths)	Aspirin, Calcium carbonate, Magnesium carbonate, Magnesium oxide (*Bristol-Myers*)	Every 4 hours; Extra Strength: Every 6 hours	Asthma, heartburn, upset stomach, stomach pain, ulcers, bleeding problems, an allergy to aspirin, last 3 months of pregnancy	Yes	Yes	Yes	No
Goody's	Acetaminophen, Aspirin, Caffeine (*Block Drug*)	Every 4 to 6 hours	An allergy to aspirin, last 3 months of pregnancy	Yes	Yes	Yes	Tablets only
Motrin IB	Ibuprofen (*Pharmacia & Upjohn*)	Every 4 to 6 hours	An allergy to aspirin, problems with other pain relievers, last 3 months of pregnancy	Caplets and tablets only	Yes	Caplets and tablets only	Yes

BRAND	ACTIVE INGREDIENTS (MANUFACTURER)	HOW OFTEN TO TAKE	GET MD APPROVAL IF YOU HAVE:	ALCOHOL-FREE	SUGAR-FREE	LACTOSE-FREE	SODIUM-FREE
Nuprin	Ibuprofen (Bristol-Myers)	Every 4 to 6 hours	An allergy to aspirin, problems with other pain relievers, last 3 months of pregnancy	Yes	Yes	Yes	Yes
Orudis KT	Ketoprofen (Whitehall-Robins)	Every 4 to 6 hours	Redness or swelling in painful area, an allergy to pain relievers, last 3 months of pregnancy	Yes	No	Yes	No
Panadol	Acetaminophen (SmithKline Beecham)	Every 4 hours	—	Yes	Yes	Yes	Yes
St. Joseph	Aspirin (Schering-Plough)	Every 4 hours	Asthma, heartburn, upset stomach, stomach pain, ulcers, bleeding problems, an allergy to aspirin, last 3 months of pregnancy	Yes	Yes	Yes	Yes
Tylenol	Acetaminophen (McNeil)	Every 4 to 6 hours; Extended Relief: Every 8 hours	—	Caplets and tablets only	Tablets, caplets, gelcaps, and geltabs only	Yes	No

FEVER, CHILDREN

Product	Generic (Company)	How Often	Check with doctor if child has				
Advil, Children's	Ibuprofen (*Whitehall-Robins*)	Every 6 to 8 hours	An allergy to aspirin, problems with other pain relievers, stomach pain, dehydration from vomiting or diarrhea	Yes	No	Yes	No
Bayer Children's Chewable	Aspirin (*Bayer*)	Every 4 hours	Arthritis, asthma, heartburn, upset stomach, stomach pain, ulcers, bleeding problems, an allergy to aspirin	Yes	No	Yes	No
Motrin (Junior Strength and Children's)	Ibuprofen (*McNeil*)	Every 6 to 8 hours	An allergy to aspirin, problems with other pain relievers, stomach pain, dehydration from vomiting or diarrhea	Yes	No	Yes	No
Panadol Children's	Acetaminophen (*SmithKline Beecham*)	Every 4 hours	—	Yes	Yes	Yes	No
Tylenol, Children's and Infants'	Acetaminophen (*McNeil*)	Every 4 hours	—	Yes	Chewables and liquid only	Yes	Chewables only

BRAND	ACTIVE INGREDIENTS (MANUFACTURER)	HOW OFTEN TO TAKE	GET MD APPROVAL IF YOU HAVE:	ALCOHOL-FREE	SUGAR-FREE	LACTOSE-FREE	SODIUM-FREE
Tylenol, Junior Strength	Acetaminophen (McNeil)	Every 4 hours	Phenylalanine intolerance (Chewable Tablets only)	Yes	Yes	Yes	Chewable tablets only

FLU (MULTI-SYMPTOM), ADULTS

BRAND	ACTIVE INGREDIENTS (MANUFACTURER)	HOW OFTEN TO TAKE	GET MD APPROVAL IF YOU HAVE:	ALCOHOL-FREE	SUGAR-FREE	LACTOSE-FREE	SODIUM-FREE
Advil Cold and Sinus	Ibuprofen, Pseudoephedrine (Whitehall-Robins)	Every 4 to 6 hours	Heart disease, high blood pressure, thyroid disease, diabetes, enlarged prostate gland, an allergy to aspirin, last 3 months of pregnancy	Yes	No	Yes	No
Alka-Seltzer Plus Cold Medicine Liqui-Gels	Acetaminophen, Chlorpheniramine, Pseudoephedrine (Bayer)	Every 4 hours	Heart disease, high blood pressure, thyroid disease, diabetes, glaucoma, enlarged prostate gland, breathing problems	Yes	Yes	Yes	Yes
Alka-Seltzer Plus Cold Medicine Tablets	Aspirin, Chlorpheniramine, Phenylpropanolamine (Bayer)	Every 4 hours	Heart disease, high blood pressure, thyroid disease, diabetes, glaucoma, enlarged prostate gland, breathing problems, bleeding problems, an allergy to aspirin, last 3 months of pregnancy	Yes	Yes	Yes	No

Alka-Seltzer Plus Cold & Cough Medicine Liqui-Gels	Acetaminophen, Chlorpheniramine, Dextromethorphan, Pseudoephedrine (*Bayer*)	Every 4 hours	Chronic cough, cough with excessive phlegm, heart disease, high blood pressure, thyroid disease, diabetes, glaucoma, enlarged prostate gland, breathing problems	Yes	Yes	Yes	Yes
Alka-Seltzer Plus Cold & Cough Medicine Tablets	Aspirin, Chlorpheniramine, Dextromethorphan, Phenylpropanolamine (*Bayer*)	Every 4 hours	Chronic cough, cough with excessive phlegm, heart disease, high blood pressure, thyroid disease, diabetes, glaucoma, enlarged prostate gland, breathing problems, bleeding problems, an allergy to aspirin, last 3 months of pregnancy	Yes	Yes	Yes	No
Alka-Seltzer Plus Flu & Body Aches Liqui-Gels	Acetaminophen, Dextromethorphan, Pseudoephedrine (*Bayer*)	Every 4 hours	Chronic cough, cough with excessive phlegm, heart disease, high blood pressure, thyroid disease, diabetes, enlarged prostate gland	Yes	Yes	Yes	Yes
Alka-Seltzer Plus Flu & Body Aches Tablets	Acetaminophen, Chlorpheniramine, Dextromethorphan, Phenylpropanolamine (*Bayer*)	Every 4 hours	Chronic cough, cough with excessive phlegm, heart disease, high blood pressure, thyroid disease, diabetes, glaucoma, enlarged prostate gland, breathing problems	Yes	Yes	Yes	No

BRAND	ACTIVE INGREDIENTS (MANUFACTURER)	HOW OFTEN TO TAKE	GET MD APPROVAL IF YOU HAVE:	ALCOHOL-FREE	SUGAR-FREE	LACTOSE-FREE	SODIUM-FREE
Alka-Seltzer Plus Night-Time Cold Medicine Liqui-Gels	Acetaminophen, Dextromethorphan, Doxylamine, Pseudoephedrine (Bayer)	Once a day	Chronic cough, cough with excessive phlegm, heart disease, high blood pressure, thyroid disease, diabetes, glaucoma, enlarged prostate gland, breathing problems	Yes	Yes	Yes	Yes
Alka-Seltzer Plus Night-Time Cold Medicine Tablets	Aspirin, Dextromethorphan, Doxylamine, Phenylpropanolamine (Bayer)	Every 4 hours	Chronic cough, cough with excessive phlegm, heart disease, high blood pressure, thyroid disease, diabetes, glaucoma, enlarged prostate gland, breathing problems, bleeding problems, an allergy to aspirin, last 3 months of pregnancy	Yes	Yes	Yes	No
Comtrex Cold & Flu Reliever Tablets and Caplets	Acetaminophen, Chlorpheniramine, Dextromethorphan, Pseudoephedrine (Bristol-Myers)	Every 6 hours	Chronic cough, cough with excessive phlegm, heart disease, high blood pressure, thyroid disease, diabetes, glaucoma, enlarged prostate gland, breathing problems	Yes	Yes	Yes	Yes

Product	Ingredients	Dosage	Do not use if you have...				
Comtrex Cold & Flu Reliever Liquid	Acetaminophen, Chlorpheniramine, Dextromethorphan, Pseudoephedrine (*Bristol-Myers*)	Every 6 hours	Chronic cough, cough with excessive phlegm, heart disease, high blood pressure, thyroid disease, diabetes, glaucoma, enlarged prostate gland, breathing problems	No	No	Yes	No
Comtrex Cold & Flu Reliever Liqui-Gels	Acetaminophen, Chlorpheniramine, Dextromethorphan, Phenylpropanolamine (*Bristol-Myers*)	Every 6 hours	Chronic cough, cough with excessive phlegm, heart disease, high blood pressure, thyroid disease, diabetes, glaucoma, enlarged prostate gland, breathing problems	Yes	Yes	Yes	Yes
Comtrex Deep Chest Cold	Acetaminophen, Dextromethorphan, Guaifenesin, Phenylpropanolamine (*Bristol-Myers*)	Every 4 hours	Chronic cough, cough with excessive phlegm, heart disease, high blood pressure, thyroid disease, diabetes, enlarged prostate gland	Yes	Yes	Yes	Yes
Comtrex Non-Drowsy Caplets	Acetaminophen, Dextromethorphan, Pseudoephedrine (*Bristol-Myers*)	Every 6 hours	Chronic cough, cough with excessive phlegm, heart disease, high blood pressure, thyroid disease, diabetes, enlarged prostate gland	Yes	Yes	Yes	Yes
Comtrex Non-Drowsy Liqui-Gels	Acetaminophen, Dextromethorphan, Phenylpropanolamine (*Bristol-Myers*)	Every 6 hours	Chronic cough, cough with excessive phlegm, heart disease, high blood pressure, thyroid disease, diabetes, enlarged prostate gland	Yes	Yes	Yes	Yes

BRAND	ACTIVE INGREDIENTS (MANUFACTURER)	HOW OFTEN TO TAKE	GET MD APPROVAL IF YOU HAVE:	ALCOHOL- FREE	SUGAR- FREE	LACTOSE- FREE	SODIUM- FREE
Contac Day & Night Cold/Flu	Day Caplets: Acetaminophen, Dextromethorphan, Pseudoephedrine; Night Caplets: Acetaminophen, Diphenhydramine, Pseudoephedrine (SmithKline Beecham)	Every 6 hours	Chronic cough, cough with excessive phlegm, heart disease, high blood pressure, thyroid disease, diabetes, glaucoma, enlarged prostate gland, breathing problems	Yes	Yes	Yes	Yes
Contac Severe Cold and Flu	Acetaminophen, Chlorpheniramine, Dextromethorphan, Phenylpropanolamine (SmithKline Beecham)	Every 6 hours	Chronic cough, cough with excessive phlegm, heart disease, high blood pressure, thyroid disease, diabetes, glaucoma, enlarged prostate gland, breathing problems	Yes	Yes	Yes	No
Contac Severe Cold and Flu Non-Drowsy	Acetaminophen, Dextromethorphan, Pseudoephedrine (SmithKline Beecham)	Every 6 hours	Chronic cough, cough with excessive phlegm, heart disease, high blood pressure, thyroid disease, diabetes, enlarged prostate gland	Yes	Yes	Yes	Yes

Product	Ingredients (Manufacturer)	Dosage	Do not take if you have...				
Coricidin Cold & Flu Tablets	Acetaminophen, Chlorpheniramine (*Schering-Plough*)	Every 4 to 6 hours	Breathing problems, glaucoma, enlarged prostate gland	Yes	No	No	Yes
Coricidin 'D'	Acetaminophen, Chlorpheniramine, Phenylpropanolamine (*Schering-Plough*)	Every 4 hours	Heart disease, high blood pressure, thyroid disease, diabetes, glaucoma, enlarged prostate gland, breathing problems	Yes	Yes	Yes	Yes
Coricidin Nighttime Cold & Cough Liquid	Acetaminophen, Diphenhydramine (*Schering-Plough*)	Every 4 hours	Chronic cough, cough with excessive phlegm, breathing problems, glaucoma, enlarged prostate gland	Yes	Yes	No	No
Drixoral Cold & Flu	Acetaminophen, Dexbrompheniramine, Pseudoephedrine (*Schering-Plough*)	Every 12 hours	Heart disease, high blood pressure, thyroid disease, diabetes, glaucoma, enlarged prostate gland, breathing problems	Yes	Yes	Yes	Yes
Robitussin Cold, Cough & Flu	Acetaminophen, Dextromethorphan, Guaifenesin, Pseudoephedrine (*Whitehall-Robins*)	Every 4 hours	Chronic cough, cough with excessive phlegm, high blood pressure, heart disease, thyroid disease, diabetes, enlarged prostate gland	Yes	Yes	Yes	Yes

BRAND	ACTIVE INGREDIENTS *(MANUFACTURER)*	HOW OFTEN TO TAKE	GET MD APPROVAL IF YOU HAVE:	ALCOHOL-FREE	SUGAR-FREE	LACTOSE-FREE	SODIUM-FREE
Robitussin Night-Time Cold Formula	Acetaminophen, Dextromethorphan, Doxylamine, Pseudoephedrine *(Whitehall-Robins)*	Every 6 hours	Chronic cough, cough with excessive phlegm, heart disease, high blood pressure, thyroid disease, diabetes, enlarged prostate gland	Yes	Yes	Yes	No
Sine-Off	Acetaminophen, Diphenhydramine, Pseudoephedrine *(Hogil)*	Every 6 hours	Heart disease, high blood pressure, thyroid disease, diabetes, glaucoma, enlarged prostate gland, breathing problems	Yes	Yes	Yes	No
Theraflu Flu and Cold Medicine	Acetaminophen, Chlorpheniramine, Pseudoephedrine *(Novartis)*	Every 4 to 6 hours	Heart disease, high blood pressure, thyroid disease, diabetes, glaucoma, enlarged prostate gland, breathing problems	Yes	No	Yes	No
Theraflu Flu, Cold & Cough (Regular and Nighttime)	Acetaminophen, Chlorpheniramine, Dextromethorphan, Pseudoephedrine *(Novartis)*	Every 6 hours	Chronic cough, cough with excessive phlegm, heart disease, high blood pressure, thyroid disease, diabetes, glaucoma, enlarged prostate gland, breathing problems	Yes	No	Hot Liquid only	No

Product	Ingredients (Manufacturer)	Dosage	Don't use if you have				
Theraflu Flu, Cold & Cough (Non-Drowsy)	Acetaminophen, Dextromethorphan, Pseudoephedrine (*Novartis*)	Every 6 hours	Chronic cough, cough with excessive phlegm, heart disease, high blood pressure, thyroid disease, diabetes, enlarged prostate gland	Yes	No	Hot Liquid only	No
Tylenol Cold Medication (Tablets and Caplets)	Acetaminophen, Chlorpheniramine, Dextromethorphan, Pseudoephedrine (*McNeil*)	Every 6 hours	Chronic cough, cough with excessive phlegm, heart disease, high blood pressure, thyroid disease, diabetes, glaucoma, enlarged prostate gland, breathing problems	Yes	Yes	Yes	No
Tylenol Cold (Hot Medication Packets)	Acetaminophen, Chlorpheniramine, Dextromethorphan, Pseudoephedrine (*McNeil*)	Every 6 hours	Chronic cough, cough with excessive phlegm, heart disease, high blood pressure, thyroid disease, diabetes, glaucoma, enlarged prostate gland, breathing problems	Yes	No	Yes	No
Tylenol Cold (No Drowsiness Caplets and Gelcaps)	Acetaminophen, Dextromethorphan, Pseudoephedrine (*McNeil*)	Every 6 hours	Chronic cough, cough with excessive phlegm, heart disease, high blood pressure, thyroid disease, diabetes, enlarged prostate gland	Caplets only	Yes	Yes	No
Tylenol Flu NightTime (Gelcaps)	Acetaminophen, Diphenhydramine, Pseudoephedrine (*McNeil*)	Every 6 hours	Heart disease, high blood pressure, thyroid disease, diabetes, glaucoma, enlarged prostate gland, breathing problems	No	Yes	Yes	No

BRAND	ACTIVE INGREDIENTS (MANUFACTURER)	HOW OFTEN TO TAKE	GET MD APPROVAL IF YOU HAVE:	ALCOHOL-FREE	SUGAR-FREE	LACTOSE-FREE	SODIUM-FREE
Tylenol Flu NightTime (Hot Medication Packets)	Acetaminophen, Diphenhydramine, Pseudoephedrine (*McNeil*)	Every 6 hours	Heart disease, high blood pressure, thyroid disease, diabetes, glaucoma, enlarged prostate gland, breathing problems	Yes	No	Yes	No
Tylenol Flu No Drowsiness Formula	Acetaminophen, Dextromethorphan, Pseudoephedrine (*McNeil*)	Every 6 hours	Chronic cough, cough with excessive phlegm, heart disease, high blood pressure, thyroid disease, diabetes, enlarged prostate gland	No	Yes	Yes	No
Vicks 44M	Acetaminophen, Chlorpheniramine, Dextromethorphan, Pseudoephedrine (*Procter & Gamble*)	Every 6 hours	Chronic cough, cough with excessive phlegm, heart disease, high blood pressure, thyroid disease, diabetes, glaucoma, enlarged prostate gland, breathing problems	No	No	Yes	No
Vicks DayQuil	Acetaminophen, Dextromethorphan, Pseudoephedrine (*Procter & Gamble*)	Every 4 hours	Chronic cough, cough with excessive phlegm, heart disease, high blood pressure, thyroid disease, diabetes, enlarged prostate gland, breathing problems	Yes	Soft-gels only	Yes	Soft-gels only

Product	Ingredients	Frequency	Warnings				
Vicks DayQuil Sinus Pressure & Pain Relief	Ibuprofen, Pseudoephedrine (*Procter & Gamble*)	Every 4 to 6 hours	Heart disease, high blood pressure, thyroid disease, diabetes, enlarged prostate gland, an allergy to aspirin, last 3 months of pregnancy	Yes	No	Yes	No
Vicks NyQuil Hot Therapy	Acetaminophen, Dextromethorphan, Doxylamine, Pseudoephedrine (*Procter & Gamble*)	Every 6 hours	Chronic cough, cough with excessive phlegm, heart disease, high blood pressure, thyroid disease, diabetes, glaucoma, enlarged prostate gland, breathing problems	Yes	No	Yes	Yes
Vicks NyQuil Liquicaps	Acetaminophen, Dextromethorphan, Doxylamine, Pseudoephedrine (*Procter & Gamble*)	Every 4 hours	Chronic cough, cough with excessive phlegm, heart disease, high blood pressure, thyroid disease, diabetes, glaucoma, enlarged prostate gland, breathing problems	Yes	Yes	Yes	Yes
Vicks NyQuil Liquid	Acetaminophen, Dextromethorphan, Doxylamine, Pseudoephedrine (*Procter & Gamble*)	Every 6 hours	Chronic cough, cough with excessive phlegm, heart disease, high blood pressure, thyroid disease, diabetes, glaucoma, enlarged prostate gland, breathing problems	No	No	Yes	No

FLU (MULTI-SYMPTOM), CHILDREN

BRAND	ACTIVE INGREDIENTS (MANUFACTURER)	HOW OFTEN TO TAKE	GET MD APPROVAL IF YOU HAVE:	ALCOHOL-FREE	SUGAR-FREE	LACTOSE-FREE	SODIUM-FREE
Tylenol Children's Flu Liquid	Acetaminophen, Chlorpheniramine, Dextromethorphan, Pseudoephedrine (McNeil)	Every 6 to 8 hours	Chronic cough, cough with excessive phlegm, heart disease, high blood pressure, thyroid disease, diabetes, glaucoma, breathing problems	Yes	No	Yes	No

GAS, ADULTS

BRAND	ACTIVE INGREDIENTS (MANUFACTURER)	HOW OFTEN TO TAKE	GET MD APPROVAL IF YOU HAVE:	ALCOHOL-FREE	SUGAR-FREE	LACTOSE-FREE	SODIUM-FREE
Beano Liquid	Alpha-D-galactosidase (AkPharma)	With meals	Galactose intolerance	Yes	Yes	Yes	Yes
Di-Gel Tablets	Calcium carbonate, Magnesium hydroxide, Simethicone (Schering-Plough)	Every 2 hours	Kidney disease	Yes	No	Yes	Yes
Di-Gel Liquid	Aluminum hydroxide, Magnesium hydroxide, Simethicone (Schering-Plough)	Every 2 hours	Kidney disease	Yes	Yes	Yes	Yes

Product	Ingredients	Dosage	Warnings				
Gas-X	Simethicone (*Novartis*)	After meals and at bedtime	—	Yes	Soft-gels only	Yes	Yes
Maalox Antacid/Anti-Gas	Aluminum hydroxide, Magnesium hydroxide, Simethicone (*Novartis*)	4 times a day	Kidney disease	Yes	Liquid only	Yes	No
Maalox Anti-Gas	Simethicone (*Novartis*)	Extra-strength: up to 3 times a day; Regular strength: up to 6 times a day	—	Yes	No	Yes	Yes
Mylanta Liquid	Aluminum hydroxide, Magnesium hydroxide, Simethicone (*J&J Merck*)	Between meals and at bedtime	Kidney disease	Yes	Yes	Yes	No
Mylanta Gas Relief	Simethicone (*J&J Merck*)	After meals and at bedtime	—	Tablets only	Gelcaps only	Yes	Tablets only

BRAND	ACTIVE INGREDIENTS (MANUFACTURER)	HOW OFTEN TO TAKE	GET MD APPROVAL IF YOU HAVE:	ALCOHOL-FREE	SUGAR-FREE	LACTOSE-FREE	SODIUM-FREE
Phazyme	Simethicone (Block Drug)	4 times a day	—	Yes	Liquid and soft-gels only	Yes	Chew-ables and soft-gels only

GAS, CHILDREN

BRAND	ACTIVE INGREDIENTS (MANUFACTURER)	HOW OFTEN TO TAKE	GET MD APPROVAL IF YOU HAVE:	ALCOHOL-FREE	SUGAR-FREE	LACTOSE-FREE	SODIUM-FREE
Infants' Mylicon	Simethicone (J&J Merck)	4 times a day	—		Yes	Yes	No
Phazyme Infant Drops	Simethicone (Block Drug)	4 times a day	—	Yes	Yes	Yes	No

HAY FEVER SYMPTOMS, ADULTS

BRAND	ACTIVE INGREDIENTS (MANUFACTURER)	HOW OFTEN TO TAKE	GET MD APPROVAL IF YOU HAVE:	ALCOHOL-FREE	SUGAR-FREE	LACTOSE-FREE	SODIUM-FREE
Actifed Cold & Allergy	Pseudoephedrine, Triprolidine (Warner-Lambert)	Every 4 to 6 hours	Heart disease, high blood pressure, thyroid disease, diabetes, glaucoma, enlarged prostate gland, breathing problems	Yes	No	No	Yes

	Ingredients	Dosage	Don't use if you have				
Actified Allergy Daytime/Nighttime Caplets	Daytime Caplets: Pseudoephedrine; Nighttime Caplets: Diphenhydramine, Pseudoephedrine (Warner-Lambert)	Daytime: Every 4 to 6 hours; Nighttime: At bedtime	Heart disease, high blood pressure, thyroid disease, diabetes, glaucoma, enlarged prostate gland, breathing problems	Yes	Yes	No	Yes
Allerest Maximum Strength	Chlorpheniramine, Pseudoephedrine (Novartis)	Every 4 to 6 hours	Heart disease, high blood pressure, thyroid disease, diabetes, glaucoma, enlarged prostate gland, breathing problems	Yes	Yes	No	Yes
Allerest No Drowsiness	Acetaminophen, Pseudoephedrine (Novartis)	Every 4 to 6 hours	Heart disease, high blood pressure, thyroid disease, diabetes, enlarged prostate gland	Yes	Yes	Yes	Yes
Benadryl Allergy Capsules and Tablets	Diphenhydramine (Warner-Lambert)	Every 4 to 6 hours	Breathing problems, glaucoma, enlarged prostate gland	Yes	Yes	Tablets only	Yes
Benadryl Allergy Chewables	Diphenhydramine (Warner-Lambert)	Every 4 to 6 hours	Breathing problems, glaucoma, enlarged prostate gland	Yes	Yes	Yes	Yes

BRAND	ACTIVE INGREDIENTS (MANUFACTURER)	HOW OFTEN TO TAKE	GET MD APPROVAL IF YOU HAVE:	ALCOHOL-FREE	SUGAR-FREE	LACTOSE-FREE	SODIUM-FREE
Benadryl Allergy Liquid	Diphenhydramine (Warner-Lambert)	Every 4 to 6 hours	Breathing problems, glaucoma, enlarged prostate gland	Yes	No	Yes	No
Benadryl Allergy/ Cold Tablets	Acetaminophen, Diphenhydramine, Pseudoephedrine (Warner-Lambert)	Every 6 hours	Heart disease, high blood pressure, thyroid disease, diabetes, glaucoma, enlarged prostate gland, breathing problems	Yes	Yes	Yes	No
Benadryl Allergy Decongestant Liquid and Tablets	Diphenhydramine, Pseudoephedrine (Warner-Lambert)	Every 4 to 6 hours	Heart disease, high blood pressure, thyroid disease, diabetes, glaucoma, enlarged prostate gland, breathing problems	Yes	Yes	Yes	No
Benadryl Allergy Sinus Headache Caplets	Acetaminophen, Diphenhydramine, Pseudoephedrine (Warner-Lambert)	Every 6 hours	Heart disease, high blood pressure, thyroid disease, diabetes, glaucoma, enlarged prostate gland, breathing problems	Yes	Yes	Yes	No

Chlor-Trimeton Allergy 4 Hour Tablets	Chlorpheniramine (*Schering-Plough*)	Every 4 to 6 hours	Breathing problems, glaucoma, enlarged prostate gland	Yes	Yes	No	Yes
Chlor-Trimeton Allergy 8 Hour Tablets	Chlorpheniramine (*Schering-Plough*)	Every 8 to 12 hours	Breathing problems, glaucoma, enlarged prostate gland	Yes	No	No	Yes
Chlor-Trimeton Allergy 12 Hour Tablets	Chlorpheniramine (*Schering-Plough*)	Every 12 hours	Breathing problems, glaucoma, enlarged prostate gland	Yes	No	No	Yes
Chlor-Trimeton Allergy/Decongestant 4 Hour Tablets	Chlorpheniramine, Pseudoephedrine (*Schering-Plough*)	Every 4 to 6 hours	Heart disease, high blood pressure, thyroid disease, diabetes, glaucoma, enlarged prostate gland, breathing problems	Yes	Yes	No	Yes

BRAND	ACTIVE INGREDIENTS (MANUFACTURER)	HOW OFTEN TO TAKE	GET MD APPROVAL IF YOU HAVE:	ALCOHOL-FREE	SUGAR-FREE	LACTOSE-FREE	SODIUM-FREE
Chlor-Trimeton Allergy/ Decongestant 12 Hour Tablets	Chlorpheniramine, Pseudoephedrine (Schering-Plough)	Every 12 hours	Heart disease, high blood pressure, thyroid disease, diabetes, glaucoma, enlarged prostate gland, breathing problems	Yes	No	No	Yes
Comtrex Allergy-Sinus	Acetaminophen, Chlorpheniramine, Pseudoephedrine (Bristol-Myers)	Every 6 hours	Heart disease, high blood pressure, thyroid disease, diabetes, glaucoma, enlarged prostate gland, breathing problems	Yes	Yes	Yes	No
Contac (Regular Strength)	Chlorpheniramine, Phenylpropanolamine (SmithKline Beecham)	Every 12 hours	Heart disease, high blood pressure, thyroid disease, diabetes, glaucoma, enlarged prostate gland, breathing problems	No	No	Yes	No
Contac (Maximum Strength)	Chlorpheniramine, Phenylpropanolamine (SmithKline Beecham)	Every 12 hours	Heart disease, high blood pressure, thyroid disease, diabetes, glaucoma, enlarged prostate gland, breathing problems	Yes	Yes	No	Yes

Coricidin Cold & Flu Tablets	Acetaminophen, Chlorpheniramine (*Schering-Plough*)	Every 4 to 6 hours	Breathing problems, glaucoma, enlarged prostate gland	Yes	No	No	Yes
Coricidin Cough & Cold Tablets	Chlorpheniramine, Dextromethorphan (*Schering-Plough*)	Every 6 hours	Chronic cough, cough with excessive phlegm, breathing problems, glaucoma, enlarged prostate gland	Yes	No	No	No
Dimetapp Elixir	Brompheniramine, Phenylpropanolamine (*Whitehall-Robins*)	Every 4 hours	Heart disease, high blood pressure, thyroid disease, diabetes, glaucoma, enlarged prostate gland, breathing problems	Yes	Yes	Yes	No
Dimetapp Extentabs	Brompheniramine, Phenylpropanolamine (*Whitehall-Robins*)	Every 12 hours	Heart disease, high blood pressure, thyroid disease, diabetes, glaucoma, enlarged prostate gland, breathing problems	No	No	Yes	Yes
Dimetapp Tablets and Liqui-Gels	Brompheniramine, Phenylpropanolamine (*Whitehall-Robins*)	Every 4 hours	Heart disease, high blood pressure, thyroid disease, diabetes, glaucoma, enlarged prostate gland, breathing problems	Yes	Yes	Yes	Yes
Dimetapp Allergy Dye-Free Elixir	Brompheniramine (*Whitehall-Robins*)	Every 4 to 6 hours	Breathing problems, glaucoma, enlarged prostate gland	Yes	Yes	Yes	No

BRAND	ACTIVE INGREDIENTS (MANUFACTURER)	HOW OFTEN TO TAKE	GET MD APPROVAL IF YOU HAVE:	ALCOHOL-FREE	SUGAR-FREE	LACTOSE-FREE	SODIUM-FREE
Dimetapp Allergy Sinus	Acetaminophen, Brompheniramine, Phenylpropanolamine (*Whitehall-Robins*)	Every 6 hours	Heart disease, high blood pressure, thyroid disease, diabetes, glaucoma, enlarged prostate gland, breathing problems	Yes	Yes	Yes	Yes
Dimetapp Cold & Cough Liqui-Gels	Brompheniramine, Dextromethorphan, Phenylpropanolamine (*Whitehall-Robins*)	Every 4 hours	Chronic cough, cough with excessive phlegm, heart disease, high blood pressure, thyroid disease, diabetes, glaucoma, enlarged prostate gland, breathing problems	Yes	Yes	Yes	Yes
Dimetapp DM Elixir	Brompheniramine, Dextromethorphan, Phenylpropanolamine (*Whitehall-Robins*)	Every 4 hours	Chronic cough, cough with excessive phlegm, heart disease, high blood pressure, thyroid disease, diabetes, glaucoma, enlarged prostate gland, breathing problems	Yes	Yes	Yes	No
Drixoral Allergy/ Sinus	Acetaminophen, Dexbrompheniramine, Pseudoephedrine (*Schering-Plough*)	Every 12 hours	Heart disease, high blood pressure, thyroid disease, diabetes, glaucoma, enlarged prostate gland, breathing problems	Yes	Yes	Yes	Yes

Product	Ingredients (Manufacturer)	Dosage	Don't take if you have				
Drixoral Cold & Allergy	Dexbrompheniramine, Pseudoephedrine (*Schering-Plough*)	Every 12 hours	Heart disease, high blood pressure, thyroid disease, diabetes, glaucoma, enlarged prostate gland, breathing problems	Yes	No	No	Yes
Drixoral Cold & Flu	Acetaminophen, Dexbrompheniramine, Pseudoephedrine (*Schering-Plough*)	Every 12 hours	Heart disease, high blood pressure, thyroid disease, diabetes, glaucoma, enlarged prostate gland, breathing problems	Yes	Yes	Yes	Yes
Nasalcrom	Cromolyn (*McNeil*)	Every 4 to 6 hours	Fever, sinus pain, wheezing, discolored nasal discharge	Yes	Yes	Yes	Yes
Nolahist	Phenindamine (*Carnrick*)	Every 4 to 6 hours	Breathing problems, glaucoma, enlarged prostate gland	Yes	NA	NA	NA
Novahistine	Chlorpheniramine, Phenylephrine (*SmithKline Beecham*)	Every 4 hours	Heart disease, high blood pressure, thyroid disease, diabetes, glaucoma, enlarged prostate gland, breathing problems, ulcers, a nursing baby, an allergy to any ingredient	No	Yes	Yes	No
Ryna Liquid	Chlorpheniramine, Pseudoephedrine (*Wallace*)	Every 4 to 6 hours	Heart disease, high blood pressure, thyroid disease, diabetes, glaucoma, enlarged prostate gland, breathing problems	Yes	Yes	Yes	No

BRAND	ACTIVE INGREDIENTS (MANUFACTURER)	HOW OFTEN TO TAKE	GET MD APPROVAL IF YOU HAVE:	ALCOHOL-FREE	SUGAR-FREE	LACTOSE-FREE	SODIUM-FREE
Ryna-C Liquid	Chlorpheniramine, Codeine, Pseudoephedrine (Wallace)	Every 4 to 6 hours	Chronic cough, cough with excessive phlegm, heart disease, high blood pressure, thyroid disease, diabetes, glaucoma, enlarged prostate gland, breathing problems	Yes	Yes	Yes	No
Sinarest (Tablets and Extra Strength Caplets)	Acetaminophen, Chlorpheniramine, Pseudoephedrine (Novartis)	Tablets: Every 4 to 6 hours; Caplets: Every 6 hours	Heart disease, high blood pressure, thyroid disease, diabetes, glaucoma, enlarged prostate gland, breathing problems	Yes	Yes	Yes	Yes
Sine-Off	Acetaminophen, Diphenhydramine, Pseudoephedrine (Hogil)	Every 6 hours	Heart disease, high blood pressure, thyroid disease, diabetes, glaucoma, enlarged prostate gland, breathing problems	Yes	Yes	Yes	No
Singlet	Acetaminophen, Chlorpheniramine, Pseudoephedrine (SmithKline Beecham)	Every 4 to 6 hours	Heart disease, high blood pressure, thyroid disease, diabetes, glaucoma, enlarged prostate gland, breathing problems	Yes	No	Yes	No

Product	Ingredients (Manufacturer)	Dosage	Do not use if you have				
Simulin	Acetaminophen, Chlorpheniramine, Phenylpropanolamine (*Carnrick*)	Every 4 to 6 hours	Heart disease, high blood pressure, thyroid disease, diabetes, glaucoma, enlarged prostate gland, breathing problems	Yes	NA	NA	NA
Sinutab Sinus Allergy	Acetaminophen, Chlorpheniramine, Pseudoephedrine (*Warner-Lambert*)	Every 6 hours	Heart disease, high blood pressure, thyroid disease, diabetes, glaucoma, enlarged prostate gland, breathing problems	Yes	Yes	Yes	No
Sudafed Cold & Allergy	Chlorpheniramine, Pseudoephedrine (*Warner-Lambert*)	Every 4 to 6 hours	Heart disease, high blood pressure, thyroid disease, diabetes, glaucoma, enlarged prostate gland, breathing problems	Yes	Yes	No	Yes
Tavist-1	Clemastine (*Novartis*)	Every 12 hours	Breathing problems, glaucoma, enlarged prostate gland	Yes	Yes	No	Yes
Tavist-D	Clemastine, Phenylpropanolamine (*Novartis*)	Every 12 hours	Heart disease, high blood pressure, thyroid disease, diabetes, glaucoma, enlarged prostate gland, breathing problems	Yes	Yes	No	Yes
Teldrin	Chlorpheniramine, Phenylpropanolamine (*Hogil*)	Every 12 hours	Heart disease, high blood pressure, thyroid disease, diabetes, glaucoma, enlarged prostate gland, breathing problems	No	No	Yes	No

BRAND	ACTIVE INGREDIENTS (MANUFACTURER)	HOW OFTEN TO TAKE	GET MD APPROVAL IF YOU HAVE:	ALCOHOL-FREE	SUGAR-FREE	LACTOSE-FREE	SODIUM-FREE
Theraflu Flu and Cold Medicine	Acetaminophen, Chlorpheniramine, Pseudoephedrine (Novartis)	Every 4 to 6 hours	Heart disease, high blood pressure, thyroid disease, diabetes, glaucoma, enlarged prostate gland, breathing problems	Yes	No	Yes	No
Tylenol Allergy Sinus	Acetaminophen, Chlorpheniramine, Pseudoephedrine (McNeil)	Every 6 hours	Heart disease, high blood pressure, thyroid disease, diabetes, glaucoma, enlarged prostate gland, breathing problems	Caplets only	Yes	Yes	No
Tylenol Allergy Sinus NightTime	Acetaminophen, Diphenhydramine, Pseudoephedrine (McNeil)	At bedtime	Heart disease, high blood pressure, thyroid disease, diabetes, glaucoma, enlarged prostate gland, breathing problems	Yes	Yes	Yes	No
Tylenol Severe Allergy	Acetaminophen, Diphenhydramine (McNeil)	Every 4 to 6 hours	Breathing problems, glaucoma, enlarged prostate gland	Yes	Yes	Yes	No

HAY FEVER SYMPTOMS, CHILDREN

Product	Ingredients (Manufacturer)	Dosage	Conditions				
Dimetapp Cold & Allergy (Chewable and Quick-Dissolving Tablets)	Brompheniramine, Phenylpropanolamine (*Whitehall-Robins*)	Every 4 hours	Heart disease, high blood pressure, thyroid disease, diabetes, glaucoma, breathing problems	Yes	Yes	Yes	Yes
Dimetapp Cold and Fever Suspension	Acetaminophen, Brompheniramine, Pseudoephedrine (*Whitehall-Robins*)	Every 4 hours	Heart disease, high blood pressure, thyroid disease, diabetes, glaucoma, breathing problems	Yes	No	Yes	No
PediaCare Cough-Cold (Liquid and Chewable Tablets)	Chlorpheniramine, Dextromethorphan, Pseudoephedrine (*McNeil*)	Every 4 to 6 hours	Chronic cough, cough with excessive phlegm, heart disease, high blood pressure, thyroid disease, diabetes, glaucoma, breathing problems	Yes	Tablets only	Tablets only	Tablets only
PediaCare Cough-Cold (NightRest Liquid)	Chlorpheniramine, Dextromethorphan, Pseudoephedrine (*McNeil*)	Every 6 to 8 hours	Chronic cough, cough with excessive phlegm, heart disease, high blood pressure, thyroid disease, diabetes, glaucoma, breathing problems	Yes	No	Yes	No

BRAND	ACTIVE INGREDIENTS (MANUFACTURER)	HOW OFTEN TO TAKE	GET MD APPROVAL IF YOU HAVE:	ALCOHOL-FREE	SUGAR-FREE	LACTOSE-FREE	SODIUM-FREE
Tylenol Children's Cold	Acetaminophen, Chlorpheniramine, Pseudoephedrine (McNeil)	Every 4 to 6 hours	Heart disease, high blood pressure, thyroid disease, diabetes, glaucoma, breathing problems	Yes	Tablets only	Yes	Tablets only
Tylenol Children's Cold Plus Cough	Acetaminophen, Chlorpheniramine, Dextromethorphan, Pseudoephedrine (McNeil)	Every 4 to 6 hours	Chronic cough, cough with excessive phlegm, heart disease, high blood pressure, thyroid disease, diabetes, glaucoma, breathing problems	Yes	Tablets only	Yes	Tablets only
Tylenol Infants' Cold Drops	Acetaminophen, Pseudoephedrine (McNeil)	Every 4 to 6 hours	Heart disease, high blood pressure, thyroid disease, diabetes	Yes	No	Yes	No
Vicks DayQuil, Children's Allergy	Chlorpheniramine, Pseudoephedrine (Procter & Gamble)	Every 6 hours	Heart disease, high blood pressure, thyroid disease, diabetes, breathing problems	Yes	No	Yes	No

HEADACHE, ADULTS

Actron	Ketoprofen (*Bayer*)	Every 4 to 6 hours	Redness or swelling in painful area, an allergy to pain relievers, last 3 months of pregnancy	Yes	Yes	No	No
Advil	Ibuprofen (*Whitehall-Robins*)	Every 4 to 6 hours	An allergy to aspirin, problems with other pain relievers, last 3 months of pregnancy	Yes	Gel caplets only	Yes	No
Aleve	Naproxen sodium (*Procter & Gamble*)	Every 8 to 12 hours (Adults over 65: Every 12 hours)	An allergy to pain relievers, last 3 months of pregnancy	Yes	Yes	Yes	Yes
Alka-Seltzer	Aspirin, Citric acid, Sodium bicarbonate (*Bayer*)	Every 4 hours; Extra Strength: Every 6 hours	Asthma, bleeding problems, an allergy to aspirin, a sodium-restricted diet, last 3 months of pregnancy, phenylalanine intolerance (Lemon Lime and Cherry only)	Yes	Yes	Yes	No

BRAND	ACTIVE INGREDIENTS (MANUFACTURER)	HOW OFTEN TO TAKE	GET MD APPROVAL IF YOU HAVE:	ALCOHOL-FREE	SUGAR-FREE	LACTOSE-FREE	SODIUM-FREE
Ascriptin	Alumina-magnesia, Aspirin, Calcium carbonate (*Novartis*)	Every 4 hours; Maximum Strength: Every 6 hours	Asthma, heartburn, upset stomach, stomach pain, ulcers, bleeding problems, an allergy to aspirin, last 3 months of pregnancy	Yes	Yes	Yes	Yes
Ascriptin Enteric	Aspirin (*Novartis*)	Every 4 hours	Asthma, heartburn, upset stomach, stomach pain, ulcers, bleeding problems, an allergy to aspirin, last 3 months of pregnancy	Yes	Yes	Yes	No
Bayer (Genuine, Extra Strength, Extended-Release)	Aspirin (*Bayer*)	Every 4 hours; Extended-Release: Every 8 hours	Asthma, heartburn, upset stomach, stomach pain, ulcers, bleeding problems, an allergy to aspirin, last 3 months of pregnancy	Yes	Yes	Yes	Yes
Bayer PM	Aspirin, Diphenhydramine (*Bayer*)	At bedtime	Asthma, bleeding problems, stomach problems, ulcers, breathing problems, glaucoma, prostate enlargement, an allergy to aspirin, last 3 months of pregnancy	Yes	Yes	Yes	Yes

BC Powder	Aspirin, Caffeine, Salicylamide (*Block Drug*)	Every 3 to 4 hours	An allergy to aspirin, last 3 months of pregnancy	Yes	Yes	Yes	Yes
Bufferin (Regular and Extra Strengths)	Aspirin, Calcium carbonate, Magnesium carbonate, Magnesium oxide (*Bristol-Myers*)	Every 4 hours; Extra Strength: Every 6 hours	Asthma, heartburn, upset stomach, stomach pain, ulcers, bleeding problems, an allergy to aspirin, last 3 months of pregnancy	Yes	Yes	Yes	No
Excedrin	Acetaminophen, Aspirin, Caffeine (*Bristol-Myers*)	Every 6 hours	Asthma, heartburn, upset stomach, stomach pain, ulcers, bleeding problems, an allergy to aspirin, last 3 months of pregnancy	Yes	Yes	Yes	No
Excedrin, Aspirin Free	Acetaminophen, Caffeine (*Bristol-Myers*)	Every 6 hours	—	Yes	Yes	Yes	No
Excedrin P.M.	Acetaminophen, Diphenhydramine (*Bristol-Myers*)	At bedtime	Breathing problems, glaucoma, prostate enlargement	Yes	Yes	Yes	No
Goody's	Acetaminophen, Aspirin, Caffeine (*Block Drug*)	Every 4 to 6 hours	An allergy to aspirin, last 3 months of pregnancy	Yes	Yes	Tablets only	Yes

BRAND	ACTIVE INGREDIENTS (MANUFACTURER)	HOW OFTEN TO TAKE	GET MD APPROVAL IF YOU HAVE:	ALCOHOL-FREE	SUGAR-FREE	LACTOSE-FREE	SODIUM-FREE
Midol Menstrual Formula	Acetaminophen, Caffeine, Pyrilamine (Bayer)	Every 4 hours	Breathing problems, glaucoma	Yes	Yes	Yes	No
Midol PMS Formula	Acetaminophen, Pamabrom, Pyrilamine (Bayer)	Every 4 hours	Breathing problems, glaucoma	Yes	Yes	Yes	No
Midol Teen Menstrual Formula	Acetaminophen, Pamabrom (Bayer)	Every 4 hours	—	Yes	Yes	Yes	No
Motrin IB	Ibuprofen (Pharmacia & Upjohn)	Every 4 to 6 hours	An allergy to aspirin, problems with other pain relievers, last 3 months of pregnancy	Caplets and tablets only	Yes	Yes	Caplets and tablets only
Nuprin	Ibuprofen (Bristol-Myers)	Every 4 to 6 hours	An allergy to aspirin, problems with other pain relievers, last 3 months of pregnancy	Yes	Yes	Yes	Yes
Orudis KT	Ketoprofen (Whitehall-Robins)	Every 4 to 6 hours	Redness or swelling in painful area, an allergy to pain relievers, last 3 months of pregnancy	Yes	No	Yes	No

Pamprin Maximum Pain Relief	Acetaminophen, Magnesium salicylate, Pamabrom (*Chattem*)	Every 4 to 6 hours	An allergy to salicylates (aspirin), last 3 months of pregnancy	Yes	Yes	Yes	No
Pamprin Multi-Symptom	Acetaminophen, Pamabrom, Pyrilamine (*Chattem*)	Every 4 to 6 hours	Breathing problems, glaucoma	Yes	Yes	Yes	No
Panadol	Acetaminophen (*SmithKline Beecham*)	Every 4 hours	—	Yes	Yes	Yes	Yes
St. Joseph	Aspirin (*Schering-Plough*)	Every 4 hours	Asthma, heartburn, upset stomach, stomach pain, ulcers, bleeding problems, an allergy to aspirin, last 3 months of pregnancy	Yes	Yes	Yes	Yes
Tylenol (Regular, Extra Strength, Extended Relief)	Acetaminophen (*McNeil*)	Every 4 to 6 hours; Extended Relief: Every 8 hours	—	Caplets and tablets only	Tablets, caplets, gelcaps, and geltabs only	Yes	No

BRAND	ACTIVE INGREDIENTS (MANUFACTURER)	HOW OFTEN TO TAKE	GET MD APPROVAL IF YOU HAVE:	ALCOHOL-FREE	SUGAR-FREE	LACTOSE-FREE	SODIUM-FREE
Tylenol PM	Acetaminophen, Diphenhydramine (McNeil)	At bedtime	Breathing problems, glaucoma, prostate enlargement	Caplets only	Yes	Yes	No
Unisom with Pain Relief	Acetaminophen, Diphenhydramine (Pfizer)	At bedtime	Breathing problems, glaucoma, prostate enlargement	Yes	Yes	Yes	Yes
Vanquish	Acetaminophen, Aluminum hydroxide, Aspirin, Caffeine, Magnesium hydroxide (Bayer)	Every 4 hours	Asthma, heartburn, upset stomach, stomach pain, ulcers, bleeding problems, an allergy to aspirin, last 3 months of pregnancy	Yes	Yes	Yes	Yes

HEADACHE, CHILDREN

BRAND	ACTIVE INGREDIENTS (MANUFACTURER)	HOW OFTEN TO TAKE	GET MD APPROVAL IF YOU HAVE:	ALCOHOL-FREE	SUGAR-FREE	LACTOSE-FREE	SODIUM-FREE
Advil, Children's	Ibuprofen (Whitehall-Robins)	Every 6 to 8 hours	An allergy to aspirin, problems with other pain relievers, stomach pain, dehydration from vomiting or diarrhea	Yes	No	Yes	No
Bayer Children's Chewable	Aspirin (Bayer)	Every 4 hours	Arthritis, asthma, heartburn, upset stomach, stomach pain, ulcers, bleeding problems, an allergy to aspirin	Yes	No	Yes	No

Product	Ingredients (Manufacturer)	Dosing	Warnings					
Motrin (Junior Strength and Children's)	Ibuprofen (*McNeil*)	Every 6 to 8 hours	An allergy to aspirin, problems with other pain relievers, stomach pain, dehydration from vomiting or diarrhea	Yes	No	No	Yes	No
Panadol Children's	Acetaminophen (*SmithKline Beecham*)	Every 4 hours	—	Yes	Yes	Yes	Yes	No
Tylenol, Junior	Acetaminophen (*McNeil*)	Every 4 hours	Phenylalanine intolerance (Chewable Tablets only)	Yes	Yes	Yes	Yes	Chewables only

HEADACHE AND INSOMNIA

Product	Ingredients (Manufacturer)	Dosing	Warnings					
Bayer PM	Aspirin, Diphenhydramine (*Bayer*)	At bedtime	Asthma, bleeding problems, stomach problems, ulcers, breathing problems, glaucoma, prostate enlargement, an allergy to aspirin, last 3 months of pregnancy	Yes	Yes	Yes	Yes	Yes
Excedrin P.M.	Acetaminophen, Diphenhydramine (*Bristol-Myers*)	At bedtime	Breathing problems, glaucoma, prostate enlargement	Yes	Yes	Yes	Yes	No
Tylenol PM	Acetaminophen, Diphenhydramine (*McNeil*)	At bedtime	Breathing problems, glaucoma, prostate enlargement	Caplets only	Yes	Yes	Yes	No

BRAND	ACTIVE INGREDIENTS (MANUFACTURER)	HOW OFTEN TO TAKE	GET MD APPROVAL IF YOU HAVE:	ALCOHOL-FREE	SUGAR-FREE	LACTOSE-FREE	SODIUM-FREE
Unisom with Pain Relief	Acetaminophen, Diphenhydramine (Pfizer)	At bedtime	Breathing problems, glaucoma, prostate enlargement	Yes	Yes	Yes	Yes

HEART ATTACK RISK REDUCTION

BRAND	ACTIVE INGREDIENTS (MANUFACTURER)	HOW OFTEN TO TAKE	GET MD APPROVAL IF YOU HAVE:	ALCOHOL-FREE	SUGAR-FREE	LACTOSE-FREE	SODIUM-FREE
Ascriptin Enteric	Aspirin (Novartis)	Once a day	Asthma, heartburn, upset stomach, stomach pain, ulcers, bleeding problems, an allergy to aspirin, last 3 months of pregnancy	Yes	Yes	Yes	No
Bayer Aspirin Regimen	Aspirin (Bayer)	Once a day	Asthma, heartburn, upset stomach, stomach pain, ulcers, bleeding problems, an allergy to aspirin, last 3 months of pregnancy	Yes	Yes	325-mg only	325-mg only
Bayer (Genuine)	Aspirin (Bayer)	Once a day	Asthma, heartburn, upset stomach, stomach pain, ulcers, bleeding problems, an allergy to aspirin, last 3 months of pregnancy	Yes	Yes	Yes	Yes

Bufferin (Regular Strength)	Aspirin, Calcium carbonate, Magnesium carbonate, Magnesium oxide (*Bristol-Myers*)	Once a day	Asthma, heartburn, upset stomach, stomach pain, ulcers, bleeding problems, an allergy to aspirin, last 3 months of pregnancy	Yes	Yes	No
Ecotrin	Aspirin (*SmithKline Beecham*)	Once a day	Asthma, heartburn, upset stomach, stomach pain, ulcers, bleeding problems, an allergy to aspirin, last 3 months of pregnancy	Yes	Yes	81-mg tablet only
Halfprin	Aspirin (*Kramer*)	Once a day	—	NA	NA	NA
St. Joseph	Aspirin (*Schering-Plough*)	4 tablets daily	Asthma, heartburn, upset stomach, stomach pain, ulcers, bleeding problems, an allergy to aspirin, last 3 months of pregnancy	Yes	Yes	Yes

IRRITABLE BOWEL SYNDROME

Konsyl Fiber Tablets	Calcium polycarbophil (*Konsyl*)	1 to 4 times a day (adults); 1 to 3 times a day (children)	Difficulty swallowing, bowel obstruction, fecal impaction	Yes	Yes	Yes

BRAND	ACTIVE INGREDIENTS (MANUFACTURER)	HOW OFTEN TO TAKE	GET MD APPROVAL IF YOU HAVE:	ALCOHOL-FREE	SUGAR-FREE	LACTOSE-FREE	SODIUM-FREE
Konsyl Powder	Psyllium (Konsyl)	1 to 3 times a day	Difficulty swallowing, bowel obstruction, fecal impaction	Yes	Yes	Yes	No
Metamucil	Psyllium (Procter & Gamble)	1 to 3 times a day	Difficulty swallowing, bowel obstruction, fecal impaction, rectal bleeding, abdominal pain, nausea, vomiting, sudden change in bowel habits lasting 2 weeks	Yes	Sugar-free varieties and powder only	Yes	No

ITCHY EYES
See Hay Fever Symptoms

ITCHY NOSE AND THROAT
See Hay Fever Symptoms

MOTION SICKNESS, ADULTS

BRAND	ACTIVE INGREDIENTS (MANUFACTURER)	HOW OFTEN TO TAKE	GET MD APPROVAL IF YOU HAVE:	ALCOHOL-FREE	SUGAR-FREE	LACTOSE-FREE	SODIUM-FREE
Bonine	Meclizine (Pfizer)	Once a day	Breathing problems, glaucoma, prostate enlargement	Yes	Yes	No	No

Dramamine Tablets	Dimenhydrinate (*Pharmacia & Upjohn*)	Every 4 to 6 hours (adults); Every 6 to 8 hours (children)	Breathing problems, glaucoma, prostate enlargement, phenylalanine intolerance (chewable tablets only)	Yes	Yes	Yes	Chewable tablets only
Dramamine II	Meclizine (*Pharmacia & Upjohn*)	1 or 2 times a day	Breathing problems, glaucoma, prostate enlargement	Yes	Yes	Yes	No

MOTION SICKNESS, CHILDREN

Dramamine Children's Liquid	Dimenhydrinate (*Pharmacia & Upjohn*)	Every 4 to 8 hours	Breathing problems	Yes	No	Yes	Yes

NASAL CONGESTION, ADULTS

4-Way Fast Acting Nasal Spray	Naphazoline, Phenylephrine, Pyrilamine (*Bristol-Myers*)	Every 6 hours	Heart disease, high blood pressure, thyroid disease, diabetes, enlarged prostate gland	Yes	Yes	Yes	No

BRAND	ACTIVE INGREDIENTS (MANUFACTURER)	HOW OFTEN TO TAKE	GET MD APPROVAL IF YOU HAVE:	ALCOHOL-FREE	SUGAR-FREE	LACTOSE-FREE	SODIUM-FREE
4-Way 12 Hour	Oxymetazoline (Bristol-Myers)	Every 10 to 12 hours	Heart disease, high blood pressure, thyroid disease, diabetes, glaucoma, enlarged prostate gland, breathing problems	Yes	No	No	Yes
Afrin-4 Hour	Phenylephrine (Schering-Plough)	Every 4 hours	Heart disease, high blood pressure, thyroid disease, diabetes, enlarged prostate gland	Yes	Yes	Yes	No
Afrin 12 Hour	Oxymetazoline (Schering-Plough)	Every 10 to 12 hours	Heart disease, high blood pressure, thyroid disease, diabetes, enlarged prostate gland	Nasal Spray, Pump, and Drops only	Yes	Yes	No
Benzedrex	Propylhexedrine (Menley & James)	Every 2 hours	—	NA	NA	NA	NA
Drixoral Nasal Decongestant	Pseudoephedrine (Schering-Plough)	Every 12 hours	Heart disease, high blood pressure, thyroid disease, diabetes, enlarged prostate gland	Yes	No	No	Yes

Duration						
12 Hour	Oxymetazoline (*Schering-Plough*)	Every 10 to 12 hours	Heart disease, high blood pressure, thyroid disease, diabetes, enlarged prostate gland	Yes	Yes	No
Neo-Synephrine (**Regular and Extra Strength**)	Phenylephrine (*Bayer*)	Every 4 hours	Heart disease, high blood pressure, thyroid disease, diabetes, enlarged prostate gland	Yes	Yes	No
Neo-Synephrine (**Maximum Strength**)	Oxymetazoline (*Bayer*)	Every 10 to 12 hours	Heart disease, high blood pressure, thyroid disease, diabetes, enlarged prostate gland	Yes	Yes	Yes
12 Hour Nostrilla	Oxymetazoline (*Novartis*)	Every 10 to 12 hours	Heart disease, high blood pressure, thyroid disease, diabetes, enlarged prostate gland	Yes	Yes	Yes
Otrivin	Xylometazoline (*Novartis*)	Every 8 to 10 hours	Heart disease, high blood pressure, thyroid disease, diabetes, enlarged prostate gland	Yes	Yes	No
Privine	Naphazoline (*Novartis*)	Every 6 hours	Heart disease, high blood pressure, thyroid disease, diabetes, enlarged prostate gland	Yes	Yes	No

BRAND	ACTIVE INGREDIENTS (MANUFACTURER)	HOW OFTEN TO TAKE	GET MD APPROVAL IF YOU HAVE:	ALCOHOL-FREE	SUGAR-FREE	LACTOSE-FREE	SODIUM-FREE
Propagest	Phenylpropanolamine (Carnrick)	Every 4 hours	Heart disease, high blood pressure, thyroid disease, diabetes, glaucoma, enlarged prostate gland	Yes	NA	NA	NA
Sudafed	Pseudoephedrine (Warner-Lambert)	Every 4 to 6 hours	Heart disease, high blood pressure, thyroid disease, diabetes, enlarged prostate gland	Yes	No	Yes	No
Sudafed 12 Hour	Pseudoephedrine (Warner-Lambert)	Every 12 hours	Heart disease, high blood pressure, thyroid disease, diabetes, enlarged prostate gland	Yes	Yes	Yes	Yes
Triaminic AM Decongestant Formula	Pseudoephedrine (Novartis)	Every 4 to 6 hours	Heart disease, high blood pressure, thyroid disease, diabetes, enlarged prostate gland	Yes	No	Yes	No
Vicks Sinex	Phenylephrine (Procter & Gamble)	Every 4 hours	Heart disease, high blood pressure, thyroid disease, diabetes, enlarged prostate gland	Yes	Yes	Yes	No
Vicks Sinex 12-Hour	Oxymetazoline (Procter & Gamble)	Every 10 to 12 hours	Heart disease, high blood pressure, thyroid disease, diabetes, enlarged prostate gland	Yes	Yes	Yes	No

NASAL CONGESTION, CHILDREN

Dimetapp Decongestant Pediatric Drops	Pseudoephedrine (*Whitehall-Robins*)	Every 4 to 6 hours	Heart disease, high blood pressure, thyroid disease, diabetes	Yes	No	Yes	No
Pediacare Infants' Drops Decongestant	Pseudoephedrine (*McNeil*)	Every 4 to 6 hours	Heart disease, high blood pressure, thyroid disease, diabetes	Yes	No	Yes	No
Sudafed Children's Nasal Decongestant (Liquid and Chewable Tablets)	Pseudoephedrine (*Warner-Lambert*)	Every 4 to 6 hours	Heart disease, high blood pressure, thyroid disease, diabetes	Yes	Yes	Yes	No
Sudafed Pediatric Nasal Decongestant Liquid Oral Drops	Pseudoephedrine (*Warner-Lambert*)	Every 4 to 6 hours	Heart disease, high blood pressure, thyroid disease, diabetes	Yes	Yes	Yes	No

BRAND	ACTIVE INGREDIENTS (MANUFACTURER)	HOW OFTEN TO TAKE	GET MD APPROVAL IF YOU HAVE:	ALCOHOL-FREE	SUGAR-FREE	LACTOSE-FREE	SODIUM-FREE
Triaminic Infant Oral Decongestant Drops	Pseudoephedrine (Novartis)	Every 4 to 6 hours	Heart disease, high blood pressure, thyroid disease, diabetes	Yes	No	Yes	No

PAIN, MENSTRUAL

BRAND	ACTIVE INGREDIENTS (MANUFACTURER)	HOW OFTEN TO TAKE	GET MD APPROVAL IF YOU HAVE:	ALCOHOL-FREE	SUGAR-FREE	LACTOSE-FREE	SODIUM-FREE
Actron	Ketoprofen (Bayer)	Every 4 to 6 hours	Redness or swelling in painful area, an allergy to pain relievers	Yes	Yes	No	No
Advil	Ibuprofen (Whitehall-Robins)	Every 4 to 6 hours	An allergy to aspirin, problems with other pain relievers	Yes	Gel caplets only	Yes	No
Aleve	Naproxen sodium (Procter & Gamble)	Every 8 to 12 hours (Adults over 65: Every 12 hours)	An allergy to pain relievers	Yes	Yes	Yes	Yes

Ascriptin	Alumina-magnesia, Aspirin, Calcium carbonate (*Novartis*)	Every 4 hours; Maximum Strength: Every 6 hours	Asthma, heartburn, upset stomach, stomach pain, ulcers, bleeding problems, an allergy to aspirin	Yes	Yes	Yes	Yes
Ascriptin Enteric	Aspirin (*Novartis*)	Every 4 hours	Asthma, heartburn, upset stomach, stomach pain, ulcers, bleeding problems, an allergy to aspirin	Yes	Yes	Yes	No
Bayer (Genuine and Extra Strength)	Aspirin (*Bayer*)	Every 4 hours	Asthma, heartburn, upset stomach, stomach pain, ulcers, bleeding problems, an allergy to aspirin	Yes	Yes	Yes	Yes
BC Powder	Aspirin, Caffeine, Salicylamide (*Block Drug*)	Every 3 to 4 hours	An allergy to aspirin	Yes	Yes	Yes	Yes
Bufferin (Regular and Extra Strengths)	Aspirin, Calcium carbonate, Magnesium carbonate, Magnesium oxide (*Bristol-Myers*)	Every 4 hours; Extra Strength: Every 6 hours	Asthma, heartburn, upset stomach, stomach pain, ulcers, bleeding problems, an allergy to aspirin	Yes	Yes	Yes	No

BRAND	ACTIVE INGREDIENTS (MANUFACTURER)	HOW OFTEN TO TAKE	GET MD APPROVAL IF YOU HAVE:	ALCOHOL-FREE	SUGAR-FREE	LACTOSE-FREE	SODIUM-FREE
Excedrin	Acetaminophen, Aspirin, Caffeine (Bristol-Myers)	Every 6 hours	Asthma, heartburn, upset stomach, stomach pain, ulcers, bleeding problems, an allergy to aspirin	Yes	Yes	Yes	No
Excedrin, Aspirin Free	Acetaminophen, Caffeine (Bristol-Myers)	Every 6 hours	—	Yes	Yes	Yes	No
Goody's	Acetaminophen, Aspirin, Caffeine (Block Drug)	Every 4 to 6 hours	An allergy to aspirin	Yes	Yes	Tablets only	Yes
Midol Menstrual Formula	Acetaminophen, Caffeine, Pyrilamine (Bayer)	Every 4 hours	Breathing problems, glaucoma	Yes	Yes	Yes	No
Midol PMS Formula	Acetaminophen, Pamabrom, Pyrilamine (Bayer)	Every 4 hours	Breathing problems, glaucoma	Yes	Yes	Yes	No
Midol Teen Menstrual Formula	Acetaminophen, Pamabrom (Bayer)	Every 4 hours	—	Yes	Yes	Yes	No

Brand	Ingredients (Manufacturer)						
Motrin IB	Ibuprofen (*Pharmacia & Upjohn*)	An allergy to aspirin, problems with other pain relievers	Every 4 to 6 hours	Caplets and tablets only	Yes	Yes	Caplets and tablets only
Nuprin	Ibuprofen (*Bristol-Myers*)	An allergy to aspirin, problems with other pain relievers	Every 4 to 6 hours	Yes	No	Yes	Yes
Orudis KT	Ketoprofen (*Whitehall-Robins*)	Redness or swelling in painful area, an allergy to pain relievers	Every 4 to 6 hours	Yes	No	Yes	No
Pamprin Maximum Pain Relief	Acetaminophen, Magnesium salicylate, Pamabrom (*Chattem*)	An allergy to salicylates (aspirin)	Every 4 to 6 hours	Yes	Yes	Yes	No
Pamprin Multi-Symptom	Acetaminophen, Pamabrom, Pyrilamine (*Chattem*)	Breathing problems, glaucoma	Every 4 to 6 hours	Yes	Yes	Yes	No
Panadol	Acetaminophen (*SmithKline Beecham*)	—	Every 4 hours	Yes	Yes	Yes	Yes
St. Joseph	Aspirin (*Schering-Plough*)	Asthma, heartburn, upset stomach, stomach pain, ulcers, bleeding problems, an allergy to aspirin	Every 4 hours	Yes	Yes	Yes	Yes

BRAND	ACTIVE INGREDIENTS (MANUFACTURER)	HOW OFTEN TO TAKE	GET MD APPROVAL IF YOU HAVE:	ALCOHOL-FREE	SUGAR-FREE	LACTOSE-FREE	SODIUM-FREE
Tylenol (Regular, Extra Strength, Extended Relief)	Acetaminophen, (McNeil)	Every 4 to 6 hours; Extended Relief: Every 8 hours	—	Caplets and tablets only	Tablets, caplets, gelcaps, and geltabs only	Yes	No
Unisom with Pain Relief	Acetaminophen, Diphenhydramine (Pfizer)	At bedtime	Breathing problems, glaucoma	Yes	Yes	Yes	Yes
Vanquish	Acetaminophen, Aluminum hydroxide, Aspirin, Caffeine, Magnesium hydroxide (Bayer)	Every 4 hours	Asthma, heartburn, upset stomach, stomach pain, ulcers, bleeding problems, an allergy to aspirin	Yes	Yes	Yes	Yes

PAIN, MUSCULAR, ADULTS

BRAND	ACTIVE INGREDIENTS (MANUFACTURER)	HOW OFTEN TO TAKE	GET MD APPROVAL IF YOU HAVE:	ALCOHOL-FREE	SUGAR-FREE	LACTOSE-FREE	SODIUM-FREE
Actron	Ketoprofen (Bayer)	Every 4 to 6 hours	Redness or swelling in painful area, an allergy to pain relievers, last 3 months of pregnancy	Yes	Yes	No	No

Advil	Ibuprofen (*Whitehall-Robins*)	Every 4 to 6 hours	An allergy to aspirin, problems with other pain relievers, last 3 months of pregnancy	Yes	Gel caplets only	No
Aleve	Naproxen sodium (*Procter & Gamble*)	Every 8 to 12 hours (Adults over 65: Every 12 hours)	An allergy to pain relievers, last 3 months of pregnancy	Yes	Yes	Yes
Alka-Seltzer	Aspirin, Citric acid, Sodium bicarbonate (*Bayer*)	Every 4 hours; Extra Strength: Every 6 hours	Asthma, bleeding problems, an allergy to aspirin, a sodium-restricted diet, last 3 months of pregnancy, phenylalanine intolerance (Lemon Lime and Cherry only)	Yes	Yes	No
Ascriptin	Alumina-magnesia, Aspirin, Calcium carbonate (*Novartis*)	Every 4 hours; Maximum Strength: Every 6 hours	Asthma, heartburn, upset stomach, stomach pain, ulcers, bleeding problems, an allergy to aspirin, last 3 months of pregnancy	Yes	Yes	Yes

BRAND	ACTIVE INGREDIENTS (MANUFACTURER)	HOW OFTEN TO TAKE	GET MD APPROVAL IF YOU HAVE:	ALCOHOL-FREE	SUGAR-FREE	LACTOSE-FREE	SODIUM-FREE
Ascriptin Enteric	Aspirin (Novartis)	Every 4 hours	Asthma, heartburn, upset stomach, stomach pain, ulcers, bleeding problems, an allergy to aspirin, last 3 months of pregnancy	Yes	Yes	Yes	No
Backache Caplets	Magnesium salicylate tetrahydrate (Bristol-Myers)	Every 6 hours	Asthma, stomach problems, ulcers, bleeding problems, allergy to salicylates (aspirin)	Yes	Yes	Yes	Yes
Bayer (Genuine, Extra Strength, Extended-Release)	Aspirin (Bayer)	Every 4 hours; Extended-Release: Every 8 hours	Asthma, heartburn, upset stomach, stomach pain, ulcers, bleeding problems, an allergy to aspirin, last 3 months of pregnancy	Yes	Yes	Yes	Yes
BC Powder	Aspirin, Caffeine, Salicylamide (Block Drug)	Every 3 to 4 hours	An allergy to aspirin, last 3 months of pregnancy	Yes	Yes	Yes	Yes

Product	Ingredients	Dosage	Conditions to avoid				
Bufferin (Regular and Extra Strengths)	Aspirin, Calcium carbonate, Magnesium carbonate, Magnesium oxide (*Bristol-Myers*)	Every 4 hours; Extra Strength: Every 6 hours	Asthma, heartburn, upset stomach, stomach pain, ulcers, bleeding problems, an allergy to aspirin, last 3 months of pregnancy	Yes	Yes	Yes	No
Excedrin	Acetaminophen, Aspirin, Caffeine (*Bristol-Myers*)	Every 6 hours	Asthma, heartburn, upset stomach, stomach pain, ulcers, bleeding problems, an allergy to aspirin, last 3 months of pregnancy	Yes	Yes	Yes	No
Excedrin, Aspirin Free	Acetaminophen, Caffeine (*Bristol-Myers*)	Every 6 hours	—	Yes	Yes	Yes	No
Goody's	Acetaminophen, Aspirin, Caffeine (*Block Drug*)	Every 4 to 6 hours	An allergy to aspirin, last 3 months of pregnancy	Yes	Yes	Yes	Yes
Midol Menstrual Formula	Acetaminophen, Caffeine, Pyrilamine (*Bayer*)	Every 4 hours	Breathing problems, glaucoma	Yes	Yes	Yes	No
Midol Teen Menstrual Formula	Acetaminophen, Pamabrom (*Bayer*)	Every 4 hours	—	Yes	Yes	Yes	No

BRAND	ACTIVE INGREDIENTS (MANUFACTURER)	HOW OFTEN TO TAKE	GET MD APPROVAL IF YOU HAVE:	ALCOHOL-FREE	SUGAR-FREE	LACTOSE-FREE	SODIUM-FREE
Motrin IB	Ibuprofen (Pharmacia & Upjohn)	Every 4 to 6 hours	An allergy to aspirin, problems with other pain relievers, last 3 months of pregnancy	Caplets and tablets only	Yes	Yes	Caplets and tablets only
Nuprin	Ibuprofen (Bristol-Myers)	Every 4 to 6 hours	An allergy to aspirin, problems with other pain relievers, last 3 months of pregnancy	Yes	Yes	Yes	Yes
Orudis KT	Ketoprofen (Whitehall-Robins)	Every 4 to 6 hours	Redness or swelling in painful area, an allergy to pain relievers, last 3 months of pregnancy	Yes	No	Yes	No
Panadol	Acetaminophen (SmithKline Beecham)	Every 4 hours	—	Yes	Yes	Yes	Yes
St. Joseph	Aspirin (Schering-Plough)	Every 4 hours	Asthma, heartburn, upset stomach, stomach pain, ulcers, bleeding problems, an allergy to aspirin, last 3 months of pregnancy	Yes	Yes	Yes	Yes

Tylenol (Regular, Extra Strength, Extended Relief)	Acetaminophen, (McNeil)	Every 4 to 6 hours; Extended Relief: Every 8 hours	—	Caplets and tablets only	Tablets, caplets, gelcaps, and geltabs only	No
Unisom with Pain Relief	Acetaminophen, Diphenhydramine (Pfizer)	At bedtime	Breathing problems, glaucoma, prostate enlargement	Yes	Yes	Yes
Vanquish	Acetaminophen, Aluminum hydroxide, Aspirin, Caffeine, Magnesium hydroxide (Bayer)	Every 4 hours	Asthma, heartburn, upset stomach, stomach pain, ulcers, bleeding problems, an allergy to aspirin, last 3 months of pregnancy	Yes	Yes	Yes

PAIN, MUSCULAR, CHILDREN

Tylenol, Junior Strength	Acetaminophen (McNeil)	Every 4 hours	Phenylalanine intolerance (Chewable Tablets only)	Yes	Yes	Yes	Chewable Tablets only

PAIN, NEURALGIA

BRAND	ACTIVE INGREDIENTS *(MANUFACTURER)*	HOW OFTEN TO TAKE	GET MD APPROVAL IF YOU HAVE:	ALCOHOL-FREE	SUGAR-FREE	LACTOSE-FREE	SODIUM-FREE
BC Powder	Aspirin, Caffeine, Salicylamide *(Block Drug)*	Every 3 to 4 hours	An allergy to aspirin, last 3 months of pregnancy	Yes	Yes	Yes	Yes

PAIN AND FEVER OF COLDS AND FLU, ADULTS

BRAND	ACTIVE INGREDIENTS *(MANUFACTURER)*	HOW OFTEN TO TAKE	GET MD APPROVAL IF YOU HAVE:	ALCOHOL-FREE	SUGAR-FREE	LACTOSE-FREE	SODIUM-FREE
Actron	Ketoprofen *(Bayer)*	Every 4 to 6 hours	Redness or swelling in painful area, an allergy to pain relievers, last 3 months of pregnancy	Yes	Yes	No	No
Advil	Ibuprofen *(Whitehall-Robins)*	Every 4 to 6 hours	An allergy to aspirin, problems with other pain relievers, last 3 months of pregnancy	Yes	Gel caplets only	Yes	No
Aleve	Naproxen sodium *(Procter & Gamble)*	Every 8 to 12 hours (Adults over 65: Every 12 hours)	An allergy to pain relievers, last 3 months of pregnancy	Yes	Yes	Yes	Yes

Ascriptin	Alumina-magnesia, Aspirin, Calcium carbonate (*Novartis*)	Every 4 hours; Maximum Strength: Every 6 hours	Asthma, heartburn, upset stomach, stomach pain, ulcers, bleeding problems, an allergy to aspirin, last 3 months of pregnancy	Yes	Yes	Yes	Yes
Bayer (Extended-Release and Extra Strength)	Aspirin (*Bayer*)	Every 4 hours; Extended-Release: Every 8 hours	Asthma, heartburn, upset stomach, stomach pain, ulcers, bleeding problems, an allergy to aspirin, last 3 months of pregnancy	Yes	Yes	Yes	Yes
BC Powder	Aspirin, Caffeine, Salicylamide (*Block Drug*)	Every 3 to 4 hours	An allergy to aspirin, last 3 months of pregnancy	NA	NA	NA	NA
Bufferin (Regular and Extra Strength)	Aspirin, Calcium carbonate, Magnesium carbonate, Magnesium oxide (*Bristol-Myers*)	Every 4 hours; Extra Strength: Every 6 hours	Asthma, heartburn, upset stomach, stomach pain, ulcers, bleeding problems, an allergy to aspirin, last 3 months of pregnancy	Yes	Yes	Yes	No

BRAND	ACTIVE INGREDIENTS (MANUFACTURER)	HOW OFTEN TO TAKE	GET MD APPROVAL IF YOU HAVE:	ALCOHOL-FREE	SUGAR-FREE	LACTOSE-FREE	SODIUM-FREE
Goody's	Acetaminophen, Aspirin, Caffeine (Block Drug)	Every 4 to 6 hours	An allergy to aspirin, last 3 months of pregnancy	Yes	Yes	Tablets only	Yes
Motrin IB	Ibuprofen (Pharmacia & Upjohn)	Every 4 to 6 hours	An allergy to aspirin, problems with other pain relievers, last 3 months of pregnancy	Caplets and tablets only	Yes	Yes	Caplets and tablets only
Nuprin	Ibuprofen (Bristol-Myers)	Every 4 to 6 hours	An allergy to aspirin, problems with other pain relievers, last 3 months of pregnancy	Yes	Yes	Yes	Yes
Orudis KT	Ketoprofen (Whitehall-Robins)	Every 4 to 6 hours	Redness or swelling in painful area, an allergy to pain relievers, last 3 months of pregnancy	Yes	No	Yes	No
Panadol	Acetaminophen (SmithKline Beecham)	Every 4 hours	—	Yes	Yes	Yes	Yes
St. Joseph	Aspirin (Schering-Plough)	Every 4 hours	Asthma, heartburn, upset stomach, stomach pain, ulcers, bleeding problems, an allergy to aspirin, last 3 months of pregnancy	Yes	Yes	Yes	Yes

Name	Ingredient (Manufacturer)	How Often	Do Not Give If Child Has			
Tylenol	Acetaminophen (*McNeil*)	Every 4 to 6 hours; Extended Relief: Every 8 hours	—	Caplets and tablets only	Tablets, caplets, gelcaps, and geltabs only — Yes	No

PAIN AND FEVER OF COLDS AND FLU, CHILDREN

Name	Ingredient (Manufacturer)	How Often	Do Not Give If Child Has			
Advil, Children's	Ibuprofen (*Whitehall-Robins*)	Every 6 to 8 hours	An allergy to aspirin, problems with other pain relievers, stomach pain, dehydration from vomiting or diarrhea	Yes	No	No
Bayer Children's Chewable	Aspirin (*Bayer*)	Every 4 hours	Arthritis, asthma, heartburn, upset stomach, stomach pain, ulcers, bleeding problems, an allergy to aspirin	Yes	No	No
Motrin (Junior Strength and Children's)	Ibuprofen (*McNeil*)	Every 6 to 8 hours	An allergy to aspirin, problems with other pain relievers, stomach pain, dehydration from vomiting or diarrhea	Yes	No	No
Panadol Children's	Acetaminophen (*SmithKline Beecham*)	Every 4 hours	—	Yes	Yes	No

BRAND	ACTIVE INGREDIENTS (MANUFACTURER)	HOW OFTEN TO TAKE	GET MD APPROVAL IF YOU HAVE:	ALCOHOL-FREE	SUGAR-FREE	LACTOSE-FREE	SODIUM-FREE
Tylenol (Children's and Infants')	Acetaminophen (McNeil)	Every 4 hours	—	Yes	Chewables and Liquid only	Yes	Chewables only
Tylenol, Junior Strength	Acetaminophen (McNeil)	Every 4 hours	Phenylalanine intolerance (Chewable Tablets only)	Yes	Yes	Yes	Chewables only
PMS							
Midol PMS Formula	Acetaminophen, Pamabrom, Pyrilamine (Bayer)	Every 4 hours	Breathing problems, glaucoma	Yes	Yes	Yes	No
QUIT SMOKING AIDS							
Nicoderm CQ	Nicotine (SmithKline Beecham)	Once a day	Heart disease, recent heart attack, irregular heartbeat, untreated high blood pressure, skin problems, an allergy to adhesive tape	Yes	Yes	Yes	Yes

Nicorette	Nicotine polacrilex (*SmithKline Beecham*)	12 to 24 times a day	Heart disease, recent heart attack, irregular heartbeat, untreated high blood pressure, ulcers	Yes	Yes	Yes	No
Nicotrol	Nicotine (*McNeil*)	Once a day	Heart disease, recent heart attack, irregular heartbeat, untreated high blood pressure, skin problems, an allergy to adhesive tape	Yes	Yes	Yes	Yes

RUNNY NOSE
See Hay Fever Symptoms

SCIATICA

BC Powder	Aspirin, Caffeine, Salicylamide (*Block Drug*)	Every 3 to 4 hours	An allergy to aspirin, last 3 months of pregnancy	Yes	Yes	Yes	Yes

SINUS CONGESTION
See Nasal Congestion

SINUS PAIN AND PRESSURE

BRAND	ACTIVE INGREDIENTS (MANUFACTURER)	HOW OFTEN TO TAKE	GET MD APPROVAL IF YOU HAVE:	ALCOHOL-FREE	SUGAR-FREE	LACTOSE-FREE	SODIUM-FREE
Actifed Sinus Daytime/ Nighttime	Daytime: Acetaminophen, Pseudoephedrine; Nighttime: Acetaminophen, Diphenhydramine, Pseudoephedrine (Warner-Lambert)	Every 6 hours	Heart disease, high blood pressure, thyroid disease, diabetes, breathing problems, glaucoma, enlarged prostate gland	Yes	Yes	Yes	Daytime only
Advil Cold and Sinus	Ibuprofen, Pseudoephedrine (Whitehall-Robins)	Every 4 to 6 hours	Heart disease, high blood pressure, thyroid disease, diabetes, enlarged prostate gland, an allergy to aspirin, last 3 months of pregnancy	Yes	No	Yes	No
Alka-Seltzer Plus Sinus Medicine Tablets	Aspirin, Phenylpropanolamine (Bayer)	Every 4 hours	Heart disease, high blood pressure, thyroid disease, diabetes, glaucoma, enlarged prostate gland, breathing problems, bleeding problems, an allergy to aspirin, last 3 months of pregnancy	Yes	Yes	Yes	No

Allerest No Drowsiness	Acetaminophen, Pseudoephedrine (*Novartis*)	Every 4 to 6 hours	Heart disease, high blood pressure, thyroid disease, diabetes, enlarged prostate gland	Yes	Yes	Yes	Yes
Benadryl Allergy Sinus Headache Caplets	Acetaminophen, Diphenhydramine, Pseudoephedrine (*Warner-Lambert*)	Every 6 hours	Heart disease, high blood pressure, thyroid disease, diabetes, glaucoma, enlarged prostate gland, breathing problems	Yes	Yes	Yes	No
Comtrex Allergy-Sinus	Acetaminophen, Chlorpheniramine, Pseudoephedrine (*Bristol-Myers*)	Every 6 hours	Heart disease, high blood pressure, thyroid disease, diabetes, glaucoma, enlarged prostate gland, breathing problems	Yes	Yes	Yes	No
Coricidin 'D'	Acetaminophen, Chlorpheniramine, Phenylpropanolamine (*Schering-Plough*)	Every 4 hours	Heart disease, high blood pressure, thyroid disease, diabetes, glaucoma, enlarged prostate gland, breathing problems	Yes	No	Yes	Yes
Dimetapp Allergy Sinus	Acetaminophen, Brompheniramine, Phenylpropanolamine (*Whitehall-Robins*)	Every 6 hours	Heart disease, high blood pressure, thyroid disease, diabetes, glaucoma, enlarged prostate gland, breathing problems	Yes	Yes	Yes	Yes

BRAND	ACTIVE INGREDIENTS (MANUFACTURER)	HOW OFTEN TO TAKE	GET MD APPROVAL IF YOU HAVE:	ALCOHOL-FREE	SUGAR-FREE	LACTOSE-FREE	SODIUM-FREE
Drixoral Allergy/ Sinus	Acetaminophen, Dexbrompheniramine, Pseudoephedrine (*Schering-Plough*)	Every 12 hours	Heart disease, high blood pressure, thyroid disease, diabetes, glaucoma, enlarged prostate gland, breathing problems	Yes	Yes	Yes	Yes
Sinarest (Tablets and Extra Strength Caplets)	Acetaminophen, Chlorpheniramine, Pseudoephedrine (*Novartis*)	Tablets: Every 4 to 6 hours; Caplets: Every 6 hours	Heart disease, high blood pressure, thyroid disease, diabetes, glaucoma, enlarged prostate gland, breathing problems	Yes	Yes	Yes	Yes
Sine-Aid	Acetaminophen, Pseudoephedrine (*McNeil*)	Every 4 to 6 hours	Heart disease, high blood pressure, thyroid disease, diabetes, enlarged prostate gland	Caplets and Tablets only	Yes	Yes	No
Sine-Off	Acetaminophen, Diphenhydramine, Pseudoephedrine (*Hogil*)	Every 6 hours	Heart disease, high blood pressure, thyroid disease, diabetes, glaucoma, enlarged prostate gland, breathing problems	Yes	Yes	Yes	No

Product	Ingredients (Manufacturer)	Dosage	Use with Caution if You Have				
Singlet	Acetaminophen, Chlorpheniramine, Pseudoephedrine (*SmithKline Beecham*)	Every 4 to 6 hours	Heart disease, high blood pressure, thyroid disease, diabetes, glaucoma, enlarged prostate gland, breathing problems	Yes	No	Yes	No
Sinulin	Acetaminophen, Chlorpheniramine, Phenylpropanolamine (*Carnrick*)	Every 4 to 6 hours	Heart disease, high blood pressure, thyroid disease, diabetes, glaucoma, enlarged prostate gland, breathing problems	Yes	NA	NA	NA
Sinutab Sinus Allergy	Acetaminophen, Chlorpheniramine, Pseudoephedrine (*Warner-Lambert*)	Every 6 hours	Heart disease, high blood pressure, thyroid disease, diabetes, glaucoma, enlarged prostate gland, breathing problems	Yes	Yes	Yes	No
Sinutab Sinus Medication	Acetaminophen, Pseudoephedrine (*Warner-Lambert*)	Every 6 hours	Heart disease, high blood pressure, thyroid disease, diabetes, enlarged prostate gland	NA	NA	NA	NA
Sudafed Cold & Sinus	Acetaminophen, Pseudoephedrine (*Warner-Lambert*)	Every 4 to 6 hours	Heart disease, high blood pressure, thyroid disease, diabetes, enlarged prostate gland	Yes	Yes	Yes	No
Sudafed Sinus	Acetaminophen, Pseudoephedrine (*Warner-Lambert*)	Every 6 hours	Heart disease, high blood pressure, thyroid disease, diabetes, enlarged prostate gland	Yes	Yes	Yes	Yes

BRAND	ACTIVE INGREDIENTS (MANUFACTURER)	HOW OFTEN TO TAKE	GET MD APPROVAL IF YOU HAVE:	ALCOHOL-FREE	SUGAR-FREE	LACTOSE-FREE	SODIUM-FREE
Theraflu Sinus	Acetaminophen, Pseudoephedrine (Novartis)	Every 6 hours	Heart disease, high blood pressure, thyroid disease, diabetes, enlarged prostate gland	Yes	Yes	No	No
Triaminicin	Acetaminophen, Chlorpheniramine, Phenylpropanolamine (Novartis)	Every 4 to 6 hours	Heart disease, high blood pressure, thyroid disease, diabetes, glaucoma, enlarged prostate gland, breathing problems	Yes	Yes	No	No
Tylenol Allergy Sinus	Acetaminophen, Chlorpheniramine, Pseudoephedrine (McNeil)	Every 6 hours	Heart disease, high blood pressure, thyroid disease, diabetes, glaucoma, enlarged prostate gland, breathing problems	Caplets only	Yes	Yes	No
Tylenol Allergy Sinus NightTime	Acetaminophen, Diphenhydramine, Pseudoephedrine (McNeil)	At bedtime	Heart disease, high blood pressure, thyroid disease, diabetes, glaucoma, enlarged prostate gland, breathing problems	Yes	Yes	Yes	No
Tylenol Sinus	Acetaminophen, Pseudoephedrine (McNeil)	Every 4 to 6 hours	Heart disease, high blood pressure, thyroid disease, diabetes, enlarged prostate gland	Caplets and Tablets only	Yes	Yes	No

Product	Ingredients	Dosage	Don't use if you have					
Vicks DayQuil Sinus Pressure & Pain Relief	Ibuprofen, Pseudoephedrine (Procter & Gamble)	Every 4 to 6 hours	Heart disease, high blood pressure, thyroid disease, diabetes, enlarged prostate gland, an allergy to aspirin, last 3 months of pregnancy	Yes	No	No	Yes	No

SLEEPLESSNESS

Product	Ingredients	Dosage	Don't use if you have					
Bayer PM	Aspirin, Diphenhydramine (Bayer)	At bedtime	Asthma, bleeding problems, stomach problems, ulcers, breathing problems, glaucoma, prostate enlargement, an allergy to aspirin, last 3 months of pregnancy	Yes	Yes	Yes	Yes	Yes
Doan's P.M.	Diphenhydramine, Magnesium salicylate tetrahydrate (Novartis)	At bedtime	Breathing problems, glaucoma, prostate enlargement, stomach problems, ulcers, bleeding problems, an allergy to salicylates (aspirin)	Yes	Yes	Yes	Yes	No
Excedrin P.M.	Acetaminophen, Diphenhydramine (Bristol-Myers)	At bedtime	Breathing problems, glaucoma, prostate enlargement	Yes	Yes	Yes	Yes	No
Legatrin PM	Acetaminophen, Diphenhydramine (Columbia)	At bedtime	Breathing problems, glaucoma, prostate enlargement	Yes	Yes	Yes	Yes	Yes

BRAND	ACTIVE INGREDIENTS (MANUFACTURER)	HOW OFTEN TO TAKE	GET MD APPROVAL IF YOU HAVE:	ALCOHOL-FREE	SUGAR-FREE	LACTOSE-FREE	SODIUM-FREE
Nytol	Diphenhydramine (Block Drug)	At bedtime	Breathing problems, glaucoma, prostate enlargement	Yes	Yes	Yes	Yes
Sleepinal	Diphenhydramine (Thompson Medical)	At bedtime	Breathing problems, glaucoma, prostate enlargement	Yes	Yes	Softgels only	Yes
Tylenol PM	Acetaminophen, Diphenhydramine (McNeil)	At bedtime	Breathing problems, glaucoma, prostate enlargement	Caplets only	Yes	Yes	No
Unisom	Doxylamine (Pfizer)	At bedtime	Breathing problems, glaucoma, prostate enlargement, pregnancy, nursing	Yes	Yes	Yes	No
Unisom Maximum Strength	Diphenhydramine (Pfizer)	At bedtime	Breathing problems, glaucoma, prostate enlargement	Yes	Yes	Yes	Yes
Unisom with Pain Relief	Acetaminophen, Diphenhydramine (Pfizer)	At bedtime	Breathing problems, glaucoma, prostate enlargement	Yes	Yes	Yes	Yes

SNEEZING
See Hay Fever Symptoms

SORE THROAT

Cepacol Sore Throat Lozenges (Regular Strength) (*J. B. Williams*)	Menthol	Every 2 hours	—	Yes	No	Yes	Yes
Cepacol Sore Throat Lozenges (Maximum Strength) (*J. B. Williams*)	Benzocaine, Menthol	Every 2 hours	—	Yes	No	Yes	Yes
Cepacol Sore Throat Spray (*J. B. Williams*)	Dyclonine	4 times a day	—	Yes	Yes	Yes	No
Cepastat Sore Throat Lozenges (*SmithKline Beecham*)	Phenol	Every 2 hours	—	Yes	Yes	Yes	No

BRAND	ACTIVE INGREDIENTS (MANUFACTURER)	HOW OFTEN TO TAKE	GET MD APPROVAL IF YOU HAVE:	ALCOHOL-FREE	SUGAR-FREE	LACTOSE-FREE	SODIUM-FREE
Halls Cough Drops (Mentho-Lyptus and Maximum Strength)	Menthol (Warner-Lambert)	Every hour as needed	Chronic cough, cough with excessive phlegm	Yes	Sugar-Free Drops only	Yes	Yes
N'Ice Sore Throat and Cough Lozenges	Menthol (SmithKline Beecham)	Every hour as needed	Chronic cough, cough with excessive phlegm	Yes	Yes	Yes	Not all flavors
Sucrets	Dyclonine (Original Mint: Hexylresorcinol) (SmithKline Beecham)	Every 2 hours	—	Yes	No	Yes	Yes
Vicks Chloraseptic Cough & Throat Drops	Menthol (Procter & Gamble)	Every hour as needed	Chronic cough, cough with excessive phlegm	Yes	No	Yes	Yes

Vicks Chloraseptic Sore Throat Lozenges (Procter & Gamble)	Benzocaine, Menthol	Every 2 hours	An allergy to "caine" anesthetics	Yes	No	Yes	Yes
Vicks Chloraseptic Sore Throat Spray (Procter & Gamble)	Phenol	Every 2 hours	—	Yes	Yes	Yes	No
Vicks Cough Drops (Oval) (Procter & Gamble)	Menthol	Every 2 hours	Chronic cough, cough with excessive phlegm	Cherry Flavor only	No	Yes	Yes
Vicks Cough Drops (Triangular) (Procter & Gamble)	Menthol	Every 2 hours	Chronic cough, cough with excessive phlegm	Yes	No	Yes	Yes

TEETHING

Bayer Children's Chewable (Bayer)	Aspirin	Every 4 hours	Arthritis, asthma, heartburn, upset stomach, stomach pain, ulcers, bleeding problems, an allergy to aspirin	Yes	No	Yes	No
Panadol Children's (SmithKline Beecham)	Acetaminophen	Every 4 hours	—	Yes	Yes	Yes	No

BRAND	ACTIVE INGREDIENTS (MANUFACTURER)	HOW OFTEN TO TAKE	GET MD APPROVAL IF YOU HAVE:	ALCOHOL-FREE	SUGAR-FREE	LACTOSE-FREE	SODIUM-FREE
Tylenol, Children's and Infants'	Acetaminophen (McNeil)	Every 4 hours	—	Yes	Chewables and liquid only	Yes	Chewables only

TOOTHACHE, ADULTS

BRAND	ACTIVE INGREDIENTS (MANUFACTURER)	HOW OFTEN TO TAKE	GET MD APPROVAL IF YOU HAVE:	ALCOHOL-FREE	SUGAR-FREE	LACTOSE-FREE	SODIUM-FREE
Actron	Ketoprofen (Bayer)	Every 4 to 6 hours	Redness or swelling in painful area, an allergy to pain relievers, last 3 months of pregnancy	Yes	Yes	No	No
Advil	Ibuprofen (Whitehall-Robins)	Every 4 to 6 hours	An allergy to aspirin, problems with other pain relievers, last 3 months of pregnancy	Yes	Gel caplets only	Yes	No
Aleve	Naproxen sodium (Procter & Gamble)	Every 8 to 12 hours (Adults over 65: Every 12 hours)	An allergy to pain relievers, last 3 months of pregnancy	Yes	Yes	Yes	Yes

Ascriptin	Alumina-magnesia, Aspirin, Calcium carbonate (*Novartis*)	Every 4 hours; Maximum Strength: Every 6 hours	Asthma, heartburn, upset stomach, stomach pain, ulcers, bleeding problems, an allergy to aspirin, last 3 months of pregnancy	Yes	Yes	Yes	Yes
Ascriptin Enteric	Aspirin (*Novartis*)	Every 4 hours	Asthma, heartburn, upset stomach, stomach pain, ulcers, bleeding problems, an allergy to aspirin, last 3 months of pregnancy	Yes	Yes	Yes	No
Bayer (Genuine and Extra Strength)	Aspirin (*Bayer*)	Every 4 hours	Asthma, heartburn, upset stomach, stomach pain, ulcers, bleeding problems, an allergy to aspirin, last 3 months of pregnancy	Yes	Yes	Yes	Yes
BC Powder	Aspirin, Caffeine, Salicylamide (*Block Drug*)	Every 3 to 4 hours	An allergy to aspirin, last 3 months of pregnancy	Yes	Yes	Yes	Yes

BRAND	ACTIVE INGREDIENTS (MANUFACTURER)	HOW OFTEN TO TAKE	GET MD APPROVAL IF YOU HAVE:	ALCOHOL-FREE	SUGAR-FREE	LACTOSE-FREE	SODIUM-FREE
Bufferin (Regular and Extra Strength)	Aspirin, Calcium carbonate, Magnesium carbonate, Magnesium oxide (*Bristol-Myers*)	Regular Strength: Every 4 hours; Extra Strength: Every 6 hours	Asthma, heartburn, upset stomach, stomach pain, ulcers, bleeding problems, an allergy to aspirin, last 3 months of pregnancy	Yes	Yes	Yes	No
Excedrin	Acetaminophen, Aspirin, Caffeine (*Bristol-Myers*)	Every 6 hours	Asthma, heartburn, upset stomach, stomach pain, ulcers, bleeding problems, an allergy to aspirin, last 3 months of pregnancy	Yes	Yes	Yes	No
Excedrin, Aspirin-Free	Acetaminophen, Caffeine (*Bristol-Myers*)	Every 6 hours	—	Yes	Yes	Yes	No
Goody's	Acetaminophen, Aspirin, Caffeine (*Block Drug*)	Every 4 to 6 hours	An allergy to aspirin, last 3 months of pregnancy	Yes	Yes	Tablets only	Yes

Motrin IB (*Pharmacia & Upjohn*)	Ibuprofen	Every 4 to 6 hours	An allergy to aspirin, problems with other pain relievers, last 3 months of pregnancy	Caplets and tablets only	Yes	Yes	Caplets and tablets only
Nuprin (*Bristol-Myers*)	Ibuprofen	Every 4 to 6 hours	An allergy to aspirin, problems with other pain relievers, last 3 months of pregnancy	Yes	Yes	Yes	Yes
Orudis KT (*Whitehall-Robins*)	Ketoprofen	Every 4 to 6 hours	Redness or swelling in painful area, an allergy to pain relievers, last 3 months of pregnancy	Yes	No	Yes	No
Panadol (*SmithKline Beecham*)	Acetaminophen	Every 4 hours	—	Yes	Yes	Yes	Yes
Tylenol (**Regular, Extra Strength, Extended Relief**) (*McNeil*)	Acetaminophen	Every 4 to 6 hours; Extended Relief: Every 8 hours	—	Caplets and tablets only	Tablets, caplets, gelcaps, and geltabs only	Yes	No

TOOTHACHE, CHILDREN

BRAND	ACTIVE INGREDIENTS (MANUFACTURER)	HOW OFTEN TO TAKE	GET MD APPROVAL IF YOU HAVE:	ALCOHOL-FREE	SUGAR-FREE	LACTOSE-FREE	SODIUM-FREE
Advil, Children's	Ibuprofen (Whitehall-Robins)	Every 6 to 8 hours	An allergy to aspirin, problems with other pain relievers, stomach pain, dehydration from vomiting or diarrhea	Yes	No	Yes	No
Motrin (Junior Strength and Children's)	Ibuprofen (McNeil)	Every 6 to 8 hours	An allergy to aspirin, problems with other pain relievers, stomach pain, dehydration from vomiting or diarrhea	Yes	No	Yes	No

TRANSIENT ISCHEMIC ATTACK, ADULT MALES

BRAND	ACTIVE INGREDIENTS (MANUFACTURER)	HOW OFTEN TO TAKE	GET MD APPROVAL IF YOU HAVE:	ALCOHOL-FREE	SUGAR-FREE	LACTOSE-FREE	SODIUM-FREE
Ascriptin Enteric	Aspirin (Novartis)	2 to 4 times a day	Asthma, heartburn, upset stomach, stomach pain, ulcers, bleeding problems, an allergy to aspirin	Yes	Yes	Yes	No
Bayer Aspirin Regimen	Aspirin (Bayer)	2 to 4 times a day	Asthma, heartburn, upset stomach, stomach pain, ulcers, bleeding problems, an allergy to aspirin	Yes	Yes	Regular strength 325-mg only	Regular strength 325-mg only

Bayer (Genuine)	Aspirin (Bayer)	2 to 4 times a day	Asthma, heartburn, upset stomach, stomach pain, ulcers, bleeding problems, an allergy to aspirin	Yes	Yes	Yes	Yes
Bufferin (Regular Strength)	Aspirin, Calcium carbonate, Magnesium carbonate, Magnesium oxide (Bristol-Myers)	2 to 4 times a day	Asthma, heartburn, upset stomach, stomach pain, ulcers, bleeding problems, an allergy to aspirin	Yes	Yes	Yes	No
Ecotrin (SmithKline Beecham)	Aspirin	2 to 4 times a day	Asthma, heartburn, upset stomach, stomach pain, ulcers, bleeding problems, an allergy to aspirin	Yes	Yes	Yes	81-mg tablet only

WATERY EYES
See Hay Fever Symptoms

2. Product Profiles

In this section you'll find complete information on each brand in the Product Selection Tables, including the problems it relieves, the way to take it, its recommended dosage and maximum daily dose, possible side effects, potential interactions with other drugs, and any special warnings that apply. The information is based on the manufacturer's own package labeling as published in *PDR for Nonprescription Drugs*, frequently augmented with additional data from the *PDR Drug Interactions Database*.

Each entry includes all information specific to the product's ingredients. The entries do *not*, however, include the type of universal warning that applies to all drug products regardless of ingredients. You can find a detailed discussion of these precautions in "Using Over-the-Counter Medications Safely" at the beginning of this book. The five most important points to remember are:

1. **When pregnant, check with your doctor before using *any* drug.**
2. **Keep *all* drugs away from children.**
3. **After an overdose, always seek medical assistance.**
4. **Never exceed the recommended dose.**
5. **Never take a drug more often than recommended.**

Brand name:

Actifed Allergy Daytime/Nighttime Caplets

Pronounced: AK-tuh-fed
Generic ingredients: Pseudoephedrine hydrochloride, Diphenhydra-
mine hydrochloride (Actifed Allergy nighttime caplets only)

What this drug is used for

The Actifed Allergy package contains two types of medicine. The day-time caplets (white) temporarily relieve stuffy nose due to hay fever or other allergies. In addition, the nighttime caplets (blue) provide temporary relief of runny nose, sneezing, itchy nose or throat, and itchy, watery eyes.

How should you take this medication?

For adults and children 12 and over, the usual dosage is 2 daytime caplets every 4 to 6 hours while you are awake, and 2 nighttime caplets at bedtime.

Do not take the daytime and nighttime caplets within 4 hours of each other. Do not take more than 8 caplets, no matter what the type, during each 24 hours. For children under 12, consult a doctor.

■ STORAGE
Store at room temperature in a dry place and protect from light.

Do not take this medication if...

Unless your doctor approves, avoid this product if you have diabetes, heart disease, high blood pressure, thyroid disease, breathing problems such as emphysema or chronic bronchitis, high pressure in the eye (glaucoma), or an enlarged prostate gland.

Special warnings about this medication

If you become nervous or dizzy, or have trouble sleeping while taking this product, stop using it and call your doctor.

If you do not feel better in 7 days, or if you have a fever, check with your doctor.

Because Actifed Allergy nighttime caplets can make you drowsy, do not take them during the day unless you are resting at home; and do not drive or operate machinery after taking them.

Be aware that the nighttime caplets sometimes cause excitability, especially in children.

**Possible food and drug interactions
when taking this medication**

Do not use Actifed Allergy within 2 weeks of taking a drug classified as an MAO inhibitor, including the antidepressants Nardil and Parnate.

If you are taking a tranquilizer such as **Valium** or **Xanax**, or a sleep aid such as **Halcion** or **Seconal**, do not take Actifed Allergy without your doctor's approval; the combination could cause extreme drowsiness. For the same reason, avoid alcohol while taking this product.

Brand name:

Actifed Cold & Allergy

Pronounced: AK-tuh-fed
Generic ingredients: Pseudoephedrine hydrochloride, Triprolidine hydrochloride

What this drug is used for

Actifed Cold & Allergy temporarily relieves the stuffy nose that often results from a common cold. It can also be used for hay fever and other allergy symptoms such as runny nose, sneezing, itchy nose or throat, and itchy, watery eyes.

How should you take this medication?

Doses may be taken every 4 to 6 hours. Do not take more than 4 doses each 24 hours.

■ ADULTS

For adults and children 12 and over, the usual dose is 1 tablet.

■ CHILDREN

For children 6 to 12, the usual dose is half a tablet. For children under 6, consult a doctor.

■ STORAGE

Store at room temperature in a dry place and protect from light.

Do not take this medication if...

Unless your doctor approves, avoid Actifed Cold & Allergy if you have diabetes, heart disease, high blood pressure, thyroid disease, breathing problems such as emphysema or chronic bronchitis, high pressure within the eye (glaucoma), or an enlarged prostate gland.

Special warnings about this medication

If you become nervous or dizzy, or have trouble sleeping while taking this product, stop using it and call your doctor. Be aware that Actifed Cold & Allergy may cause excitability, especially in children.

If you do not feel better in 7 days, or if you have a fever, see your doctor.

Actifed Cold & Allergy can cause drowsiness. Be especially careful when driving or operating machinery.

Possible food and drug interactions when taking this medication

Do not use Actifed Cold & Allergy within 2 weeks of taking a drug classified as an MAO inhibitor, including the antidepressants Nardil and Parnate.

If you are taking a tranquilizer such as **Valium** or **Xanax**, or a sleep aid such as **Halcion** or **Seconal**, do not take Actifed Cold & Allergy without your doctor's approval; the combination could cause extreme drowsiness. For the same reason, avoid alcohol while taking this product.

Brand name:

Actifed Cold & Sinus

Pronounced: AK-tuh-fed
Generic ingredients: Acetaminophen, Pseudoephedrine hydrochloride, Triprolidine hydrochloride

What this drug is used for

Actifed Cold & Sinus temporarily relieves the stuffy nose caused by a cold, as well as the congestion and pressure of sinusitis. It can also be used for the minor aches and pains, headaches, and fever that accompany a cold, and for the runny nose, sneezing, itchy nose or throat, and itchy, watery eyes that mark a case of hay fever.

Actifed Cold & Sinus is available in tablet and caplet form.

How should you take this medication?

For adults and children 12 and over, the usual dose is 2 pills every 6 hours while you still have symptoms. Do not take more than 8 pills each 24 hours. For children under 12, consult a doctor.

■ STORAGE

Store at room temperature in a dry place and protect from light.

Do not take this medication if...

Unless your doctor approves, avoid Actifed Cold & Sinus if you have diabetes, heart disease, high blood pressure, thyroid disease, breathing problems such as emphysema or chronic bronchitis, high pressure within the eye (glaucoma), or an enlarged prostate gland.

Special warnings about this medication

Do not take Actifed Cold & Sinus for more than 10 days. If you do not feel better, or if you develop new symptoms or a fever that lasts more than 3 days, see your doctor.

If you become nervous or dizzy, or have trouble sleeping while taking this product, stop using it and call your doctor. Be aware that Actifed Cold & Sinus may cause excitement, especially in children.

Actifed Cold & Sinus can cause drowsiness. Be especially careful when driving or operating machinery.

Possible food and drug interactions
when taking this medication

Do not use Actifed Cold & Sinus within 2 weeks of taking a drug classified as an MAO inhibitor, including the antidepressants **Nardil** and **Parnate**.

If you are taking a tranquilizer such as **Valium** or **Xanax**, or a sleep aid such as **Halcion** or **Seconal**, do not take Actifed Cold & Sinus without your doctor's approval; the combination could cause extreme drowsiness. For the same reason, avoid alcohol while taking this product.

Brand name:

Actifed Sinus Daytime/Nighttime

Pronounced: AK-tuh-fed

Generic ingredients: Acetaminophen, Pseudoephedrine hydrochloride, Diphenhydramine hydrochloride (Actifed Sinus Nighttime only)

What this drug is used for

Actifed Sinus temporarily relieves stuffy nose, pressure and congestion in the sinuses, and the minor aches, pains, and headaches that often come with a cold.

The package contains two kinds of pills—white Daytime pills and blue Nighttime pills. The Nighttime pills contain an extra ingredient that can cause drowsiness, but also provides relief from runny nose, sneezing, itchy nose or throat, and itchy, watery eyes due to hay fever.

This product is available in tablet or caplet form.

How should you take this medication?
The usual dosage for adults and children 12 years and over is 2 Daytime pills every 6 hours while you are awake and 2 Nighttime pills at bedtime. If you are staying in bed or resting at home, you may take 2 Nighttime pills every 6 hours throughout the day. Otherwise, do not take this form of Actifed Sinus while you are awake because of the risk of drowsiness.

Do not take either type of pill within 6 hours of the other. Take no more than 8 pills in each 24 hours.

For children under 12, consult your doctor.

■ STORAGE
Store at room temperature in a dry place and protect from light.

Do not take this medication if...
Avoid either form of Actifed Sinus if you have diabetes, heart disease, high blood pressure, an enlarged prostate gland, or thyroid disease.

In addition, do not take the Nighttime pills without your doctor's approval if you have breathing problems (such as emphysema and chronic bronchitis) or high pressure within the eye (glaucoma).

Special warnings about this medication
If you become nervous or dizzy, or if you have trouble sleeping while taking this product, stop using it and call your doctor.

If you do not feel better, or if you have new symptoms or a fever that lasts more than 3 days, call your doctor. In any event, do not take Actifed Sinus for more than 10 days.

Be especially careful when driving or operating machinery after taking the Nighttime pills. Also, you should be aware that the Nighttime pills can make children—and some adults—excitable.

Possible food and drug interactions
when taking this medication

Do not use Actifed Sinus within 2 weeks of taking a drug classified as an MAO inhibitor, such as the antidepressants **Nardil** and **Parnate**.

If you are taking a tranquilizer such as **Valium** or **Xanax**, or a sleep aid such as **Halcion** or **Seconal**, do not take Actifed Sinus Nighttime pills without your doctor's approval; the combination could cause extreme drowsiness. For the same reason, avoid combining alcohol with the Nighttime pills.

Brand name:

Actron

See Orudis KT

Brand name:

Acutrim

Pronounced: ACK-you-trim
Generic name: Phenylpropanolamine
Other brand name: Dexatrim

What this drug is used for

Acutrim and Dexatrim are used to help control appetite as part of an overall weight-loss program. Both products are timed-release formulations. Dexatrim is available alone and in "Dexatrim Plus Vitamins" combination packages that include a vitamin/mineral supplement. Acutrim comes in tablet form; Dexatrim as tablets and caplets.

How should you take this medication?

Take 1 pill at mid-morning with a full glass of water. Swallow the pill whole. Do not divide, crush, chew, or dissolve it.

■ STORAGE
Store at room temperature.

Do not take this medication if...

Unless your doctor approves, avoid these products if you have high blood pressure, depression, or an eating disorder. Also check with your doctor if you have an enlarged prostate gland, diabetes, heart disease, or thyroid disease. Do not take either product if one of them has given you an allergic reaction in the past.

These products should not be given to children under age 12. Consult your doctor before giving them to a teenager.

Special warnings about this medication

Do not take more than 1 tablet or caplet a day. Increasing the dosage will not help you lose more weight, and this medication has been known to cause serious health problems, including heart attack, irregular heartbeat, mental disorders, seizures, and stroke.

Stop taking this product and call your doctor if you develop:

Dizziness
Headache
Nervousness
Pounding heartbeat
Problems sleeping

Remember that these products do not automatically reduce weight; to shed excess pounds, you must cut back your intake of calories. Do not take either of these products for more than 3 months. That should be enough time to establish new, healthier eating habits.

If you are over age 60, or are pregnant or nursing a baby, check with your doctor before taking either product.

Possible food and drug interactions
when taking this medication

Do not take Acutrim or Dexatrim if you are using any of the following:

Any other product that contains phenylpropanolamine, such as **Dimetane**, **Dura-Vent**, **Sinuvent**, and **Triaminic**

Drugs containing phenylephrine, such as **Atrohist**, **Neo-Synephrine**, and **Phenergan VC**

Ephedrine preparations such as **Quadrinal**, **Broncholate**, and **Mudrane**

Medications containing pseudoephedrine, such as **Claritin-D** and **Trinalin**

Also avoid taking **Acutrim** or **Dexatrim** within 2 weeks of taking any drug classified as an MAO inhibitor, including the antidepressants **Nardil** and **Parnate**. Check with your doctor about any other prescription drugs you are taking.

Brand name:

Advil

Pronounced: ADD-vill
Generic name: Ibuprofen
Other brand names: Motrin, Nuprin

What this drug is used for

These ibuprofen-based pain relievers can be used by both adults and children for headache, toothache, and the type of minor aches and pains that accompany a cold or flu. Adults can also use them for muscular aches, backache, minor arthritis pain, and menstrual cramps. The products also reduce fever.

The adult formulations—Advil, Motrin IB, and Nuprin—are available in tablet, caplet, and gelcap form. Two of the children's products—Children's Advil and Children's Motrin—are liquids. The third—Junior Strength Motrin—comes in caplet form.

How should you take this medication?

If you find that this medication causes mild heartburn, upset stomach, or stomach pain, try taking it with food or milk.

■ ADULTS

For adults and children 12 years and over, the usual dosage is 1 pill every 4 to 6 hours. If you do not feel better, you may increase the dosage to 2 pills, but do not take more than 6 pills each 24 hours.

■ CHILDREN

Doses may be repeated every 6 to 8 hours, up to a maximum of 4 times a day. Shake liquid products well before using. A measuring cup is provided for accurate dosing of Children's Advil and Children's Motrin Oral Suspension. Children's Motrin Drops come with a calibrated dropper.

Children 11 to 12

The usual dosage is 3 teaspoonfuls of Children's Advil or Children's Motrin Oral Suspension, or 3 caplets of Junior Strength Motrin.

Children 9 to 10

The usual dosage is 2.5 teaspoonfuls of Children's Advil or Children's Motrin Oral Suspension, or 2.5 caplets of Junior Strength Motrin.

Children 6 to 8

The usual dosage is 2 teaspoonfuls of Children's Advil or Children's Motrin Oral Suspension, or 2 caplets of Junior Strength Motrin.

Children 4 to 5

The usual dosage is 1.5 teaspoonfuls of Children's Advil or Children's Motrin Oral Suspension. Consult your doctor if giving Junior Strength Motrin.

Children 2 to 3

The usual dosage is 1 teaspoonful of Children's Advil or Children's Motrin Oral Suspension, or 2 dropperfuls of Children's Motrin Drops.

Children under 2

Consult your doctor.

■ STORAGE

Store at room temperature. Protect from high temperatures.

Do not take this medication if...

If aspirin has ever given you a severe allergic reaction (asthma, swelling, shock, or hives), do not take these products. They could have a similar effect. Check with your doctor before using these products if you've had any side effects from other over-the-counter pain relievers.

Do not give these products to a child who has lost a great deal of fluid through vomiting or diarrhea. Unless your doctor approves, do not use these products for stomach pain in a child.

Special warnings about this medication

Stop taking this medication and call your doctor if you develop any unusual or unexpected new symptoms. Do likewise if the drug causes significant or lasting stomach problems.

Do not take this medication for more than 10 days for pain or 3 days for fever without your doctor's approval. (Limit its use in children to 3 days.) If the pain or fever won't go away or gets worse, or if you develop new symptoms or notice any redness or swelling, check with your doctor; you might have a serious condition.

You should also check with your doctor immediately if you have a severe sore throat that lasts for more than 2 days, or if your sore throat is accompanied or followed by fever, headache, rash, nausea, or vomiting.

Do not take this medication during the last 3 months of pregnancy. It could harm the baby or cause complications during delivery. Earlier during pregnancy, and while nursing a baby, check with your doctor before taking any of these products.

Possible food and drug interactions when taking this medication

Unless your doctor approves, do not combine this medication with other pain relievers, including aspirin-containing products such as **Ecotrin**, **Empirin**, and **Excedrin**, acetaminophen-containing products such as **Tylenol**, **Panadol**, and **TheraFlu**, and other ibuprofen-containing products such as **Sine-Aid IB**.

Also check with your doctor before combining this medication with any of the following prescription drugs:

Blood pressure medications known as ACE inhibitors, including
Vasotec and **Capoten**
Blood-thinning drugs such as **Coumadin**
Diuretics such as **Lasix** and **HydroDIURIL**
Lithium (**Lithonate**)
Methotrexate (**Rheumatrex**)

Overdosage

■ *Symptoms of ibuprofen overdose may include:*
Abdominal pain, breathing difficulties, coma, drowsiness, headache, irregular heartbeat, kidney failure, low blood pressure, nausea, ringing in the ears, seizures, sluggishness, vomiting

If you suspect an overdose, seek medical attention immediately.

Brand name:

Advil Cold and Sinus

Pronounced: ADD-vill
Generic ingredients: Ibuprofen, Pseudoephedrine hydrochloride
Other brand name: Vicks Dayquil Sinus Pressure & Pain Relief

What this drug is used for

Both these sinus products temporarily relieve symptoms of the common cold, sinusitis (swelling and pain in the sinuses), and flu, including stuffy nose, fever, headache, and body aches and pains.

The Advil product comes in tablet and caplet forms. The Vicks Dayquil product is available in caplets only.

How should you take this medication?

Take 1 pill every 4 to 6 hours as long as you have symptoms. If you do not feel better, you can take 2 pills, but do not take more than 6 pills in 24 hours unless your doctor tells you to.

If you have occasional mild heartburn, upset stomach, or stomach pain while using this product, take it with food or milk. If your stomach problems continue or get worse, call your doctor.

■ STORAGE

Store at room temperature. Protect from excessive heat.

Do not take this medication if...

Unless your doctor approves, avoid these products if you have high blood pressure, heart disease, diabetes, thyroid disease, or an enlarged prostate gland.

If you are allergic to aspirin, do not take these products. They could cause a similar reaction even though they contain no aspirin. If you have had serious side effects from *any* nonprescription pain reliever, or you are taking any prescription drugs, check with your doctor before taking either of these products.

Do not give these products to children under 12 without your doctor's approval.

Special warnings about this medication

Avoid these products during the last 3 months of pregnancy. They could harm the unborn child or cause problems during delivery. Check with your doctor before taking either product at any time during pregnancy. Check, too, if you are under a doctor's care for any serious medical problem.

Do not use either product for cold symptoms for more 7 days. If you are taking it to lower a fever, do not use it for more than 3 days. If your cold or fever continues or gets worse, or if you have new symptoms, call your doctor.

If you become nervous or dizzy, or have trouble sleeping while taking one of these products, stop using it and call your doctor. In fact, if you have any symptoms that are unusual or seem to have nothing to do with the condition for which you took the product, talk to your doctor before taking any more of this medicine.

Possible food and drug interactions when taking this medication

Do not use either of these products within 2 weeks of taking a drug classified as an MAO inhibitor, such as the antidepressants **Nardil** and **Parnate**.

Do not combine these products with others containing ibuprofen, such as **Motrin** or **Nuprin**, or with other nonprescription pain relievers such as **Aspirin** or **Tylenol**.

Brand name:

Afrin 4 Hour

See Neo-Synephrine

Brand name:

Afrin 12 Hour

Pronounced: A-frin
Generic name: Oxymetazoline hydrochloride
Other brand names: 4-Way 12 Hour, 12 Hour Nostrilla, Duration 12 Hour, Neo-Synephrine 12 Hour, Vicks Sinex 12-Hour

What this drug is used for

These products provide temporary relief of stuffy nose caused by colds, inflamed sinuses, or allergies such as hay fever. Three of these products—Afrin, Neo-Synephrine, and Vicks Sinex—also come in a shorter-acting, 4-hour formulation based on a different active ingredient. (See the profile on *Neo-Synephrine*.)

How should you use this medication?

Squeeze Bottles: Squeeze the bottle quickly and firmly while you inhale. Do not tilt your head backward while spraying. Wipe the nozzle clean after use.

Pump Spray: Remove the cap and prime the pump by pressing it down firmly several times. Hold the bottle with your thumb at the base and the nozzle between your first and second fingers. With your head held upright, put the nozzle into your nostril, depress the pump 2 or 3 times, and sniff deeply.

■ ADULTS

For adults and children 6 and over, the usual dose is 2 or 3 sprays in each nostril. Do not use any of these products more often than every 10 to 12 hours or take more than 2 doses in any 24-hour period. Children need adult supervision.

■ CHILDREN

For children under 6, consult your doctor.

■ STORAGE

Store at room temperature.

Do not take this medication if...

Unless your doctor approves, do not use any of these products if you have diabetes, heart disease, high blood pressure, thyroid disease, or an enlarged prostate gland.

Special warnings about this medication

These products may cause temporary burning, stinging, sneezing, or runny nose.

Do not take more than the recommended dosage or use for more than 3 days. If you use these products too often or too long, your stuffy nose may come back or get worse. Do not share this medication, since this could spread infection. If your stuffy nose doesn't clear up, call your doctor.

Brand name:

Aleve

Pronounced: ah-LEEV
Generic name: Naproxen sodium

What this drug is used for

Aleve reduces fever and gives temporary relief from pain. It can be used for:

Aches and pains of the common cold
Headache
Toothache
Muscle aches

Backache
Minor arthritis pain
Menstrual cramps

Aleve is available in tablet and caplet form.

How should you take this medication?

Take each dose with a full glass of liquid. Use the minimum amount needed to provide relief.

■ ADULTS

The usual dose is 1 pill every 8 to 12 hours. Some people find the drug works better when they take 2 pills for the first dose, followed by 1 pill 12 hours later. Do not take more than 3 pills in 24 hours.

■ OLDER ADULTS

If you are over age 65, do not take more than 1 pill every 12 hours.

■ CHILDREN

Not for use in children under 12.

■ STORAGE

Aleve may be stored at room temperature. Protect from excessive heat.

Do not take this medication if...

Avoid Aleve if any other pain reliever has given you hives or a severe allergic reaction. People who are allergic to one type of pain reliever are often allergic to others.

Special warnings about this medication

Do not take Aleve for more than 10 days for pain or 3 days for fever.

Do not take Aleve during the last 3 months of pregnancy. It could harm the baby or cause complications during delivery. Earlier in pregnancy, and while nursing, consult your doctor before taking Aleve.

If you generally drink 3 or more alcoholic beverages per day, check with your doctor before taking Aleve.

Also check with a doctor if:

■ Your pain or fever gets worse or won't go away
■ The painful area is red or swollen
■ You have had serious side effects from any other pain reliever
■ Any new or unusual symptoms appear

■ You develop significant heartburn, upset stomach, or stomach pain, or if even mild digestive problems persist

Possible food and drug interactions when taking this medication

Unless your doctor directs, do not combine Aleve with aspirin, ibuprofen (**Motrin, Advil**), or acetaminophen (**Tylenol**). Also avoid other products that contain Aleve's active ingredient, naproxen. Medications containing naproxen include the prescription painkillers **Anaprox** and **Naprosyn**.

Naproxen can also interact with a number of other prescription drugs. It is especially important to check with your doctor before taking Aleve with the following:

Blood-thinning drugs such as **Coumadin**
Furosemide (**Lasix**)
Heart and blood pressure medications classified as ACE inhibitors,
  including **Capoten, Vasotec**, and **Zestril**
Heart and blood pressure medications known as beta blockers,
  including **Inderal, Lopressor**, and **Tenormin**
Lithium (**Lithonate**)
Methotrexate
Oral diabetes drugs such as **Diabinese** and **Micronase**
Phenytoin (**Dilantin**)
Probenecid (**Benemid**)
Sulfa drugs such as **Bactrim** and **Septra**

Brand name:
Alka-Mints

See Tums

Brand name:
Alka-Seltzer

Pronounced: AL-ka-SELL-tser
Generic ingredients: Aspirin, Citric acid, Sodium bicarbonate

What this drug is used for

Alka-Seltzer relieves heartburn, acid indigestion, and sour stomach with headache. It can also be used for pain alone, including headaches and muscular aches and pains.

Alka-Seltzer is available in regular- and extra-strength effervescent tablets. Regular-strength Alka-Seltzer comes in three flavors: "original," lemon-lime, and cherry.

How should you take this medication?

Do not swallow Alka-Seltzer tablets whole. They must be dissolved in water. For regular-strength tablets, doses can be repeated every 4 hours, up to a maximum of 8 tablets each 24 hours. For extra-strength tablets, doses can be repeated every 6 hours, up to a maximum of 7 tablets each 24 hours. Those over the age of 60 should take no more than 4 tablets a day of either type.

The usual dose is 2 tablets dissolved in 4 ounces of water.

Do not take this medication if...

Do not take this product if you are allergic to aspirin, have asthma or a bleeding disorder, or are on a sodium-restricted diet.

Special warnings about this medication

The aspirin in Alka-Seltzer has been known to trigger a serious illness called Reye's syndrome in children and teenagers who catch a virus. If your child gets chickenpox or flu, do not treat the symptoms with this product.

Do not take the maximum dosage every day for more than 10 days. If you are using the product for pain relief, stop after 10 days unless your doctor recommends otherwise. Call your doctor if you develop new symptoms, your pain gets worse, or you notice redness or swelling. These could be signs of a serious condition. Also check with your doctor if your stomach problems won't go away or tend to come back, or if you're being treated for an ulcer.

Do not take this product during the last 3 months of pregnancy. It could harm the baby or cause complications during delivery. Earlier during pregnancy, and while nursing a baby, check with your doctor before taking Alka-Seltzer.

If you develop ringing in the ears or notice a loss of hearing, stop taking this product and contact your doctor.

Possible food and drug interactions
when taking this medication

Aspirin-containing products such as Alka-Seltzer can interact with a number of prescription drugs. Check with your doctor before combining it with any of the following:

Acetazolamide (**Diamox**)

ACE-inhibitor-type blood pressure medications such as **Capoten**

Anti-gout drugs such as **Anturane**, **Benemid**, and **Zyloprim**

Arthritis preparations such as **Aleve**, **Anaprox**, **Ecotrin**, **Indocin**, **Motrin**, **Naprosyn**, and **Orudis**

Blood-thinning drugs such as **Coumadin**

Certain diuretics (water pills), including **Lasix**

Diabetes medications, including **DiaBeta**, **Diabinese**, **Micronase**, and **Glucotrol**

Diltiazem (**Cardizem**)

Dipyridamole (**Persantine**)

Seizure medications such as **Depakene**

Steroids such as prednisone (**Deltasone**, **Orasone**)

Brand name:

Alka-Seltzer Gold

Pronounced: AL-kah SELL-tser

Generic ingredients: Citric acid, Potassium bicarbonate, Sodium bicarbonate

What this drug is used for

Alka-Seltzer Gold relieves heartburn, upset stomach, and indigestion. Unlike regular Alka-Seltzer, it contains no aspirin, and therefore will not relieve pain.

How should you take this medication?

Do not swallow Alka-Seltzer Gold tablets whole. They must be dissolved in water.

■ ADULTS

The usual dose is 2 tablets completely dissolved in water every 4 hours. Do not take more than 8 tablets in 24 hours. (Those age 60 or older should take no more than 7 tablets in 24 hours.)

■ CHILDREN

The usual dose is 1 tablet dissolved in water. Children should not take more than 4 tablets in 24 hours.

Do not take this medication if...

Avoid Alka-Seltzer Gold if you are on a sodium-restricted diet.

Special warnings about this medication

Do not use the maximum dosage of this product for more than 2 weeks.

Possible food and drug interactions
when taking this medication

When taken at the same time, antacids such as Alka-Seltzer Gold can interfere with a number of prescription drugs. It is especially important to check with your doctor before combining it with the following:

Cellulose sodium phosphate (**Calcibind**)
Isoniazid (**Rifamate**)
Ketoconazole (**Nizoral**)
Mecamylamine (**Inversine**)
Methenamine (**Mandelamine**)
Sodium polystyrene sulfonate resin (**Kayexalate**)
Tetracycline antibiotics (**Sumycin, Minocin**)

Brand name:

Alka-Seltzer Plus Cold & Cough Medicine Liqui-Gels

Pronounced: AL-ka SELL-tser
Generic ingredients: Acetaminophen, Chlorpheniramine maleate,
* Dextromethorphan hydrobromide, Pseudoephedrine hydrochloride*

What this drug is used for

All members of the Alka-Seltzer Plus family of products relieve cold and flu symptoms such as fever, headache, and body aches and pains. (The tablets contain aspirin for this purpose; the liquigels use acetaminophen.) In addition, the Cold & Cough liquigels unclog stuffy nose and sinuses, combat coughing, and relieve runny nose, sneezing, and sore throat.

How should you take this medication?

Alka-Seltzer Plus liquigels should be swallowed with a glass of water. Doses of the Cold & Cough liquigels may be repeated every 4 hours if needed—but don't take more than 4 doses per day.

■ ADULTS

For adults and children 12 years and over, the usual dosage is 2 liquigels.

■ CHILDREN

For children 6 to 12, the usual dose is 1 liquigel. For children under 6, consult your doctor.

Do not take this medication if...

Unless your doctor approves, do not take this product if you have heart disease, high blood pressure, thyroid disease, diabetes, high pressure within the eye (glaucoma), an enlarged prostate gland, or a breathing problem such as emphysema or chronic bronchitis.

Also check with your doctor before using the Cold & Cough liquigels for the type of chronic cough that results from smoking or asthma, or for a cough that brings up lots of phlegm.

Special warnings about this medication

If you become dizzy or nervous, or have trouble sleeping, stop taking this product and check with your doctor.

Alka-Seltzer Plus liquigels contain an antihistamine that may cause drowsiness. Be especially cautious when driving, and when operating machinery. The antihistamine can also cause excitability, especially in children.

Do not take this product for more than 7 days. If your symptoms do not improve or include a fever, call your doctor.

You should also check with your doctor immediately if you have a severe sore throat that lasts for more than 2 days, or if your sore throat is accompanied or followed by fever, headache, rash, nausea, or vomiting.

Likewise, call your doctor if you have a cough that lasts for more than 7 days or tends to come back, or a cough accompanied by rash, lasting headache, and fever.

Possible food and drug interactions
when taking this medication

Do not use this product within 2 weeks of taking a drug classified as an MAO inhibitor, such as the antidepressants **Nardil** and **Parnate**.

If you are taking a tranquilizer such as **Valium** or **Xanax**, or a sleep aid such as **Halcion** or **Seconal**, do not take this product without your doctor's approval; the combination could cause extreme drowsiness. For the same reason, avoid alcohol while taking this product.

Brand name:

Alka-Seltzer Plus Cold & Cough Medicine Tablets

Pronounced: AL-ka SELL-tser
Generic ingredients: Aspirin, Chlorpheniramine maleate, Dextro-methorphan hydrobromine, Phenylpropanolamine bitartrate

What this drug is used for

All members of the Alka-Seltzer Plus family of products relieve cold and flu symptoms such as fever, headache, and body aches and pains. (The tablets contain aspirin for this purpose; the liquigels use acetaminophen.) In addition, the Cold & Cough tablets include ingredients to unclog stuffy nose and sinuses, combat coughing, and relieve runny nose, sneezing, and scratchy throat.

How should you take this medication?

The usual dose for adults and children 12 years and over is 2 tablets dissolved in 4 ounces of water. Do not swallow Alka-Seltzer Plus Cold & Cough tablets whole. Doses can be repeated every 4 hours if needed, to a maximum of 8 tablets each 24 hours. For children under 12, consult your doctor.

Do not take this medication if...

Do not take this product if you are allergic to aspirin, must avoid phenylalanine, or need to limit your intake of sodium. Unless your doctor approves, also avoid the product if you have bleeding problems, heart disease, high blood pressure, thyroid disease, diabetes, high pressure within the eye (glaucoma), an enlarged prostate gland, or a breathing problem such as asthma, emphysema, or chronic bronchitis.

Likewise, check with your doctor before using this product for the type of chronic cough that results from smoking or asthma, or for a cough that brings up lots of phlegm.

Special warnings about this medication

The aspirin in this product has been known to trigger a serious illness called Reye's syndrome in children and teenagers who catch a virus. If your child gets chickenpox or flu, do not treat the symptoms with this formulation of Alka-Seltzer Plus.

If you become dizzy or nervous, or have trouble sleeping, stop taking this product and check with your doctor.

This variety of Alka-Seltzer Plus contains an antihistamine that can cause drowsiness. Be especially cautious when driving, and when operating machinery. The antihistamine can also cause excitability, especially in children.

Do not take this product for more than 7 days. If your symptoms do not improve or include a fever that lasts more than 3 days, call your doctor.

You should also check with your doctor immediately if you have a severe sore throat that lasts for more than 2 days, or if your sore throat is accompanied or followed by fever, headache, nausea, or vomiting.

Likewise, call your doctor if you have a cough that lasts for more than 7 days or tends to come back, or a cough accompanied by rash, lasting headache, and fever.

Do not take this product during the last 3 months of pregnancy. It could harm the baby or cause complications during delivery. Earlier during pregnancy, and while nursing a baby, check with your doctor before taking this type of Alka-Seltzer Plus.

Possible food and drug interactions when taking this medication

Do not use this product within 2 weeks of taking a drug classified as an MAO inhibitor, such as the antidepressants **Nardil** and **Parnate**.

Aspirin-containing products such as this can also interact with a number of other prescription drugs. Check with your doctor before combining this product with any of the following:

Acetazolamide (**Diamox**)
ACE-inhibitor-type blood pressure medications such as **Capoten**
Anti-gout drugs such as **Anturane**, **Benemid**, and **Zyloprim**
Arthritis preparations such as **Aleve**, **Anaprox**, **Ecotrin**, **Indocin**, **Motrin**, **Naprosyn**, and **Orudis**
Blood-thinning drugs such as **Coumadin**
Certain diuretics (water pills), including **Lasix**
Diabetes medications, including **DiaBeta**, **Diabinese**, **Micronase**, and **Glucotrol**
Diltiazem (**Cardizem**)

Dipyridamole (**Persantine**)

Seizure medications such as **Depakene**

Steroids such as prednisone (**Deltasone, Orasone**)

If you are taking a tranquilizer such as **Valium** or **Xanax**, or a sleep aid such as **Halcion** or **Seconal**, do not take this form of Alka-Seltzer Plus without your doctor's approval; the combination could cause extreme drowsiness. For the same reason, avoid alcohol while taking this product.

Brand name:

Alka-Seltzer Plus Cold Medicine Liqui-Gels

Pronounced: AL-ka SELL-tser

Generic ingredients: Acetaminophen, Chlorpheniramine maleate, Pseudoephedrine hydrochloride

What this drug is used for

All members of the Alka-Seltzer Plus family of products relieve cold and flu symptoms such as fever, headache, and body aches and pains. (The tablets contain aspirin for this purpose; the liquigels use acetaminophen.) In addition, the Cold Medicine liquigels unclog stuffy nose and sinuses, and relieve runny nose, sneezing, and sore throat. They do not contain an ingredient for cough.

How should you take this medication?

Alka-Seltzer Plus liquigels should be swallowed with a glass of water. Doses of the Cold Medicine liquigels may be repeated every 4 hours if needed—but don't take more than 4 doses per day.

■ ADULTS

For adults and children 12 years and over, the usual dosage is 2 liquigels.

■ CHILDREN

For children 6 to 12, the usual dose is 1 liquigel. For children under 6, consult your doctor.

Do not take this medication if...

Unless your doctor approves, do not take this product if you have heart disease, high blood pressure, thyroid disease, diabetes, high pressure within the eye (glaucoma), an enlarged prostate gland, or a breathing problem such as emphysema or chronic bronchitis.

Special warnings about this medication

If you become dizzy or nervous, or have trouble sleeping, stop taking this product and check with your doctor.

Alka-Seltzer Plus liquigels contain an antihistamine that may cause drowsiness. Be especially cautious when driving, and when operating machinery. The antihistamine can also cause excitability, especially in children.

Do not take this product for more than 7 days. If your symptoms do not improve or include a fever, call your doctor.

You should also check with your doctor immediately if you have a severe sore throat that lasts for more than 2 days, or if your sore throat is accompanied or followed by fever, headache, rash, nausea, or vomiting.

Possible food and drug interactions when taking this medication

Do not use this product within 2 weeks of taking a drug classified as an MAO inhibitor, such as the antidepressants **Nardil** and **Parnate**.

If you are taking a tranquilizer such as **Valium** or **Xanax**, or a sleep aid such as **Halcion** or **Seconal**, do not take this product without your doctor's approval; the combination could cause extreme drowsiness. For the same reason, avoid alcohol while taking this product.

Brand name:

Alka-Seltzer Plus Cold Medicine Tablets

Pronounced: AL-ka SELL-tser
Generic ingredients: Aspirin, Chlorpheniramine maleate, Phenyl-
propanolamine bitartrate

What this drug is used for

All members of the Alka-Seltzer Plus family of products relieve cold and flu symptoms such as fever, headache, and body aches and pains. (The tablets contain aspirin for this purpose; the liquigels use acetaminophen.) In addition, the Cold tablets include ingredients to unclog stuffy nose and sinuses, and relieve runny nose, sneezing, and scratchy throat. They do not contain an ingredient for cough.

How should you take this medication?

The usual dose for adults and children 12 years and over is 2 tablets dissolved in 4 ounces of water. Do not swallow Alka-Seltzer Plus Cold tablets whole. Doses can be repeated every 4 hours if needed, to a maximum of 8 tablets each 24 hours. For children under 12, consult your doctor.

Do not take this medication if...

Do not take this product if you are allergic to aspirin, must avoid phenylalanine, or have to limit your intake of sodium. Unless your doctor approves, also avoid the product if you have bleeding problems, heart disease, high blood pressure, thyroid disease, diabetes, high pressure within the eye (glaucoma), an enlarged prostate gland, or a breathing problem such as asthma, emphysema, or chronic bronchitis.

Special warnings about this medication

The aspirin in this product has been known to trigger a serious illness called Reye's syndrome in children and teenagers who catch a virus. If your child gets chickenpox or flu, do not treat the symptoms with Alka-Seltzer Plus Cold Medicine Tablets.

If you become dizzy or nervous, or have trouble sleeping, stop taking this product and check with your doctor.

This variety of Alka-Seltzer Plus contains an antihistamine that can cause drowsiness. Be especially cautious when driving, and when operating machinery. The antihistamine can also cause excitability, especially in children.

Do not take this product for more than 7 days. If your symptoms do not improve or include a fever that lasts more than 3 days, call your doctor.

You should also check with your doctor immediately if you have a severe sore throat that lasts for more than 2 days, or if your sore throat is accompanied or followed by fever, headache, nausea, or vomiting.

Do not take this product during the last 3 months of pregnancy. It could harm the baby or cause complications during delivery. Earlier during pregnancy, and while nursing a baby, check with your doctor before taking Alka-Seltzer Plus Cold Medicine Tablets.

Possible food and drug interactions when taking this medication

Do not use this product within 2 weeks of taking a drug classified as an MAO inhibitor, such as the antidepressants **Nardil** and **Parnate**.

Aspirin-containing products such as this can also interact with a number of other prescription drugs. Check with your doctor before combining this product with any of the following:

Acetazolamide (**Diamox**)
ACE-inhibitor-type blood pressure medications such as **Capoten**
Anti-gout drugs such as **Anturane, Benemid,** and **Zyloprim**
Arthritis preparations such as **Aleve, Anaprox, Ecotrin, Indocin, Motrin, Naprosyn,** and **Orudis**
Blood-thinning drugs such as **Coumadin**
Certain diuretics (water pills), including **Lasix**
Diabetes medications, including **DiaBeta, Diabinese, Micronase,** and **Glucotrol**
Diltiazem (**Cardizem**)
Dipyridamole (**Persantine**)
Seizure medications such as **Depakene**
Steroids such as prednisone (**Deltasone, Orasone**)

If you are taking a tranquilizer such as **Valium** or **Xanax**, or a sleep aid such as **Halcion** or **Seconal**, do not take this form of Alka-Seltzer Plus without your doctor's approval; the combination could cause extreme drowsiness. For the same reason, avoid alcohol while taking this product.

Brand name:

Alka-Seltzer Plus Flu & Body Aches Liqui-Gels

Pronounced: AL-kah SELL-tser
Generic ingredients: Acetaminophen, Dextromethorphan hydrobromide, Pseudoephedrine hydrochloride

What this drug is used for

Alka-Seltzer Plus Flu & Body Aches liquigels provide temporary relief from common flu and cold symptoms such as fever, head and body aches, minor sore throat pain, cough, and stuffy nose and sinuses.

Unlike the regular Alka-Seltzer Flu & Body Aches Formula—which contains an antihistamine for sneezing and runny nose, and therefore may cause drowsiness—the liquigels will not put you to sleep.

How should you take this medication?

The liquigels must be swallowed with water. Doses can be repeated every 4 hours, up to a maximum of 4 doses a day.

■ ADULTS
The usual dose is 2 liquigels.

■ CHILDREN
For children 6 to 12, the usual dose is 1 liquigel. For children under 6, consult your doctor.

Do not take this medication if...

Unless your doctor approves, do not take this product if you have heart disease, high blood pressure, thyroid disease, diabetes, or an enlarged prostate gland.

Also check with your doctor before using this product for the type of chronic cough that results from smoking, asthma, or emphysema, or for a cough that brings up lots of phlegm.

Special warnings about this medication

If you become dizzy or nervous, or have trouble sleeping, stop taking this product and call your doctor.

Also check with your doctor if cough and other symptoms don't improve within 7 days or tend to come back—or if you also have a fever, rash, or lasting headache. A lingering cough could signal a serious condition.

Call your doctor immediately if you have a severe sore throat that lasts for more than 2 days, or if your sore throat is accompanied or followed by fever, headache, rash, nausea, or vomiting.

Possible food and drug interactions
when taking this medication

Do not use this product within 2 weeks of taking a drug classified as an MAO inhibitor, such as the antidepressants **Nardil** and **Parnate**.

Brand name:

Alka-Seltzer Plus Flu & Body Aches Tablets

Pronounced: ALK-ah SELL-tser
Generic ingredients: Acetaminophen, Chlorpheniramine maleate,
  Dextromethorphan hydrobromide, Phenylpropanolamine bitartrate

What this drug is used for

Alka-Seltzer Plus Flu & Body Aches tablets provides temporary relief from common flu and cold symptoms such as head and body aches, fever, minor sore throat pain, cough, and stuffy nose and sinuses.

This version of Alka-Seltzer Plus Flu & Body Aches includes an antihistamine for sneezing and runny nose, and can therefore make you drowsy. The Flu & Body Aches liquigels are antihistamine-free.

How should you take this medication?

The tablets must be dissolved in 4 ounces of hot (but not boiling) water. Sip the mixture while it's still hot.

The usual dose is 2 tablets. Doses can be repeated every 4 hours, up to a maximum of 4 doses a day. For children under 12, consult your doctor.

Do not take this medication if...

Unless your doctor approves, do not take this product if you have heart disease, high blood pressure, thyroid disease, diabetes, high pressure within the eye (glaucoma), an enlarged prostate gland, or a breathing problem such as emphysema or chronic bronchitis.

Also check with your doctor before using this product for the type of chronic cough that results from smoking, asthma, or emphysema, or for a cough that brings up lots of phlegm.

Special warnings about this medication

If you become dizzy or nervous, or have trouble sleeping, stop taking this product and check with your doctor.

The antihistamine in this product can cause overexcitement, especially in children. It also tends to make some people drowsy. Be especially cautious when driving and when operating machinery.

If cough and other symptoms don't improve within 7 days or tend to come back—or if you also have a fever, rash, or lasting headache—check with your doctor. A lingering cough could signal a serious condition.

You should also check with your doctor immediately if you have a severe sore throat that lasts for more than 2 days, or if your sore throat is accompanied or followed by fever, headache, rash, nausea, or vomiting.

If you must avoid phenylalanine, do not take this variety of Alka-Seltzer. If you are on a sodium-restricted diet, remember that each tablet contains 111 milligrams of sodium.

Possible food and drug interactions when taking this medication

Do not use Alka-Seltzer Plus Flu & Body Aches tablets within 2 weeks of taking a drug classified as an MAO inhibitor, such as the antidepressants **Nardil** and **Parnate**.

If you are taking a tranquilizer such as **Valium** or **Xanax**, or a sleep aid such as **Halcion** or **Seconal,** do not take this product without your doctor's approval; the combination could cause extreme drowsiness. For the same reason, avoid alcohol while taking this medication.

Brand name:

Alka-Seltzer Plus Night-Time Cold Medicine Liqui-Gels

Pronounced: AL-ka SELL-tser
Generic ingredients: Acetaminophen, Dextromethorphan hydrobromide, Doxylamine succinate, Pseudoephedrine hydrochloride

What this drug is used for

All members of the Alka-Seltzer Plus family of products relieve cold and flu symptoms such as fever, headache, and body aches and pains. (The tablets contain aspirin for this purpose; the liquigels use acetaminophen.) In addition, the Night-Time liquigels unclog stuffy nose and sinuses, combat coughing, and relieve runny nose, sneezing, and sore throat.

How should you take this medication?

The usual dose for adults and children 12 years and over is 2 liquigels swallowed with a glass of water at bedtime. Take only once a day.

Do not take this medication if...

Unless your doctor approves, do not take this product if you have heart disease, high blood pressure, thyroid disease, diabetes, high pressure within the eye (glaucoma), an enlarged prostate gland, or a breathing problem such as emphysema or chronic bronchitis.

Also check with your doctor before using the Night-Time liquigels for the type of chronic cough that results from smoking or asthma, or for a cough that brings up lots of phlegm.

Not for children under 12.

Special warnings about this medication

If you become dizzy or nervous, or have trouble sleeping, stop taking this product and check with your doctor.

The antihistamine in this product is likely to cause drowsiness. Be especially cautious when driving, and when operating machinery. The antihistamine can also cause excitability, especially in children.

Do not take this product for more than 7 days. If your symptoms do not improve or include a fever, call your doctor.

You should also check with your doctor immediately if you have a severe sore throat that lasts for more than 2 days, or if your sore throat is accompanied or followed by fever, headache, rash, nausea, or vomiting.

Likewise, call your doctor if you have a cough that lasts for more than 7 days or tends to come back, or a cough accompanied by rash, lasting headache, and fever.

Possible food and drug interactions
when taking this medication

Do not use this product within 2 weeks of taking a drug classified as an MAO inhibitor, such as the antidepressants **Nardil** and **Parnate**.

If you are taking a tranquilizer such as **Valium** or **Xanax**, or a sleep aid such as **Halcion** or **Seconal**, do not take the Night-Time liquigels without your doctor's approval; the combination could cause extreme drowsiness. For the same reason, avoid alcohol while taking this product.

Brand name:

Alka-Seltzer Plus Night-Time Cold Medicine Tablets

Pronounced: AL-ka SELL-tser
Generic ingredients: Aspirin, Dextromethorphan hydrochloride, Doxylamine succinate, Phenylpropanolamine bitartrate

What this drug is used for

All members of the Alka-Seltzer Plus family of products relieve cold and flu symptoms such as fever, headache, and body aches and pains.

(The tablets contain aspirin for this purpose; the liquigels use acetaminophen.) In addition, the Night-Time Cold tablets include ingredients to unclog stuffy nose and sinuses and combat cough, and a strong antihistamine to relieve runny nose, sneezing, and scratchy throat.

How should you take this medication?

The usual dose for adults and children 12 years and over is 2 tablets dissolved in 4 ounces of water. Do not swallow Alka-Seltzer Plus Night-Time Cold tablets whole. Doses can be repeated every 4 hours if needed, to a maximum of 8 tablets each 24 hours. For children under 12, consult your doctor.

Do not take this medication if...

Do not take this product if you are allergic to aspirin, must avoid phenylalanine, or have to limit your intake of sodium. Unless your doctor approves, also avoid the product if you have bleeding problems, heart disease, high blood pressure, thyroid disease, diabetes, high pressure within the eye (glaucoma), an enlarged prostate gland, or a breathing problem such as asthma, emphysema, or chronic bronchitis.

Also check with your doctor before using this product for the type of chronic cough that results from smoking or asthma, or for a cough that brings up lots of phlegm.

Special warnings about this medication

The aspirin in this product has been known to trigger a serious illness called Reye's syndrome in children and teenagers who catch a virus. If your child gets chickenpox or flu, do not treat the symptoms with this type of Alka-Seltzer Plus.

If you become dizzy or nervous, or have trouble sleeping, stop taking this product and check with your doctor.

The antihistamine in this variety of Alka-Seltzer Plus is likely to cause drowsiness. Be especially cautious when driving and when operating machinery. The antihistamine can also cause excitability, especially in children.

Do not take this product for more than 7 days. If your symptoms do not improve or include a fever that lasts more than 3 days, call your doctor.

You should also check with your doctor immediately if you have a severe sore throat that lasts for more than 2 days, or if your sore throat is accompanied or followed by fever, headache, nausea, or vomiting.

Likewise, call your doctor if you have a cough that lasts for more than

7 days or tends to come back, or a cough accompanied by rash, lasting headache, and fever.

Do not take this product during the last 3 months of pregnancy. It could harm the baby or cause complications during delivery. Earlier during pregnancy, and while nursing a baby, check with your doctor before taking this variety of Alka-Seltzer Plus.

**Possible food and drug interactions
when taking this medication**
Do not use this product within 2 weeks of taking a drug classified as an MAO inhibitor, such as the antidepressants **Nardil** and **Parnate**.

Aspirin-containing products such as this can also interact with a number of other prescription drugs. Check with your doctor before combining this product with any of the following:

Acetazolamide (**Diamox**)
ACE-inhibitor-type blood pressure medications such as **Capoten**
Anti-gout drugs such as **Anturane**, **Benemid**, and Zyloprim
Arthritis preparations such as **Aleve**, **Anaprox**, **Ecotrin**, **Indocin**, **Motrin**, **Naprosyn**, and **Orudis**
Blood-thinning drugs such as **Coumadin**
Certain diuretics (water pills), including **Lasix**
Diabetes medications, including **DiaBeta**, **Diabinese**, **Micronase**, and **Glucotrol**
Diltiazem (**Cardizem**)
Dipyridamole (**Persantine**)
Seizure medications such as **Depakene**
Steroids such as prednisone (**Deltasone**, **Orasone**)

If you are taking a tranquilizer such as **Valium** or **Xanax**, or a sleep aid such as **Halcion** or **Seconal**, do not take this form of Alka-Seltzer Plus without your doctor's approval; the combination could cause extreme drowsiness. For the same reason, avoid alcohol while taking this product.

Brand name:

Alka-Seltzer Plus Sinus Medicine Tablets

Pronounced: AL-ka SELL-tser
Generic ingredients: Aspirin, Phenylpropanolamine bitartrate

What this drug is used for
All members of the Alka-Seltzer Plus family of products relieve cold and flu symptoms such as fever, headache, and body aches and pains.

(The tablets contain aspirin for this purpose; the liquigels use acetaminophen.) In addition, the Sinus Medicine contains an ingredient to unclog stuffy nose and sinuses.

How should you take this medication?

The usual dose for adults and children 12 years and over is 2 tablets dissolved in 4 ounces of water. Do not swallow Alka-Seltzer Plus Sinus tablets whole. Doses can be repeated every 4 hours if needed, to a maximum of 8 tablets each 24 hours. For children under 12, consult your doctor.

Do not take this medication if...

Do not take this product if you are allergic to aspirin, must avoid phenylalanine, or have to limit your intake of sodium. Unless your doctor approves, also avoid the product if you have bleeding problems, heart disease, high blood pressure, thyroid disease, diabetes, high pressure within the eye (glaucoma), an enlarged prostate gland, or a breathing problem such as asthma, emphysema, or chronic bronchitis.

Special warnings about this medication

The aspirin in this product has been known to trigger a serious illness called Reye's syndrome in children and teenagers who catch a virus. If your child gets chickenpox or flu, do not treat the symptoms with Alka-Seltzer Plus Sinus Tablets.

If you become dizzy or nervous, or have trouble sleeping, stop taking this product and check with your doctor.

Do not take this product for more than 7 days. If your symptoms do not improve or include a fever that lasts more than 3 days, call your doctor.

Do not take this product during the last 3 months of pregnancy. It could harm the baby or cause complications during delivery. Earlier during pregnancy, and while nursing a baby, check with your doctor before taking this variety of Alka-Seltzer Plus.

Possible food and drug interactions
when taking this medication

Do not use this product within 2 weeks of taking a drug classified as an MAO inhibitor, such as the antidepressants **Nardil** and **Parnate**.

Aspirin-containing products such as this can also interact with a number of other prescription drugs. Check with your doctor before combining this product with any of the following:

Acetazolamide (**Diamox**)
ACE-inhibitor-type blood pressure medications such as **Capoten**
Anti-gout drugs such as **Anturane, Benemid**, and **Zyloprim**
Arthritis preparations such as **Aleve, Anaprox, Ecotrin, Indocin,
Motrin, Naprosyn**, and **Orudis**
Blood-thinning drugs such as **Coumadin**
Certain diuretics (water pills), including **Lasix**
Diabetes medications, including **DiaBeta, Diabinese, Micronase,**
and **Glucotrol**
Diltiazem (**Cardizem**)
Dipyridamole (**Persantine**)
Seizure medications such as **Depakene**
Steroids such as prednisone (**Deltasone, Orasone**)

Brand name:

Allerest

Pronounced: AL-er-est
*Generic ingredients: Pseudoephedrine, Chlorpheniramine maleate
(Maximum Strength only), Acetaminophen (No Drowsiness only)*

What this drug is used for

Allerest is available in Maximum Strength and No Drowsiness formulations. Both provide temporary relief from stuffy nose and
clogged sinuses.

In addition, Maximum Strength Allerest relieves allergy and hay fever
symptoms such as runny nose, sneezing, itchy nose or throat, and
itchy, watery eyes.

No Drowsiness Allerest does not relieve these additional symptoms,
but does work against headache and minor aches and pains.

Maximum Strength Allerest comes in tablet form; the No Drowsiness
formulation comes as a caplet.

How should you take this medication?

■ ADULTS

For adults and children 12 years and over, the usual dose of either formulation is 2 pills every 4 to 6 hours. Do not take more than 8 pills
each 24 hours.

■ CHILDREN

For children 6 to 12 years of age, the usual dose is 1 pill every 4 to 6 hours, not to exceed 4 pills each 24 hours. For children under 6, consult a doctor.

■ STORAGE

Store Allerest at room temperature.

Do not take this medication if...

If you have heart disease, high blood pressure, thyroid disease, diabetes, or an enlarged prostate gland, do not take either form of Allerest unless your doctor approves. Avoid Maximum Strength Allerest if you have high pressure within the eye (glaucoma) or a breathing problem such as emphysema or chronic bronchitis.

Special warnings about this medication

With either form of Allerest, if you become nervous or dizzy, or have trouble sleeping, stop taking the product and call your doctor.

Maximum Strength Allerest: If symptoms do not improve within 7 days or you have a fever, call your doctor. This form of Allerest can make you drowsy, so be especially careful when driving or operating machinery. This form can also cause excitability, especially in children.

No Drowsiness Allerest: Do not take this form of Allerest for more than 10 days (for adults) or 5 days (for children). If symptoms don't improve or are accompanied by fever that lasts for more than 3 days, check with your doctor. Also call the doctor if any new symptoms develop.

Possible food and drug interactions
when taking this medication

Do not use either form of Allerest within 2 weeks of taking a drug classified as an MAO inhibitor, such as the antidepressants **Nardil** and **Parnate**.

Do not use Maximum Strength Allerest without your doctor's approval if you are taking a tranquilizer such as **Valium** or **Xanax**, or a sleep aid such as **Halcion** or **Seconal**; the combination could cause extreme drowsiness. For the same reason, avoid alcohol while taking this product.

Brand name:

ALternaGEL

Pronounced: all-TERN-uh-jel
Generic name: Aluminum hydroxide
Other brand name: Amphojel

What this drug is used for

These products relieve symptoms caused by excess stomach acid, including heartburn, upset stomach, sour stomach, and acid indigestion.

ALternaGEL is available only as a liquid. Amphojel is available in liquid or tablet form.

How should you take this medication?

Take doses between meals and at bedtime. Do not use the maximum dosage of either product for more than 2 weeks.

Shake liquids well before using. You may wish to follow liquid doses with a sip of water.

■ ALTERNAGEL

The usual dose is 1 or 2 teaspoonfuls. Do not take more than 18 teaspoonfuls in a 24-hour period.

■ AMPHOJEL

Liquid

The usual dosage is 2 teaspoonfuls 5 or 6 times a day. Do not take more than 12 teaspoonfuls in a 24-hour period.

Tablets

For the 0.3-gram tablets, the usual dose is 2 tablets 5 or 6 times a day. Swallow the tablets with water; it is not necessary to chew them. Do not take more than 12 tablets in a 24-hour period.

For the 0.6-gram tablets, the usual dose is 1 tablet 5 or 6 times a day. Chew the tablet and then sip about half a glass of water. Do not take more than 6 tablets in a 24-hour period.

■ STORAGE

These products may be stored at room temperature. Keep the bottle tightly closed. Protect liquid forms from freezing.

Special warnings about this medication

These products may cause constipation.

Possible food and drug interactions when taking this medication

Antacids interact with a variety of prescription drugs when taken at the same time. An interaction is unlikely, however, if you keep doses of the two at least 2 or 3 hours apart. Drugs that may interact include the following:

Alendronate (**Fosamax**)
Allopurinol (**Zyloprim**)
Antibiotics classified as quinolones, such as **Cipro**, **Floxin**, and **Noroxin**
Aspirin
Atenolol (**Tenormin**)
Captopril (**Capoten**)
Chlordiazepoxide (**Librium**)
Cimetidine (**Tagamet**)
Digoxin (**Lanoxin**)
Doxycycline (**Vibramycin**)
Fosfomycin (**Monurol**)
Gabapentin (**Neurontin**)
Glipizide (**Glucotrol**)
Glyburide (**Micronase**, **DiaBeta**)
Isoniazid (**Rifamate**)
Ketoconazole (**Nizoral**)
Levothyroxine (**Synthroid**)
Methenamine (**Urised**)
Metronidazole (**Flagyl**)
Misoprostol (**Cytotec**)
Mycophenolate mofetil (**CellCept**)
Nonsteroidal anti-inflammatory drugs such as **Dolobid**, **Motrin**, **Naprosyn**, and **Voltaren**
Penicillamine (**Cuprimine**)
Phenytoin (**Dilantin**)
Quinidine (**Quinidex**)
Sodium polystyrene sulfonate (**Kayexalate**)
Sucralfate (**Carafate**)
Tetracycline antibiotics such as **Achromycin V** and **Minocin**
Tilodronate (**Skelid**)
Ursodiol (**Actigall**)

A high-protein meal, such as a steak dinner, can reduce the effectiveness of aluminum-containing antacids such as ALternaGEL and Amphojel.

Overdosage

Heavy long-term use of aluminum antacids can lead to symptoms such as loss of appetite, a general feeling of uneasiness, muscle weakness, and bone pain. If you suspect an overdose, call your doctor immediately.

Brand name:

Amphojel

See ALternaGEL

Brand name:

Arco-Lase

Pronounced: AHR-koh-lais
Generic ingredients: Lipase, Trizyme

What this drug is used for

Arco-Lase is taken for symptoms of poor digestion such as gas, bloating, fullness, sour stomach, and heartburn.

How should you take this medication?

Take 1 tablet with or immediately after meals. The tablet may be swallowed or chewed.

Special warnings about this medication

With digestive enzymes as its active ingredients, Arco-Lase has no side effects.

Brand name:

Ascriptin

Pronounced: a-SKRIP-tin
Generic ingredients: Aspirin, Calcium carbonate, Maalox (Alumina-magnesia)

What this drug is used for

Ascriptin provides temporary relief from minor aches and pains, including headaches, muscle aches, toothaches, menstrual cramps, and arthritis pain. It can also be used to reduce fever and to combat the discomforts of the common cold.

The product comes in three varieties. Regular Strength and Arthritis Pain Ascriptin both contain 325 milligrams of aspirin. Maximum Strength Ascriptin contains 500 milligrams.

How should you take this medication?

Drink a full glass of water with each dose.

■ REGULAR STRENGTH AND ARTHRITIS PAIN ASCRIPTIN

For adults and children 12 years and over, the usual dose is 2 pills every 4 hours as needed. Do not take more than 12 pills each 24 hours. For children under 12, consult your doctor.

■ MAXIMUM STRENGTH ASCRIPTIN

For adults and children 12 years and over, the usual dose is 2 caplets every 6 hours as needed. Do not take more than 8 caplets in 24 hours. For children under 12, consult your doctor.

Do not take this medication if...

Unless your doctor approves, avoid Ascriptin if you are allergic to aspirin; have asthma, ulcers, or bleeding problems; or suffer from stomach problems—heartburn, upset stomach, or stomach pain—that continue a long time or that go away and come back.

Special warnings about this medication

The aspirin in Ascriptin has been known to trigger a serious illness called Reye's syndrome in children and teenagers who've come down with a virus. If your child gets chickenpox or flu, do not treat the symptoms with Ascriptin.

Do not take Ascriptin for more than 10 days for pain or 3 days for fever, unless your doctor recommends. Call your doctor if you develop new symptoms, your pain or fever continues or gets worse, or you notice redness or swelling.

Do not take Ascriptin during the last 3 months of pregnancy. It could harm the baby or cause complications during delivery. Earlier during pregnancy, and while nursing a baby, check with your doctor before taking Ascriptin.

If you develop ringing in the ears or loss of hearing, consult your doctor before taking any more Ascriptin.

Possible food and drug interactions when taking this medication

Aspirin-containing products such as Ascriptin can interact with a number of prescription drugs. Check with your doctor before combining with any of the following:

Acetazolamide (**Diamox**)
ACE-inhibitor-type blood pressure medications such as **Capoten**
Anti-gout drugs such as **Anturane**, **Benemid**, and **Zyloprim**
Arthritis preparations such as **Aleve**, **Anaprox**, **Ecotrin**, **Indocin**,
 Motrin, **Naprosyn**, and **Orudis**
Blood-thinning drugs such as **Coumadin**
Certain diuretics (water pills), including **Lasix**
Diabetes medications, including **DiaBeta**, **Diabinese**, **Micronase**,
 and **Glucotrol**
Diltiazem (**Cardizem**)
Dipyridamole (**Persantine**)
Seizure medications such as **Depakene**
Steroids such as prednisone (**Deltasone**, **Orasone**)

Also avoid combining Ascriptin with tetracycline antibiotics such as **Sumycin**.

Brand name:

Ascriptin Enteric

See Aspirin

Generic name:

Aspirin

Pronounced: ASS-pih-rin
Brand names: Ascriptin Enteric, Bayer, Ecotrin, Halfprin, St. Joseph

What this drug is used for

Aspirin relieves pain and reduces fever. It is used for headaches, toothaches, and the minor aches and pains of arthritis, colds, and flu. It can also be used for muscle aches, menstrual discomfort, and teething pain; and it is often prescribed for the long-term treatment of various forms of arthritis and related diseases.

For men, small daily doses of aspirin have proven effective in reducing the chances of mini-strokes (in which clogged blood vessels prevent sufficient oxygen from reaching the brain). Aspirin is also used to reduce the risk of heart attack in people with clogged coronary arteries, and in those who've already had an attack.

Aspirin comes in several strengths and varieties, including chewable tablets. Several brands have a special "enteric" coating to protect the stomachs of people who are sensitive to other forms of the medication. One brand has calcium to help strengthen bones.

How should you take this medication?

Do not chew or crush sustained-release brands, such as Bayer time-release aspirin, or pills coated to delay breakdown of the drug, such as Ecotrin. To make them easier to swallow, take them with a full glass of water. The usual dosages are as follows.

◼ ADULTS AND CHILDREN 12 YEARS AND OVER
Relief of minor pain and fever

◼ **Ascriptin Enteric Regular Strength:** 2 pills every 4 hours; no more than 12 pills a day

◼ **Ascriptin Enteric Low Strength:** 4 to 8 pills every 4 hours, no more than 48 pills a day

◼ **Genuine Bayer:** 1 or 2 pills every 4 hours; no more than 12 pills a day

◼ **Extra Strength Bayer:** 1 or 2 pills every 4 hours; no more than 8 pills a day

◼ **Extended Release Bayer:** 2 pills every 8 hours, no more than 6 pills a day

◼ **Aspirin Regimen Bayer (81-milligram tablets):** A maximum of 8 pills every 4 hours or 12 pills every 6 hours

◼ **Aspirin Regimen Bayer (325-milligram caplets):** A maximum of 2 pills every 4 hours or 3 pills every 6 hours

◼ **Aspirin Regimen Bayer with Calcium:** 4 to 8 pills every 4 hours; no more than 32 pills a day

◼ **Ecotrin:** Up to 650 milligrams every 4 hours, or 1,000 milligrams every 6 hours

◼ **St. Joseph Adult Chewable Aspirin:** Chew 4 to 8 pills every 4 hours; no more than 48 pills a day. Drink a full glass of water with each dose.

Treatment of arthritis
■ Extra Strength Bayer Arthritis Pain Regimen Formula: 2 caplets every 6 hours; no more than 8 caplets a day

Prevention of heart attack
The usual daily dosage ranges from one-half to one conventional 325-milligram aspirin tablet, one 162-milligram tablet, or two to four 81-milligram aspirin tablets. Your doctor may recommend a larger dose.

Prevention of mini-strokes (transient ischemic attacks)
The usual dose is 1 conventional 325-milligram tablet 4 times daily, or 2 tablets 2 times a day.

■ CHILDREN
All doses are for Bayer Children's Chewable Tablets, which may be chewed, swallowed, or dissolved on the tongue. (The tablets may also be crushed in a teaspoonful of water.) Doses may be given every 4 hours. Follow with half a glass of liquid. Do not give more than 5 doses a day.

11 to 12 years: 4 to 6 tablets
9 to 11 years: 4 to 5 tablets
6 to 9 years: 4 tablets
4 to 6 years: 3 tablets
2 to 4 years: 2 tablets
Under 2 years: Consult your doctor

For dosage of other brands in children under 12, check with your doctor.

■ STORAGE
Store at room temperature in a dry place. Keep container tightly closed. Protect from heat.

Do not take this medication if...
Unless your doctor approves, do not take aspirin if it has ever given you an allergic reaction, or if you have asthma, ulcers, bleeding problems, or stomach complaints—heartburn, upset stomach, or stomach pain—that fail to get better or keep coming back.

Special warnings about this medication
Aspirin has been known to trigger a serious illness called Reye's syndrome in children and teenagers who catch a virus. If your child gets chickenpox or flu, do not treat the symptoms with aspirin.

When taken for long periods, as it is for arthritis and prevention of mini-strokes and heart attacks, aspirin sometimes causes stomach problems, including pain, heartburn, nausea, vomiting, and bleeding. It can also cause ringing in the ears or a loss of hearing. If you notice any hearing changes, check with your doctor before taking any more aspirin.

Do not take aspirin for more than 10 days for pain or 3 days for fever, unless your doctor recommends. Call your doctor if you develop new symptoms, your pain or fever continues or gets worse, or you notice redness or swelling. (In children, do not use aspirin for pain relief for more than 5 days.)

Do not take aspirin during the last 3 months of pregnancy. It could harm the baby or cause complications during delivery. Earlier during pregnancy, and while nursing a baby, check with your doctor before taking aspirin.

Bayer Children's Chewable Tablets should not be given for arthritis pain without your doctor's approval. Also, wait at least 7 days after a tonsillectomy or oral surgery before giving the tablets. Check with your doctor immediately if the child has a severe sore throat that lasts for more than 2 days, or has a sore throat accompanied or followed by fever, headache, rash, nausea, or vomiting.

Possible food and drug interactions when taking this medication

Aspirin can interact with a number of prescription drugs. Check with your doctor before combining it with any of the following:

Acetazolamide (**Diamox**)
ACE-inhibitor-type blood pressure medications such as **Capoten**
Antacids such as **Rolaids, Tums**, and **Titrilac**
Anti-gout drugs such as **Anturane, Benemid**, and **Zyloprim**
Arthritis preparations such as **Aleve, Anaprox, Indocin, Motrin, Naprosyn**, and **Orudis**
Blood-thinning drugs such as **Coumadin**
Certain diuretics (water pills), including **Lasix**
Diabetes medications, including **DiaBeta, Diabinese, Micronase**, and **Glucotrol**
Diltiazem (**Cardizem**)
Dipyridamole (**Persantine**)
Seizure medications such as **Depakene**
Steroids such as prednisone (**Deltasone, Orasone**)

Brand name:

Axid AR

Pronounced: AK-sid
Generic name: Nizatidine

What this drug is used for

When taken before eating, Axid AR prevents heartburn, acid indigestion, and sour stomach caused by food and beverages.

Axid AR is part of a family of acid-blocking prescription drugs recently released in over-the-counter formulations. Others in the family are Mylanta AR, Pepcid AC, Tagamet HB, and Zantac 75.

How should you take this medication?

Swallow 1 tablet with water one-half to 1 hour before enjoying food or beverages that might cause you trouble. Take no more than 2 tablets a day.

■ STORAGE

Store at room temperature and protect from light. Keep the bottle tightly closed.

Do not take this medication if...

Not for children under 12, unless your doctor approves.

Special warnings about this medication

See your doctor promptly if you have trouble swallowing or develop stomach pain that won't go away. You might have a serious problem. Also check with your doctor if you find you need 2 tablets every day continuously for 2 weeks.

Possible food and drug interactions
when taking this medication

Unless your doctor approves, do not combine Axid AR with aspirin, especially in high doses.

Brand name:

Backache Caplets

See Doan's

Brand name:

Basaljel

Pronounced: BAY-zuhl-jel
Generic name: Basic aluminum carbonate

What this drug is used for

Basaljel relieves symptoms associated with the excess stomach acid that often accompanies an ulcer, stomach inflammation, inflammation of the food canal (the esophagus), or a weakened stomach diaphragm (a hiatal hernia).

Basaljel is available in liquid, capsule, and tablet form.

How should you take this medication?

The usual dose is 2 teaspoonfuls, capsules, or tablets. You may take Basaljel as often as every 2 hours and up to 12 times a day. Mix the liquid with water or fruit juice.

Special warnings about this medication

Do not use the maximum dosage of Basaljel for more than 2 weeks unless your doctor recommends it.

Basaljel may cause constipation. Be sure to drink plenty of liquid while you are taking it.

Possible food and drug interactions when taking this medication

Antacids interact with a variety of prescription drugs when taken at the same time. An interaction is unlikely, however, if you keep doses of the two at least 2 or 3 hours apart. Drugs that may interact include the following:

Alendronate (**Fosamax**)
Allopurinol (**Zyloprim**)
Antibiotics classified as quinolones, such as **Cipro**, **Floxin**, and
  Noroxin
Aspirin
Atenolol (**Tenormin**)
Captopril (**Capoten**)
Chlordiazepoxide (**Librium**)
Cimetidine (**Tagamet**)
Digoxin (**Lanoxin**)

Doxycycline (**Vibramycin**)

Fosfomycin (**Monurol**)

Gabapentin (**Neurontin**)

Glipizide (**Glucotrol**)

Glyburide (**Micronase, DiaBeta**)

Isoniazid (**Rifamate**)

Ketoconazole (**Nizoral**)

Levothyroxine (**Synthroid**)

Methenamine (**Urised**)

Metronidazole (**Flagyl**)

Misoprostol (**Cytotec**)

Mycophenolate mofetil (**CellCept**)

Nonsteroidal anti-inflammatory drugs such as **Dolobid, Motrin, Naprosyn,** and **Voltaren**

Penicillamine (**Cuprimine**)

Phenytoin (**Dilantin**)

Quinidine (**Quinidex**)

Sodium polystyrene sulfonate (**Kayexalate**)

Sucralfate (**Carafate**)

Tetracycline antibiotics such as **Achromycin V** and **Minocin**

Tilodronate (**Skelid**)

Ursodiol (**Actigall**)

A high-protein meal, such as a steak dinner, can reduce the effectiveness of aluminum-containing antacids such as Basaljel.

Overdosage

Heavy long-term use of aluminum antacids can lead to symptoms such as loss of appetite, a general feeling of uneasiness, muscle weakness, and bone pain. If you suspect an overdose, call your doctor immediately.

Brand name:

Bayer

See Aspirin

Brand name:

Bayer PM

Pronounced: BAY-er
Generic ingredients: Aspirin, Diphenhydramine hydrochloride

What this drug is used for

This product combines aspirin, for relief of headaches and other minor pains, with an antihistamine to help you sleep.

How should you take this medication?

The usual dose is 2 caplets with water at bedtime.

■ STORAGE

Store at room temperature.

Do not take this medication if...

Unless your doctor approves, do not take Bayer PM if you are allergic to aspirin, or if you have ulcers, bleeding problems, or stomach complaints—heartburn, upset stomach, or stomach pain—that fail to get better or keep coming back. Also avoid Bayer PM if you have high pressure within the eye (glaucoma), an enlarged prostate gland, or a breathing problem such as asthma, emphysema, or chronic bronchitis.

Not for children under 12.

Special warnings about this medication

The aspirin in Bayer PM has been known to trigger a serious illness called Reye's syndrome in children and teenagers who catch a virus. If your child gets chickenpox or flu, do not treat the symptoms with Bayer PM.

If you develop ringing in the ears or notice a loss of hearing, stop taking this product and call your doctor.

Do not take Bayer PM for more than 10 days for pain or 3 days for fever, unless your doctor recommends. Call your doctor if you develop new symptoms, your pain or fever continues or gets worse, or you notice any redness or swelling. These symptoms could signal a serious problem. Likewise, check with your doctor if your sleep problem lasts more than 2 weeks.

Do not take this product during the last 3 months of pregnancy. It could harm the baby or cause complications during delivery. Earlier during pregnancy, and while nursing a baby, check with your doctor before taking Bayer PM.

Possible food and drug interactions when taking this medication

Aspirin-containing products such as Bayer PM can interact with a number of prescription drugs. Check with your doctor before combining this product with any of the following:

Acetazolamide (**Diamox**)
ACE-inhibitor-type blood pressure medications such as **Capoten**
Anti-gout drugs such as **Anturane**, **Benemid**, and **Zyloprim**
Arthritis preparations such as **Aleve**, **Anaprox**, **Ecotrin**, **Indocin**, **Motrin**, **Naprosyn**, and **Orudis**
Blood-thinning drugs such as **Coumadin**
Certain diuretics (water pills), including **Lasix**
Diabetes medications, including **DiaBeta**, **Diabinese**, **Micronase**, and **Glucotrol**
Diltiazem (**Cardizem**)
Dipyridamole (**Persantine**)
Seizure medications such as **Depakene**
Steroids such as prednisone (**Deltasone**, **Orasone**)

Also, if you are taking a tranquilizer such as **Valium** or **Xanax**, or a sleep aid such as **Halcion** or **Seconal**, do not take Bayer PM without your doctor's approval; the antihistamine it contains can interact with such drugs and cause extreme drowsiness. For the same reason, avoid alcohol while taking this product.

Brand name:

BC Powder

Generic ingredients: Aspirin, Caffeine, Salicylamide

What this drug is used for

BC Powder comes in regular and arthritis strengths. Both provide temporary relief from minor arthritis pain, pain from inflamed nerves, and low back pain radiating down the leg (sciatica). They can also be used to relieve the muscle aches, fever, and discomfort of a cold, as well as the pain of tooth extraction. Regular strength BC powder is also recommended for headache and normal menstrual pain.

How should you take this medication?

For adults and children 12 years and over, the usual dose is 1 powder placed on your tongue and followed with a glass of water or other liquid. If you prefer, you may stir 1 powder into a glass of liquid. Take a dose every 3 to 4 hours, if needed. Do not take more than 4 powders in 24 hours. For children under 12, consult your doctor.

Do not take this medication if...

Avoid BC Powder if you are allergic to aspirin.

Special warnings about this medication

The aspirin in BC Powder has been known to trigger a serious illness called Reye's syndrome in children and teenagers who catch a virus. If your child gets chickenpox or flu, do not treat the symptoms with BC Powder.

If pain lasts more than 10 days or you notice redness, stop taking BC and call your doctor.

Do not take this product during the last 3 months of pregnancy. It could harm the baby or cause complications during delivery. Earlier during pregnancy, and while nursing a baby, check with your doctor before taking BC.

Possible food and drug interactions when taking this medication

Aspirin-containing products such as BC Powder can interact with a number of prescription drugs. Check with your doctor before combining BC with any of the following:

Acetazolamide (**Diamox**)
ACE-inhibitor-type blood pressure medications such as **Capoten**
Anti-gout drugs such as **Anturane**, **Benemid**, and **Zyloprim**
Arthritis preparations such as **Aleve**, **Anaprox**, **Ecotrin**, **Indocin**, **Motrin**, **Naprosyn**, and **Orudis**
Blood-thinning drugs such as **Coumadin**
Certain diuretics (water pills), including **Lasix**
Diabetes medications, including **DiaBeta**, **Diabinese**, **Micronase**, and **Glucotrol**
Diltiazem (**Cardizem**)
Dipyridamole (**Persantine**)
Seizure medications such as **Depakene**
Steroids such as prednisone (**Deltasone**, **Orasone**)

Brand name:

BC Sinus Cold Powders

Generic ingredients: Aspirin, Phenylpropanolamine hydrochloride,
  Chlorpheniramine maleate (Allergy Sinus Cold Powder only)

What this drug is used for

BC Sinus Cold Powder and Allergy Sinus Cold Powder both contain a
pain reliever and a decongestant for temporary relief of body aches,
fever, and stuffy nose. The Allergy Sinus Cold Powder also contains an
antihistamine for relief of sneezing, runny nose, and watery, itchy eyes.

How should you take this medication?

■ ADULTS

For adults and children 12 years and over, the usual dose is 1 powder
placed on your tongue and followed with a glass of water or other liquid. If you prefer, you may stir 1 powder into a glass of liquid. Take a
dose every 3 to 4 hours, if needed. Do not take more than 4 powders
in 24 hours.

■ CHILDREN

For children under 12, consult your doctor.

Do not take this medication if...

Avoid both types of BC Sinus Cold Powder if you are allergic to
aspirin. Unless your doctor approves, do not take either product if you
have asthma, emphysema, chronic lung disease, breathing problems,
heart disease, high blood pressure, thyroid disease, diabetes, high
pressure within the eye (glaucoma), or an enlarged prostate gland.

Special warnings about this medication

The aspirin in these products has been known to trigger a serious illness called Reye's syndrome in children and teenagers who catch a
virus. If your child gets chickenpox or flu, do not treat the symptoms
with either type of BC Sinus Cold Powder.

Do not take either product during the last 3 months of pregnancy. It
could harm the baby or cause complications during delivery. Earlier
during pregnancy, and while nursing a baby, check with your doctor
before taking either of these products.

Taking more than the recommended dose of these products could
make you nervous or dizzy, or interfere with your sleep.

The antihistamine in BC Allergy Sinus Cold Powder can cause
excitability, especially in children. It also tends to make some people

drowsy. When taking this type of BC, be especially careful when driving, and when operating machinery.

If symptoms do not improve within 7 days or new ones appear—or if you run a fever for more than 3 days—check with your doctor before using any more of either product.

Possible food and drug interactions when taking this medication

Do not use either of these products within 2 weeks of taking a drug classified as an MAO inhibitor, such as the antidepressants Nardil and Parnate. Check with your doctor before combining these products with a prescription blood pressure medicine.

Aspirin-containing products such as BC can interact with a number of additional prescription drugs. Check with your doctor before combining either of these products with any of the following:

Acetazolamide (**Diamox**)
ACE-inhibitor-type blood pressure medications such as **Capoten**
Anti-gout drugs such as **Anturane**, **Benemid**, and **Zyloprim**
Arthritis preparations such as **Aleve**, **Anaprox**, **Ecotrin**, **Indocin**, **Motrin**, **Naprosyn**, and **Orudis**
Blood-thinning drugs such as **Coumadin**
Certain diuretics (water pills), including **Lasix**
Diabetes medications, including **DiaBeta**, **Diabinese**, **Micronase**, and **Glucotrol**
Diltiazem (**Cardizem**)
Dipyridamole (**Persantine**)
Seizure medications such as **Depakene**
Steroids such as prednisone (**Deltasone**, **Orasone**)

Brand name:

Benadryl Allergy

Pronounced: BEH-na-drill
Generic name: Diphenhydramine hydrochloride

What this drug is used for

Benadryl Allergy temporarily relieves symptoms of hay fever such as itchy nose or throat, runny nose, sneezing, and itchy, watery eyes. It also can be used for the runny nose and sneezing that accompany the common cold.

Benadryl Allergy is available in a variety of forms, including tablets and capsules, dye-free softgels, chewable tablets, and regular and dye-free liquid.

How should you take this medication?

■ ADULTS AND CHILDREN 12 YEARS AND OLDER

Tablets, Capsules, and Softgels

The usual dosage is 1 or 2 pills every 4 to 6 hours. Do not take more than 12 pills each 24 hours.

Chewables

Chew 2 to 4 tablets every 4 to 6 hours. Do not take more than 24 tablets in 24 hours. Chew tablets thoroughly before swallowing.

Liquid

The usual dosage is 2 to 4 teaspoonfuls every 4 to 6 hours. Do not take more than 24 teaspoonfuls in 24 hours.

■ CHILDREN 6 TO 12 YEARS OF AGE

For children under 6, consult your doctor.

Tablets, Capsules, and Softgels

The usual dose is 1 pill every 4 to 6 hours. Do not give children this age more than 6 pills in 24 hours.

Chewables

Children should chew 1 or 2 tablets every 4 to 6 hours. They should not have more than 12 tablets in 24 hours.

Liquid

The usual dose is 1 or 2 teaspoonfuls every 4 to 6 hours, but not more than 12 teaspoonfuls in 24 hours.

■ STORAGE

Store at room temperature in a dry place. Protect chewables and softgels from heat. Protect liquids from freezing.

Do not take this medication if...

Unless your doctor approves, avoid this product if you have high pressure within the eye (glaucoma), an enlarged prostate gland, or a breathing problem such as emphysema or chronic bronchitis.

If you must avoid phenylalanine, do not use the chewable tablets.

Special warnings about this medication

This product may make you drowsy. Be especially careful when driving or operating machinery. Benadryl Allergy can also cause excitability in some people, especially in children.

**Possible food and drug interactions
when taking this medication**

Do not take Benadryl Allergy if you are using any other products containing the active ingredient diphenhydramine, including **Actifed Allergy** or **Sinus, Tylenol Flu NightTime, PM,** or **Severe Allergy Medication,** and **Unisom with Pain Relief.**

If you are taking a tranquilizer such as **Valium** or **Xanax,** or a sleep aid such as **Halcion** or **Seconal,** do not take Benadryl Allergy without your doctor's approval; the combination could cause extreme drowsiness. For the same reason, avoid alcohol while taking this product.

Brand name:

Benadryl Allergy Decongestant

Pronounced: BEH-na-drill
*Generic ingredients: Diphenhydramine hydrochloride, Pseudo-
    ephedrine hydrochloride*

What this drug is used for

Like other Benadryl products, Benadryl Allergy Decongestant temporarily relieves symptoms of hay fever such as itchy nose or throat, runny nose, sneezing, and itchy, watery eyes. It also can be used for the runny nose and sneezing that accompany the common cold.

In addition, Benadryl Allergy Decongestant contains an extra ingredient, pseudoephedrine, that relieves stuffy nose.

This product is available in tablet and liquid form

How should you take this medication?

■ ADULTS

For adults and children 12 years and older, the usual dosage is 1 tablet or 2 teaspoonfuls every 4 to 6 hours. Do not take more than 4 tablets or 8 teaspoonfuls each 24 hours.

■ CHILDREN

For children 6 to 12, the usual dosage is 1 teaspoonful of liquid every 4 to 6 hours. Do not give children more than 4 teaspoonfuls in 24 hours.

Consult your doctor before giving the tablets to children under 12 and the liquid to children under 6.

■ STORAGE

Store at room temperature. Protect tablets from moisture. Protect liquid from freezing.

Do not take this medication if...

Unless your doctor approves, avoid this product if you have diabetes, an enlarged prostate gland, high pressure within the eye (glaucoma), heart disease, high blood pressure, thyroid disease, or a breathing problem such as emphysema or chronic bronchitis.

Special warnings about this medication

This product may make you drowsy. Be especially careful when driving or operating machinery.

Benadryl Allergy Decongestant can also cause excitability in some people, especially in children. If you become nervous or dizzy, or if you have trouble sleeping, stop taking this product and call your doctor.

If you do not feel better in 7 days, or if you develop a fever, check with your doctor.

Possible food and drug interactions when taking this medication

Do not take Benadryl Allergy Decongestant if you are using any other products containing the active ingredient diphenhydramine, including **Actifed Allergy** or **Sinus**, **Tylenol Flu NightTime**, **PM**, or **Severe Allergy Medication**, and **Unisom with Pain Relief**.

In addition, do not use Benadryl Allergy Decongestant within 2 weeks of taking a drug classified as an MAO inhibitor, such as the antidepressants **Nardil** and **Parnate**.

If you are taking a tranquilizer such as **Valium** or **Xanax**, or a sleep aid such as **Halcion** or **Seconal**, do not take Benadryl Allergy Decongestant without your doctor's approval; the combination could cause extreme drowsiness. For the same reason, avoid alcohol while taking this product.

Brand name:

Benadryl Allergy Sinus and Cold Products

Pronounced: BEH-na-drill
Generic ingredients: Acetaminophen, Diphenhydramine hydrochloride, Pseudoephedrine hydrochloride

What this drug is used for

Two Benadryl products—Benadryl Allergy/Cold Tablets and Benadryl Allergy Sinus Headache Caplets—share the same ingredients. The acetaminophen in these products relieves symptoms such as minor aches and pains, muscle aches, headache, sore throat, and fever. Diphenhydramine relieves runny nose and sneezing, itchy nose or throat, and itchy, watery eyes. Pseudoephedrine helps unclog stuffy nose and sinuses.

How should you take this medication?

For adults and children 12 years and older, the usual dosage is 2 pills every 6 hours until you feel better. Do not take more than 8 pills each 24 hours. For children under 12, consult your doctor.

■ STORAGE
Store at room temperature. Protect from moisture.

Do not take this medication if...

Unless your doctor approves, avoid these products if you have heart disease, high blood pressure, thyroid disease, diabetes, high pressure within the eye (glaucoma), an enlarged prostate gland, or a breathing problem such as emphysema or chronic bronchitis.

Special warnings about this medication

If you become nervous or dizzy, or have trouble sleeping, stop taking this medication and call your doctor.

Do not take either of these products for more than 10 days. Check with your doctor if:

■ You develop a sore throat that is severe, lasts more than 2 days, or is accompanied by fever, headache, rash, nausea, or vomiting

■ Your symptoms do not improve, or you have a fever for more than 3 days
■ You develop new symptoms

These products may make you drowsy. Be especially careful when driving or operating machinery. They can also cause excitability in some people, especially in children.

Possible food and drug interactions when taking this medication

Do not take Benadryl Allergy Sinus and Cold products if you are using any other medications containing the active ingredient diphenhydramine, including **Actifed Allergy** or **Sinus**, **Tylenol Flu NightTime**, **PM**, or **Severe Allergy Medication**, and **Unisom with Pain Relief**.

In addition, do not use these products within 2 weeks of taking a drug classified as an MAO inhibitor, such as the antidepressants **Nardil** and **Parnate**.

If you are taking a tranquilizer such as **Valium** or **Xanax**, or a sleep aid such as **Halcion** or **Seconal**, do not take these products without your doctor's approval; the combination could cause extreme drowsiness. For the same reason, avoid alcohol while using either of these products.

Brand name:

Benylin Adult Formula Cough Suppressant

Pronounced: BEN-uh-lin
Generic name: Dextromethorphan
Other brand names: Delsym Cough Formula, Diabe-Tuss DM, Pertussin DM, Robitussin Cough Suppressant, Vicks 44 Cough Relief

What this drug is used for

All these dextromethorphan-based liquids—typically labeled "adult formula," "extra strength," or "maximum strength"—contain a relatively high dose of the active ingredient. They provide temporary relief of cough due to sore throat or irritated bronchial tubes, as brought on by the common cold.

Many of these products are also available in a weaker strength, usually labeled "pediatric" or "children's strength" (see *Benylin Pediatric*

Cough Suppressant). Dextromethorphan is also available in lozenge form (see *Sucrets 4 Hour Cough Suppressant*).

How should you take this medication?

These medications may be taken every 6 to 8 hours, up to a maximum of 4 doses each 24 hours (every 12 hours for Delsym, with a 2-dose daily maximum).

■ ADULTS

For adults and children 12 years and over, the usual dose is 2 teaspoonfuls (3 teaspoonfuls for Vicks 44).

■ CHILDREN

Age 6 to 12

The usual dose is 1 teaspoonful (1½ teaspoonfuls for Vicks 44).

Age 2 to 6

The usual dose is half a teaspoonful (for Pertussin DM and Vicks 44, consult your doctor).

Less than 2

Consult your doctor.

■ STORAGE

Store at room temperature.

Do not take this medication if...

Unless your doctor tells you otherwise, do not use these products for cough due to smoking, asthma, or emphysema, or for coughs that bring up a lot of phlegm.

Special warnings about this medication

A persistent cough may be a sign of a serious illness. If you have a cough that lasts for more than 1 week, goes away and comes back, or is accompanied by a fever, rash, or long-lasting headache, call your doctor.

Possible food and drug interactions
when taking this medication

Do not use any of these products within 2 weeks of taking a drug classified as an MAO inhibitor, including the antidepressants **Nardil** and **Parnate**.

Brand name:

Benylin Cough Suppressant Expectorant

Pronounced: BEN-uh-lin
Generic ingredients: Dextromethorphan hydrobromide, Guaifenesin

What this drug is used for

Benylin Cough Suppressant Expectorant temporarily relieves cough due to the minor throat and bronchial irritation that occurs with the common cold. It also helps loosen and thin mucus, making it easier to bring up with a cough.

This product comes as a liquid.

How should you take this medication?

You may take a dose every 4 hours. Do not take more than 6 doses each 24 hours.

■ ADULTS

For adults and children 12 years and over, the usual dose is 4 teaspoonfuls.

■ CHILDREN

Age 6 to 12 years
The usual dose is 2 teaspoonfuls.

Age 2 to 6 years
The usual dose is 1 teaspoonful.

Under age 2
Consult a doctor.

■ STORAGE

Store at room temperature.

Do not take this medication if...

Do not use this product for a chronic cough due to smoking, asthma, chronic bronchitis, or emphysema, or for a cough that produces excessive phlegm, unless your doctor advises it.

Special warnings about this medication

Check with your doctor if a cough lasts more than 1 week, tends to come back, or is accompanied by a fever, rash, or persistent headache. A lingering cough could signal a serious condition.

Possible food or drug interactions
when taking this medication

Do not use Benylin Cough Suppressant Expectorant within 2 weeks of taking a drug classified as an MAO inhibitor, such as the antidepressants **Nardil** and **Parnate**.

Brand name:

Benylin Multisymptom

Pronounced: BEN-uh-lin
Generic ingredients: Dextromethorphan hydrobromide, Guaifenesin,
  Pseudoephedrine hydrochloride

What this drug is used for

Benylin Multisymptom relieves cough due to minor throat and bronchial irritation. It also helps loosen and thin phlegm, making it easier to cough up, and relieves stuffy nose due to the common cold.

This product comes in liquid form.

How should you take this medication?

Benylin Multisymptom can be taken every 4 hours. Do not take more than 4 doses each 24 hours.

■ ADULTS

For adults and children 12 years and over, the usual dose is 4 teaspoonfuls.

■ CHILDREN

Age 6 to 12
The usual dose is 2 teaspoonfuls.

Age 2 to 6
The usual dose is 1 teaspoonful.

Under age 2
Consult a doctor.

■ STORAGE

Store at room temperature.

Do not take this medication if...

Unless your doctor approves, do not take this product if you have heart disease, high blood pressure, thyroid disease, diabetes, or an enlarged prostate gland.

Do not use Benylin Multisymptom for a chronic cough due to smoking, asthma, chronic bronchitis, or emphysema, or for a cough that produces excessive phlegm, unless your doctor advises it.

Special warnings about this medication

If you become dizzy or nervous, or have trouble sleeping, stop taking this product and check with your doctor.

If symptoms do not improve within 7 days or you have a fever, call your doctor. Also check with your doctor if a cough lasts more than 1 week, tends to come back, or is accompanied by a fever, rash, or persistent headache. A lingering cough could signal a serious condition.

Possible food and drug interactions when taking this medication

Do not use Benylin Multisymptom within 2 weeks of taking a drug classified as an MAO inhibitor, such as the antidepressants **Nardil** and **Parnate**.

Brand name:

Benylin Pediatric Cough Suppressant

Pronounced: BEN-uh-lin
Generic name: Dextromethorphan
Other brand names: Pertussin CS, Robitussin Pediatric Cough Suppressant

What this drug is used for

These pediatric and CS (children's strength) liquids contain less of the active ingredient dextromethorphan than do the adult-, extra-, and maximum-strength formulations (see *Benylin Adult Formula Cough Suppressant*). All dextromethorphan products provide temporary relief of cough due to sore throat or irritated bronchial tubes, as brought on by the common cold.

Dextromethorphan is also available in lozenge form (see *Sucrets 4 Hour Cough Suppressant*).

How should you take this medication?

These products may be given every 6 to 8 hours, up to a maximum of 4 doses each 24 hours (every 4 hours for Pertussin CS, with a 6-dose maximum).

■ ADULTS

For adults and children 12 years and over, the usual dose is 4 teaspoonfuls.

■ CHILDREN

Age 6 to 12

The usual dose is 2 teaspoonfuls.

Age 2 to 6

The usual dose is 1 teaspoonful.

Under 2 years

Consult your doctor.

■ STORAGE

Store at room temperature.

Do not take this medication if...

Unless your doctor tells you otherwise, do not use these products for cough due to smoking, asthma, or emphysema, or for coughs that bring up a lot of phlegm. Avoid them if they've ever given you an allergic reaction.

Special warnings about this medication

A persistent cough may be a sign of a serious illness. If a cough lasts for more than 1 week, goes away and comes back, or is accompanied by a fever, rash, or long-lasting headache, call your doctor.

Possible food and drug interactions
when taking this medication

Do not use any of these products within 2 weeks of taking a drug classified as an MAO inhibitor, including the antidepressants **Nardil** and **Parnate**.

Brand name:

Benzedrex

Pronounced: BEN-zuh-drex
Generic name: Propylhexedrine

What this drug is used for

Benzedrex temporarily relieves stuffy nose caused by the common cold, hay fever, or sinusitis (swelling and pain in the sinuses). The product comes in an inhaler.

How should you take this medication?

For adults and children 6 years and over, the usual dose is 2 sprays in each nostril every 2 hours, as needed. Do not take more often. For children under 6, seek your doctor's advice.

▮ STORAGE

Benzedrex may be stored at room temperature. Keep the inhaler tightly closed between uses. The medication will stay good for at least 3 months after it is first opened.

Special warnings about this medication

Do not use this product for more than 3 days. If you take Benzedrex too often or use it for longer than the recommended time, your stuffy nose may come back or get worse. If your clogged nose does not improve, call your doctor.

Benzedrex may cause temporary discomfort such as a burning sensation, runny nose, sneezing, or stinging.

Do not share your Benzedrex inhaler with anyone. It could spread infection.

Brand name:

Bonine

Pronounced: BOW-neen
Generic name: Meclizine hydrochloride
Other brand name: Dramamine II

What this drug is used for

Bonine and Dramamine II prevent the dizziness, nausea, and vomiting that accompany motion sickness.

How should you take this medication?

To prevent motion sickness, take 1 or 2 tablets 1 hour before travel starts. Do not take more than 2 tablets in 24 hours. After that, you may take 1 or 2 tablets every 24 hours while traveling.

Chew the tablet and, if you choose, follow with water; or swallow the tablet whole with water.

Do not take this medication if...

Unless your doctor approves, avoid these products if you have a breathing problem such as chronic bronchitis or emphysema, an enlarged prostate gland, or high pressure within the eye (glaucoma).

Do not give this medication to children under 12; it has not been tested in this age group.

Special warnings about this medication

These products can make you drowsy. Do not drive or operate machinery while taking either of them. Other possible side effects are blurry vision and a dry mouth. For use only when traveling.

Possible food and drug interactions
when taking this medication

If you are taking a tranquilizer such as **Valium** or **Xanax**, or a sleep aid such as **Halcion** or **Seconal**, do not take either of these products without your doctor's approval; the combination could cause extreme drowsiness. For the same reason, avoid alcohol.

Brand name:

Bufferin

Pronounced: BUF-fer-in
Generic ingredients: Aspirin, Calcium Carbonate, Magnesium carbonate, Magnesium oxide

What this drug is used for

Both Bufferin and Extra Strength Bufferin provide fast, temporary relief of:

Headaches
Minor arthritis pain and inflammation
Muscle aches

Pain and fever of colds
Menstrual pain
Toothaches

Bufferin is also used to lower the risk of both mini-strokes (TIAs) and full-blown strokes in men who have had previous TIAs resulting from the partial blockage of an artery by cholesterol buildup or by a blood clot.

Aspirin, the main ingredient in Bufferin, has been proven to reduce the risk of both mild and serious heart attacks in people who have had previous heart attacks or who suffer from angina (chest pain that occurs when clogged arteries prevent the heart muscle from getting enough oxygen).

Arthritis Strength Bufferin, which contains the same amount of aspirin as Extra Strength Bufferin, is sold for the temporary relief of minor aches and pain, stiffness, swelling, redness, and heat in arthritic joints.

How should you take this medication?
Dosages are for adults and children 12 years and older. For children under 12, consult your doctor.

■ REGULAR STRENGTH BUFFERIN
For Relief of Aches, Pain, and Fever
The usual dose is 2 tablets with water every 4 hours while you still have symptoms. Do not take more than 12 tablets in 24 hours unless your doctor approves.

To Prevent Recurrent TIA's
For men, the usual dosage is 2 tablets twice a day or 1 tablet 4 times a day.

To Reduce the Risk of Heart Attacks
The recommended daily dosage is 300 to 325 milligrams (1 tablet).

■ EXTRA STRENGTH AND ARTHRITIS STRENGTH BUFFERIN
Swallow 2 pills with water every 6 hours while your symptoms last. Do not take more than 8 pills in 24 hours unless your doctor tells you to.

■ STORAGE
Store at room temperature.

Do not take this medication if...
Unless your doctor approves, do not use Bufferin if you are allergic to aspirin, or if you have asthma, ulcers or bleeding problems, or stom-

ach problems—heartburn, upset stomach, or stomach pain—that do not get better or that go away and come back again.

Special warnings about this medication

The aspirin in Bufferin has been known to trigger a serious illness called Reye's syndrome in children and teenagers who catch a virus. If your child gets chickenpox or flu, do not treat the symptoms with Bufferin.

Do not take Bufferin for more than 10 days for pain or 3 days for fever, unless your doctor recommends. Call your doctor if you develop new symptoms, your pain or fever continues or gets worse, or you have redness or swelling.

Do not take Bufferin during the last 3 months of pregnancy. It could harm the baby or cause complications during delivery. Earlier during pregnancy, and while nursing a baby, check with your doctor before taking Bufferin.

If you develop ringing in the ears or loss of hearing, consult your doctor before taking any more of this product.

High doses of aspirin—about 3 regular-strength or 2 extra-strength tablets a day—occasionally cause side effects such as heartburn, stomach pain, stomach and intestinal bleeding, nausea, vomiting, and a small increase in blood pressure.

Possible food and drug interactions
when taking this medication

Check with your doctor before combining Bufferin with any of the following:

Acetazolamide (**Diamox**)
ACE-inhibitor-type blood pressure medications such as **Capoten**
Anti-gout drugs such as **Anturane, Benemid**, and **Zyloprim**
Arthritis preparations such as **Aleve, Anaprox, Ecotrin, Indocin, Motrin, Naprosyn**, and **Orudis**
Blood-thinning drugs such as **Coumadin**
Certain diuretics (water pills), including **Lasix**
Diabetes medications, including **DiaBeta, Diabinese, Glucotrol,** and **Micronase**
Diltiazem (**Cardizem**)
Dipyridamole (**Persantine**)
Seizure medications such as **Depakene**
Steroids such as prednisone (**Deltasone, Orasone**)

Brand name:

Cepacol Sore Throat Lozenges

See Halls Cough Suppressant

Brand name:

Cepacol Sore Throat Spray

See Sucrets

Brand name:

Cepastat

Pronounced: SEE-puh-stat
Generic name: Phenol
Other brand name: Vicks Chloraseptic Sore Throat Spray

What this drug is used for

Cepastat and Vicks Chloraseptic Sore Throat Spray provide temporary relief from minor irritation and pain in the mouth and throat. Cepastat is available in regular-strength cherry-flavor and extra-strength lozenges. Vicks Chloraseptic is a liquid spray.

How should you take this medication?

■ CEPASTAT LOZENGES

The usual dosage for adults and children 6 years and over is 1 lozenge every 2 hours. Allow the lozenge to dissolve slowly in the mouth. For children 6 to 12, the maximum dosage is 20 cherry-flavor or 10 extra-strength lozenges per day. For children under 6, consult your doctor.

■ CHLORASEPTIC SORE THROAT SPRAY
Adults and children 12 years and over
The usual dosage is 5 sprays directly into the throat or other painful area every 2 hours.

Children 2 to 11 years
The usual dosage is 3 sprays every 2 hours. Have the child swallow.

Children under 2
Consult your doctor.

■ STORAGE

Store lozenges at room temperature, and protect from humidity.

Special warnings about this medication

Check with your doctor immediately if you have a severe sore throat that lasts for more than 2 days or is accompanied by difficult breathing, or if your sore throat is accompanied or followed by fever, headache, rash, nausea, or vomiting.

Likewise, see your doctor or dentist if a sore mouth does not improve in 7 days; or if the irritation, pain, or redness gets worse.

If you have diabetes, remember that each Cepastat lozenge contains approximately 2 grams of sugar.

Brand name:

Cerose DM

Pronounced: se-ROHS
Generic ingredients: Chlorpheniramine maleate, Dextromethorphan
  hydrobromide, Phenylephrine hydrochloride

What this drug is used for

Cerose DM temporarily relieves coughing caused by a cold or irritants that reach your throat and bronchial tubes. It is also useful for the stuffy, runny nose and sneezing that accompany colds, hay fever, and other allergies.

How should you take this medication?

Do not take more than 6 doses in 24 hours.

■ ADULTS

For adults and children 12 and older, the usual dosage is 1 teaspoonful every 4 hours as needed.

■ CHILDREN

For children 6 to 12, the usual dosage is half a teaspoonful every 4 hours as needed. For children under 6, consult your doctor.

■ STORAGE

Keep tightly closed. May be stored at room temperature.

Do not take this medication if...

Unless your doctor approves, avoid Cerose DM if you have a breathing problem such as emphysema or chronic bronchitis, diabetes, high pressure within the eye (glaucoma), heart disease, high blood pressure, an enlarged prostate gland, or thyroid disease.

Also check with your doctor before using Cerose DM for the type of chronic cough that results from smoking or asthma, or for a cough that brings up lots of phlegm.

Special warnings about this medication

If you become nervous or dizzy, or if you have trouble sleeping while taking this product, stop using it and contact your doctor.

Cerose DM can make you very drowsy. Be especially careful when driving, and when operating machinery. Be aware that Cerose DM may also cause overexcitement—especially in children.

If coughing or other symptoms last more than 1 week without getting better, or they tend to come back, check with your doctor. Also call your doctor if you develop a fever, a rash, or a headache that doesn't improve.

**Possible food and drug interactions
when taking this medication**

Do not use Cerose DM within 2 weeks of taking a drug classified as an MAO inhibitor, including the antidepressants **Nardil** and **Parnate**.

If you are taking a tranquilizer such as **Valium** or **Xanax**, or a sleep aid such as **Halcion** or **Seconal**, do not take Cerose DM without your doctor's approval; the combination could cause extreme drowsiness. For the same reason, avoid alcohol while taking this product.

Brand name:

Cheracol D

Pronounced: CHAIR-uh-call
Generic ingredients: Dextromethorphan hydrobromide, Guaifenesin

What this drug is used for

Cheracol D liquid helps quiet dry, hacking coughs and helps loosen phlegm.

How should you take this medication?

■ ADULTS

For adults and children 12 and over, the usual dose is 2 teaspoonfuls every 4 hours. Do not take more than 12 teaspoonfuls in 24 hours.

■ CHILDREN

For children 6 to 12, the usual dosage is 1 teaspoonful every 4 hours. Do not give children this age more than 6 teaspoonfuls in 24 hours. For children under 6, consult a doctor.

Do not take this medication if...

Unless your doctor approves, do not use Cheracol D for the type of chronic cough that results from smoking, asthma, or emphysema, or for a cough that brings up lots of phlegm.

Special warnings about this medication

If your cough lasts more than 1 week without getting better, or goes away and comes back, check with your doctor. Also call your doctor if you develop a high fever, a rash, or a headache that doesn't improve.

Possible food and drug interactions
when taking this medication

Do not use Cheracol D within 2 weeks of taking a drug classified as an MAO inhibitor, including the antidepressants **Nardil** and **Parnate**.

Brand name:

Cheracol Plus

Pronounced: CHAIR-uh-call
Generic ingredients: Chlorpheniramine maleate, Dextromethorphan
*   hydrobromide, Phenylpropanolamine hydrochloride*

What this drug is used for

Cheracol Plus temporarily stops a cough and clears up head-cold symptoms such as congestion and a runny nose.

How should you take this medication?

The usual dosage is 1 tablespoonful every 4 hours. Do not take more than 6 tablespoonfuls in 24 hours.

Do not take this medication if...

Unless your doctor approves, avoid Cheracol Plus if you have high blood pressure, asthma, diabetes, high pressure within the eye (glaucoma), heart disease, an enlarged prostate gland, or thyroid disease.

If you cough a great deal because of smoking, asthma, or emphysema, or if you bring up a great deal of mucus when you cough, do not take this product without your doctor's approval.

Do not give this product to children under 12.

Special warnings about this medication

If coughing or other symptoms last more than 7 days without getting better, or if you develop a high fever, stop taking this product and call your doctor.

Be aware that Cheracol Plus may cause overexcitement, especially in children.

This product can make you drowsy. While taking it, avoid driving or operating machinery.

Possible food and drug interactions when taking this medication

Do not use this product within 2 weeks of taking a drug classified as an MAO inhibitor, including the antidepressants **Nardil** and **Parnate**.

Because both can make you drowsy, avoid alcoholic beverages while taking Cheracol Plus.

Brand name:

Children's Mylanta

See Tums

Brand name:

Chlor-Trimeton Allergy

Pronounced: klor-TRI-muh-ton
Generic name: Chlorpheniramine maleate

What this drug is used for

Chlor-Trimeton Allergy tablets contain an antihistamine that temporarily relieves the sneezing, runny nose, itchy throat, and itchy, watery eyes caused by allergies such as hay fever.

The tablets come in 4-, 8-, and 12-hour formulations.

How should you take this medication?

■ 4-HOUR TABLETS

Adults

The usual dose for adults and children 12 years and over is 1 tablet every 4 to 6 hours. Do not take more than 6 tablets each 24 hours.

Children

For children 6 to 12, break a tablet in half and give half a tablet every 4 to 6 hours. Do not give more than 3 whole tablets in 24 hours. For children under 6, consult your doctor.

■ 8-HOUR TABLETS

The usual dose for adults and children 12 years and over is 1 tablet every 8 to 12 hours. Allow at least 8 hours between doses, and do not take more than 3 tablets each 24 hours. For children under 12, consult your doctor.

■ 12-HOUR TABLETS

The usual dose for adults and children 12 years and over is 1 tablet every 12 hours. Do not take more than 2 tablets each 24 hours. For children under 12, consult your doctor.

■ STORAGE

Store at room temperature. Protect from too much moisture.

Do not take this medication if...

Unless your doctor approves, avoid Chlor-Trimeton Allergy tablets if you have high pressure within the eye (glaucoma), an enlarged prostate gland, or a breathing problem such as emphysema or chronic bronchitis.

Special warnings about this medication

The antihistamine in this product can make you drowsy. Be especially careful when driving, and when operating machinery. It can also cause excitability, especially in children.

Possible food and drug interactions
when taking this medication

If you are taking a tranquilizer such as **Valium** or **Xanax**, or a sleep aid such as **Halcion** or **Seconal**, do not take Chlor-Trimeton Allergy tablets without your doctor's approval; the combination could cause extreme drowsiness. For the same reason, avoid alcohol while taking this product.

Brand name:

Chlor-Trimeton Allergy/Decongestant

Pronounced: klor-TRI-muh-ton
Generic ingredients: Chlorpheniramine maleate, Pseudoephedrine sulfate

What this drug is used for

Like regular Chlor-Trimeton Allergy tablets, these tablets temporarily relieve the sneezing, itchy and watery eyes, itchy throat, and runny nose caused by allergies such as hay fever. In addition, they contain an ingredient to unclog stuffy nose and sinuses.

The tablets come in 4-hour and 12-hour formulations. The 12-hour tablets are twice the strength of the 4-hour variety.

How should you take this medication?

■ 4-HOUR ALLERGY/DECONGESTANT TABLETS
Adults
The usual dose for adults and children 12 and over is 1 tablet every 4 to 6 hours. Do not take more than 4 tablets in 24 hours.

Children
For children 6 to 12, break a tablet in half and give half a tablet every 4 to 6 hours. Do not give more than 2 whole tablets in 24 hours. For children under 6, consult your doctor.

■ 12-HOUR ALLERGY/DECONGESTANT TABLETS
Adults
The usual dose for adults and children 12 and over is 1 tablet every 12 hours. Do not take more than 2 tablets in 24 hours.

Children
Do not give to children under 12 unless your doctor approves.

■ STORAGE
Store at room temperature. Protect from too much moisture.

Do not take this medication if...

Unless your doctor approves, avoid Chlor-Trimeton Allergy/Decongestant if you have a breathing problem such as emphysema or chronic bronchitis, high pressure within the eye (glaucoma), heart disease, high blood pressure, thyroid disease, diabetes, or an enlarged prostate gland.

Special warnings about this medication

If you become nervous or dizzy, or if you have trouble sleeping while taking this product, stop using it and call your doctor.

If you do not feel better in 7 days, or if you develop a fever, contact your doctor.

Be aware that Chlor-Trimeton Allergy/Decongestant may cause over-excitement—especially in children.

Because Chlor-Trimeton Allergy/Decongestant can make you drowsy, be especially careful when driving or operating machinery while taking this product.

**Possible food and drug interactions
when taking this medication**

Do not use Chlor-Trimeton Allergy/Decongestant within 2 weeks of taking a drug classified as an MAO inhibitor, including the antidepressants **Nardil** and **Parnate**.

If you are taking a tranquilizer such as **Valium** or **Xanax**, or a sleep aid such as **Halcion** or **Seconal**, do not take Chlor-Trimeton Allergy/Decongestant without your doctor's approval; the combination could cause extreme drowsiness. For the same reason, avoid alcohol while taking this product.

Brand name:

Citrucel

Pronounced: SIT-ruh-sel
Generic name: Methylcellulose
Other brand name: Unifiber (cellulose)

What this drug is used for

Citrucel and Unifiber provide additional fiber (bulk) to the diet, thus relieving constipation.

They can be used for constipation associated with irritable bowel syndrome, diverticular disease (a pouch in the wall of the bowel), and hemorrhoids. They will also help keep bowel movements regular after surgery or delivery, and during convalescence.

Citrucel comes in regular and sugar-free forms, and is available in bulk containers and single-dose packets. Unifiber is available only in containers.

How should you take this medication?
■ CITRUCEL

Mix each dose of Citrucel with *at least* 8 ounces of cold water or other liquid. Another 8 ounces of liquid is strongly recommended. It takes 12 to 72 hours for full results to be felt.

Adults

The usual dose is 1 rounded tablespoonful up to 3 times daily.

Children 6 to 12

The usual dose is half a tablespoonful once a day.

Children under 6

Consult a doctor.

■ UNIFIBER

The usual dose is 1 or 2 tablespoonfuls once or twice a day. Unifiber should be mixed with a glass of liquid or a soft food such as mashed potatoes, applesauce, or pudding. Full results won't be felt for 7 to 10 days.

■ STORAGE

Store at room temperature in a tightly closed container. Keep dry.

Do not take this medication if...

Avoid both these products if you have an intestinal blockage or a fecal impaction. Do not take Citrucel if you have any trouble swallowing, or the product gives you an allergic reaction.

Unless your doctor approves, do not use either of these products if you have nausea, vomiting, or abdominal pain, or if you've noticed a sudden change in bowel habits lasting 2 weeks or more.

Special warnings about this medication

Always take Citrucel with plenty of fluid. Otherwise, it could swell, block your throat, and make you choke.

If you develop chest pain, have trouble swallowing or breathing, or start vomiting after a dose of Citrucel, call your doctor immediately.

If you notice rectal bleeding or fail to have a bowel movement after taking one of these products, stop using it and call your doctor.

Do not take Citrucel for more than 1 week without your doctor's approval. If you must avoid phenylalanine, do not use Sugar-free Citrucel.

Brand name:

Colace

Pronounced: KO-lase
Generic ingredient: Docusate
Other brand names: Correctol Stool Softener, Dialose, Ex-Lax Stool Softener, Fleet Sof-Lax, Surfak

What this drug is used for

All these products soften stool to make bowel movements easier, thus easing constipation and painful straining. They are not stimulant laxatives, which may become habit-forming.

The products are available in a variety of forms, including capsule, softgel, tablet, liquigel, caplet, gelcap, liquid, and syrup.

How should you take this medication?

Generally, it's better to start at the high end of the recommended dosage range, then reduce the dose until you find the minimum amount that works for you. You should feel results within 1 to 3 days.

Take the pill forms with a glass of water. Mix liquid and syrup forms with 6 to 8 ounces of milk, juice, or infant formula to prevent throat irritation. Colace liquid also can be added to an enema. Check the package for directions.

■ ADULTS AND CHILDREN 12 AND OVER
Capsules: 1 to 4 of the 50-milligram capsules, or 1 to 2 of the 100-milligram capsules daily
Softgels, caplets, or tablets: 1 to 3 pills daily
Gelcaps: 1 or 2 pills daily
Liquigels: 1 pill daily
Liquid or syrup: 50 to 200 milligrams daily

■ CHILDREN 6 TO 12
Softgels, caplets, gelcaps, or tablets: 1 pill daily
Liquid, syrup, or capsules: 40 to 120 milligrams daily
Liquigels: Check with your doctor.

■ CHILDREN 3 TO 6
Liquid, syrup, or capsules: 20 to 60 milligrams daily
Softgels or caplets: 1 pill daily
Liquigels, gelcaps, or tablets: Check with your doctor.

■ CHILDREN UNDER 3
The usual daily dose of capsules, liquid, or syrup is 10 to 40 milligrams. For all other forms, consult a doctor.

■ STORAGE
These products may be stored at room temperature in a dry place. Protect Correctol softgels from freezing.

Do not take this medication if...
Unless your doctor approves, do not use any of these medications if you have abdominal pain, nausea, or vomiting. Also check first if you have noticed a sudden change in bowel habits that has continued for 2 weeks.

Special warnings about this medication
If you notice bleeding from the rectum or fail to have a bowel movement after using one of these products, stop taking it and check with your doctor. Do not use any of these products for more than 1 week unless your doctor approves.

Throat irritation and nausea are rare side effects, usually seen only with the liquid and syrup. Rash is also a remote possibility.

**Possible food and drug interactions
when taking this medication**
Do not take any of these products if you are also taking mineral oil, unless your doctor approves.

Brand name:

Comtrex Allergy-Sinus

Pronounced: CAHM-trecks
*Generic ingredients: Acetaminophen, Chlorpheniramine maleate,
Pseudoephedrine hydrochloride*

What this drug is used for
Comtrex Allergy-Sinus temporarily relieves symptoms of sinus inflammation and allergies such as hay fever. It can be used for stuffy

nose, sinus pressure, headache pain, sneezing, runny nose, itchy nose or throat, and itchy, watery eyes.

Comtrex is available in tablet and caplet form.

How should you take this medication?
The usual dose for adults and children 12 years and older is 2 pills every 6 hours. Do not take more than 8 pills each 24 hours. For children under 12, consult your doctor.

■ STORAGE
Store at room temperature.

Do not take this medication if...
Unless your doctor approves, do not take this product if you have heart disease, high blood pressure, thyroid disease, diabetes, high pressure within the eye (glaucoma), an enlarged prostate gland, or a breathing problem such as emphysema or chronic bronchitis.

Special warnings about this medication
Do not take Comtrex Allergy-Sinus for more than 7 days unless your doctor approves. If symptoms do not improve or you develop a fever that lasts for more than 3 days, check with your doctor. Also call your doctor if any new symptoms appear.

Comtrex Allergy-Sinus may cause excitability, especially in children. If you become nervous or dizzy, or have trouble sleeping, stop taking this product and check with your doctor.

Comtrex Allergy-Sinus can also cause drowsiness. Be especially careful when driving or operating machinery.

Possible food and drug interactions
when taking this medication
Do not use Comtrex Allergy-Sinus within 2 weeks of taking a drug classified as an MAO inhibitor, such as the antidepressants **Nardil** and **Parnate**.

If you are taking a tranquilizer such as **Valium** or **Xanax**, or a sleep aid such as **Halcion** or **Seconal**, do not take Comtrex Allergy-Sinus without your doctor's approval; the combination could cause extreme drowsiness. For the same reason, avoid alcohol while taking this product.

Overdosage

The acetaminophen in Comtrex Allergy-Sinus can damage the liver if taken in massive amounts. Early signs of a dangerous overdose include sweating, a generally uneasy feeling, nausea, and vomiting.

If you suspect an overdose, seek medical help immediately, even if symptoms have not yet appeared.

Brand name:

Comtrex Cold & Flu Reliever

Pronounced: CAHM-trecks
Generic ingredients: Acetaminophen, Chlorpheniramine maleate,
  Dextromethorphan hydrobromide, Phenylpropanolamine
  hydrochloride, Pseudoephedrine hydrochloride

What this drug is used for

Like Non-Drowsy Comtrex, this product temporarily relieves such cold and flu symptoms as minor aches, pains, headache, sore throat, fever, cough, and stuffy nose. However, Comtrex Cold & Flu Reliever also contains an antihistamine to relieve sneezing and runny nose, and therefore may cause drowsiness.

The product is available in tablet, caplet, liquigel, and liquid form.

How should you take this medication?

Doses may be repeated every 6 hours, up to a maximum of 4 times a day. For children under 12, check dosage with your doctor.

Tablets, caplets, and liquigels: The usual dosage is 2 pills.
Liquid: The usual dose is 1 ounce or 2 tablespoonfuls.

■ STORAGE
Store at room temperature. Protect liquigels from high temperatures and freezing.

Do not take this medication if...

Unless your doctor approves, do not take Comtrex Cold & Flu Reliever if you have heart disease, high blood pressure, thyroid disease, diabetes, high pressure within the eye (glaucoma), an enlarged prostate gland, or a breathing problem such as emphysema or chronic bronchitis.

Also check with your doctor before using Comtrex Cold & Flu Reliever for the type of chronic cough that results from smoking or asthma, or for a cough that brings up lots of phlegm.

Special warnings about this medication

If you become dizzy or nervous, or have trouble sleeping, stop taking Comtrex Cold & Flu Reliever and check with your doctor.

This variety of Comtrex can cause excitability, especially in children. It can also make some people drowsy. Be especially cautious when driving and when operating machinery.

Do not take this product for more than 7 days. If your symptoms won't go away, get worse, or include a fever—or if you develop new symptoms—check with your doctor.

You should also check with your doctor immediately if you have a severe sore throat that lasts for more than 2 days, or if your sore throat is accompanied or followed by fever, headache, rash, nausea, or vomiting.

Likewise, call your doctor if you have a cough that lasts for more than 7 days or tends to come back, or your cough is accompanied by rash, lasting headache, or a 3-day fever.

Possible food and drug interactions when taking this medication

Do not use Comtrex Cold & Flu Reliever within 2 weeks of taking a drug classified as an MAO inhibitor, such as the antidepressants **Nardil** and **Parnate**.

If you are taking a tranquilizer such as **Valium** or **Xanax**, or a sleep aid such as **Halcion** or **Seconal**, do not take this product without your doctor's approval; the combination could cause extreme drowsiness. For the same reason, avoid alcohol while taking this product.

Overdosage

A massive overdose of the acetaminophen in this product could conceivably cause liver damage. Early signs of an overdose include a generally uneasy feeling, sweating, nausea, and vomiting. If you suspect an overdose, seek medical attention immediately.

Brand name:

Comtrex Deep Chest Cold

Pronounced: CAHM-trecks
Generic ingredients: Acetaminophen, Dextromethorphan hydrobro-
  mide, Guaifenesin, Phenylpropanolamine hydrochloride

What this drug is used for

Comtrex Deep Chest Cold temporarily relieves the minor aches, pains, headache, sore throat, cough, fever, and stuffy nose associated with the common cold and flu. It also helps loosen phlegm, making it easier to cough up.

How should you take this medication?

For adults and children 12 years and over, the usual dose is 2 liquigels every 4 hours. Do not take more than 12 liquigels each 24 hours. For children under 12, consult your doctor.

Do not take this medication if...

Unless your doctor approves, do not take Comtrex Deep Chest Cold if you have heart disease, high blood pressure, thyroid disease, diabetes, or an enlarged prostate gland.

Also check with your doctor before using this product for the type of chronic cough that results from smoking, emphysema, chronic bronchitis, or asthma, or for a cough that brings up lots of phlegm.

Special warnings about this medication

If you become dizzy or nervous, or have trouble sleeping, stop taking this product and check with your doctor.

Do not take this product for more than 7 days (3 days for fever) without your doctor's approval. If your pain or fever won't go away or gets worse, or if you develop new symptoms, check with your doctor.

You should also check with your doctor immediately if you have a severe sore throat that lasts for more than 2 days, or if your sore throat is accompanied or followed by fever, headache, rash, nausea, or vomiting.

Likewise, call your doctor if you have a cough that lasts for more than 7 days or tends to come back, or a cough accompanied by rash, lasting headache, or fever.

**Possible food and drug interactions
when taking this medication**

Do not use Comtrex Deep Chest Cold within 2 weeks of taking a drug classified as an MAO inhibitor, such as the antidepressants **Nardil** and **Parnate.**

Combined with heavy drinking, the acetaminophen in this product could conceivably cause liver damage. Check with your doctor before taking this product if you generally have more than 3 alcoholic beverages a day.

Overdosage

■ *Symptoms of an overdose of Comtrex Deep Chest Cold may include:* Nausea, vomiting, sweating, and a generally uneasy feeling

Particularly in heavy drinkers, a massive overdose of acetaminophen could cause liver damage. Even if you have no symptoms, when you suspect an overdose, seek medical attention immediately.

Brand name:

Comtrex Non-Drowsy

Pronounced: CAHM-trecks
Generic ingredients: Acetaminophen, Dextromethorphan hydrobromide, Phenylpropanolamine hydrochloride, Pseudoephedrine hydrochloride

What this drug is used for

Non-Drowsy Comtrex temporarily relieves symptoms of the common cold and flu, including minor aches and pains, headache, muscular aches, fever, cough, and stuffy nose.

Non-Drowsy Comtrex is available in caplet and liquigel form.

How should you take this medication?

For adults and children 12 years and older, the usual dose is 2 pills every 6 hours. Do not take more than 8 pills each 24 hours. For children under 12, consult your doctor.

■ STORAGE
Store at room temperature.

Do not take this medication if...

Unless your doctor approves, do not take Non-Drowsy Comtrex for a persistent cough due to smoking, asthma, or emphysema, or for a cough accompanied by lots of mucus. You should also seek your doctor's approval before using Non-Drowsy Comtrex if you have heart disease, high blood pressure, thyroid disease, diabetes, or an enlarged prostate gland.

Special warnings about this medication

Do not take Non-Drowsy Comtrex for more than 7 days. If symptoms last for 7 days, or you develop a fever, call your doctor. Also check with your doctor if any new symptoms appear, or if you have a cough that lasts more than 7 days, tends to come back, or is accompanied by rash, persistent headache, and fever that lasts more than 3 days. A lingering cough may signal a more serious condition.

If you become nervous or dizzy, or have trouble sleeping, stop taking this product and call your doctor.

Possible food and drug interactions
when taking this medication

Do not use Non-Drowsy Comtrex within 2 weeks of taking a drug classified as an MAO inhibitor, such as the antidepressants **Nardil** and **Parnate**.

If you generally drink more than 3 alcoholic beverages a day, there is a remote possibility that the acetaminophen in this product could harm your liver. You may want to ask your doctor whether you should be concerned.

Brand name:

Contac

Pronounced: KON-tack
Generic ingredients: Chlorpheniramine maleate,
  Phenylpropanolamine hydrochloride

What this drug is used for

Contac temporarily relieves stuffy nose and clogged sinuses due to the common cold, allergies such as hay fever, and inflammation of the sinuses. It also helps clear up cold and allergy symptoms such as runny nose, sneezing, itchy nose or throat, and itchy, watery eyes.

Contac is available in two forms: regular-strength capsules and maximum-strength caplets. Both provide timed-release continuous action.

How should you take this medication?

For adults and children 12 years and over, the dosage is 1 pill every 12 hours. Do not take more than 2 pills each 24 hours unless your doctor recommends. For children under 12, consult a doctor.

■ STORAGE

Store in a dry place at room temperature.

Do not take this medication if...

Unless your doctor approves, do not take Contac if you have diabetes, heart disease, high blood pressure, thyroid disease, high pressure within the eye (glaucoma), an enlarged prostate gland, or breathing problems such as emphysema or chronic bronchitis.

Special warnings about this medication

Contac sometimes causes excitability, especially in children. If you become nervous or dizzy, or have trouble sleeping while taking this product, stop using it and call your doctor.

If you do not feel better within 7 days, or if you have a fever, get in touch with your doctor.

Because Contac may make you feel sleepy, be especially careful when you are driving or operating machinery.

If you are taking maximum-strength Contac, you may notice a soft mass in your stool. It's the remains of the caplet and is nothing to worry about.

Possible food and drug interactions
when taking this medication

Do not take Contac while using any other medication that contains the active ingredient phenylpropanolamine, including **Dimetane-DC**, **Ornade**, **Sinulin**, and **Triaminic**.

In addition, do not use Contac within 2 weeks of taking a drug classified as an MAO inhibitor, such as the antidepressants **Nardil** and **Parnate**.

If you are taking a tranquilizer such as **Valium** or **Xanax**, or a sleep aid such as Halcion or Seconal, do not take Contac without your doctor's approval; the combination could cause extreme drowsiness. For the same reason, avoid alcohol while taking this product.

Brand name:

Contac Day & Night Cold/Flu

Pronounced: CON-tak

Generic ingredients: Acetaminophen, Pseudoephedrine hydrochloride, Dextromethorphan hydrobromide (Day Caplets),
*   Diphenhydramine hydrochloride (Night Caplets)*

What this drug is used for

Each Contac Day & Night Cold/Flu package contains 15 Day Caplets and 5 Night Caplets. Both types of caplet relieve stuffy nose, fever, headache, and minor aches and pains. The Day Caplets also quiet a cough. The Night Caplets, which contain an antihistamine that can make you drowsy, also combat sneezing and runny nose.

How should you take this medication?

For adults and children 12 years and over, the usual dosage is 1 yellow Day Caplet every 6 hours during the day, and 1 blue Night Caplet every 6 hours at night. Allow at least 6 hours between doses and do not take a total of more than 4 caplets—no matter what the type—each 24 hours. For children under 12, consult your doctor.

■ STORAGE

Store at room temperature.

Do not take this medication if...

Unless your doctor approves, do not take Contac Day & Night Cold/Flu if you have heart disease, high blood pressure, thyroid disease, diabetes, high pressure within the eye (glaucoma), an enlarged prostate gland, or a breathing problem such as emphysema or chronic bronchitis.

Also check with your doctor before using the Day Caplets for the type of chronic cough that results from smoking or asthma, or for a cough that brings up lots of phlegm.

Special warnings about these medications

If you become dizzy or nervous, or have trouble sleeping, stop taking Contac Day & Night Cold/Flu and check with your doctor.

Do not take this product for more than 10 days. If your symptoms do not improve or include a fever that lasts more than 3 days—or if new symptoms appear—call your doctor.

You should also check with your doctor if you have a cough that lasts for more than 7 days or tends to come back, or a cough accompanied by rash, lasting headache, and a 3-day fever.

If you take a Night Caplet during the day, be cautious when driving and when operating machinery, since drowsiness could become a problem. The Night Caplets may also cause excitability, especially in children.

Possible food and drug interactions when taking this medication

Do not use Contac Day & Night Cold/Flu within 2 weeks of taking a drug classified as an MAO inhibitor, such as the antidepressants **Nardil** and **Parnate**.

If you are taking a tranquilizer such as **Valium** or **Xanax**, or a sleep aid such as **Halcion** or **Seconal**, do not take the Night Caplets without your doctor's approval; the combination could cause extreme drowsiness. For the same reason, avoid alcohol while using the Night Caplets.

Brand name:

Contac Severe Cold and Flu

Pronounced: CON-tak
Generic ingredients: Acetaminophen, Chlorpheniramine maleate, Dextromethorphan hydrobromide, Phenylpropanolamine hydrochloride

What this drug is used for

This version of Contac Severe Cold and Flu contains antihistamines to fight sneezing and runny nose, and therefore may cause drowsiness. (The Non-Drowsy version omits these ingredients.) Contac Severe Cold and Flu also provides temporary relief from nasal and sinus congestion, coughing, fever, headache, and minor aches and pains.

How should you take this medication?

The usual dose for adults and children 12 years and over is 2 caplets every 6 hours. Do not take more than 8 caplets each 24 hours.

■ STORAGE
Protect from temperatures higher than 100 degrees Fahrenheit.

Do not take this medication if...

Unless your doctor approves, do not take if you have heart disease, high blood pressure, thyroid disease, diabetes, high pressure within the eye (glaucoma), an enlarged prostate gland, or a breathing problem such as emphysema or chronic bronchitis.

Also check with your doctor before using Contac Severe Cold and Flu for the type of chronic cough that results from smoking or asthma, or for a cough that brings up lots of phlegm.

Special warnings about this medication

If you become dizzy or nervous, or have trouble sleeping, stop taking Contac Severe Cold and Flu and check with your doctor.

Do not take this product for more than 10 days. If your symptoms do not improve or include a fever that lasts more than 3 days—or if new symptoms appear—call your doctor.

You should also check with your doctor immediately if you have a severe sore throat that lasts for more than 2 days, or if your sore throat is accompanied or followed by fever, headache, rash, nausea, or vomiting.

Likewise, call your doctor if you have a cough that lasts for more than 7 days or tends to come back, or a cough accompanied by rash, lasting headache, and a 3-day fever.

Because of the possibility of drowsiness, be especially cautious when driving and when operating machinery. This product can also cause excitability, especially in children.

Possible food and drug interactions when taking this medication

Do not use Contac Severe Cold and Flu within 2 weeks of taking a drug classified as an MAO inhibitor, such as the antidepressants **Nardil** and **Parnate**.

If you are taking a tranquilizer such as **Valium** or **Xanax**, or a sleep aid such as Halcion or Seconal, do not take Contac Severe Cold and Flu without your doctor's approval; the combination could cause extreme drowsiness. For the same reason, avoid alcohol while taking this product.

Brand name:

Contac Severe Cold and Flu Non-Drowsy

Pronounced: CON-tak

Generic ingredients: Acetaminophen, Dextromethorphan hydrobro-
mide, Pseudoephedrine hydrochloride

What this drug is used for

This version of Contac Severe Cold and Flu does not contain antihistamines, which can make you drowsy. The product temporarily
relieves the stuffy nose and coughing of a cold, as well the fever, sore
throat, headache, and minor aches that often accompany a cold or the
flu. Because it is antihistamine-free, it does NOT help sneezing or a
runny nose.

How should you take this medication?

The usual dose for adults and children 12 years and over is 2 caplets
every 6 hours. Do not take more than 8 caplets each 24 hours. For children under 12, consult your doctor.

■ STORAGE
Store at room temperature.

Do not take this medication if...

Unless your doctor approves, do not take this product if you have heart
disease, high blood pressure, thyroid disease, diabetes, or an enlarged
prostate gland.

Also check with your doctor before using this product for the type of
chronic cough that results from smoking, asthma, or emphysema, or
for a cough that brings up lots of phlegm.

Special warnings about this medication

If you become dizzy or nervous, or have trouble sleeping, stop taking
this product and check with your doctor.

Do not take this product for more than 10 days. If your symptoms do
not improve or include a fever that lasts more than 3 days—or if new
symptoms appear—call your doctor.

You should also check with your doctor immediately if you have a severe sore throat that lasts for more than 2 days, or if your sore throat is accompanied or followed by fever, headache, rash, nausea, or vomiting.

Likewise, call your doctor if you have a cough that lasts for more than 7 days or tends to come back, or a cough accompanied by rash, lasting headache, and a 3-day fever. A lingering cough could signal a serious condition

Possible food and drug interactions when taking this medication

Do not use this product within 2 weeks of taking a drug classified as an MAO inhibitor, such as the antidepressants **Nardil** and **Parnate**.

Brand name:

Coricidin 'D'

Pronounced: kor-i-SEE-din
Generic ingredients: Acetaminophen, Chlorpheniramine maleate,
 Phenylpropanolamine hydrochloride

What this drug is used for

Coricidin 'D' tablets temporarily relieve the minor aches, pains, sneezing, runny nose, and fever associated with a cold or flu. Unlike other Coricidin products, they also contain an ingredient to unclog stuffy nose and sinuses, which makes them less safe for people with high blood pressure.

How should you take this medication?

■ ADULTS

For adults and children 12 years and over, the usual dosage is 2 tablets every 4 hours. Do not take more than 12 tablets in 24 hours.

■ CHILDREN

For children 6 to 12, the usual dose is 1 tablet every 4 hours, up to a maximum of 5 tablets a day. For children under 6, consult your doctor.

■ STORAGE

Store at room temperature.

Do not take this medication if...

Unless your doctor approves, do not take Coricidin 'D' if you have heart disease, high blood pressure, thyroid disease, diabetes, high pressure within the eye (glaucoma), an enlarged prostate gland, or a breathing problem such as emphysema or chronic bronchitis.

Special warnings about this medication

If you become dizzy or nervous, or have trouble sleeping, stop taking Coricidin 'D' and check with your doctor.

Do not take this product for more than 10 days for pain (5-day limit for children) or 3 days for fever without your doctor's approval. If your pain or fever won't go away or gets worse, or if you develop new symptoms or notice any redness or swelling, check with your doctor; you might have a serious condition. Check after 7 days if your congestion doesn't improve.

Coricidin 'D' may cause marked drowsiness; use caution when driving and when operating machinery. It can also cause excitability, especially in children.

Possible food and drug interactions
when taking this medication

Do not use Coricidin 'D' within 2 weeks of taking a drug classified as an MAO inhibitor, such as the antidepressants **Nardil** and **Parnate**. Also avoid Coricidin 'D' if you are taking other products that contain the active ingredient phenylpropanolamine, such as the diet drugs **Acutrim** and **Dexatrim**.

If you are taking a tranquilizer such as **Valium** or **Xanax**, or a sleep aid such as **Halcion** or **Seconal**, do not take Coricidin 'D' without your doctor's approval; the combination could cause extreme drowsiness. For the same reason, avoid alcohol while taking this product.

Brand name:

Coricidin Cold & Flu Tablets

Pronounced: kor-i-SEE-din
Generic ingredients: Acetaminophen, Chlorpheniramine maleate

What this drug is used for

Coricidin Cold & Flu Tablets temporarily relieve minor aches, pains, and headache, and reduce the fever associated with colds or flu. They also relieve the sneezing, runny nose, and itchy, watery eyes that accompany colds and allergies such as hay fever. Because Coricidin Cold & Flu Tablets do not contain an ingredient to combat stuffy nose, they are safe to use if you have high blood pressure.

How should you take this medication?
■ ADULTS

For adults and children 12 years and over, the usual dose is 2 tablets every 4 to 6 hours. Do not take more than 12 tablets each 24 hours.

■ CHILDREN

For children 6 to 12, the usual dose is 1 tablet every 4 to 6 hours, up to a maximum of 5 tablets a day. For children under 6, consult your doctor.

■ STORAGE

Store at room temperature.

Do not take this medication if...
Unless your doctor approves, do not take Coricidin Cold & Flu Tablets if you have high pressure within the eye (glaucoma), an enlarged prostate gland, or a breathing problem such as emphysema or chronic bronchitis.

Special warnings about this medication
Do not take this product for more than 10 days for pain (5-day limit for children) or 3 days for fever without your doctor's approval. If your pain or fever won't go away or gets worse, or if you develop new symptoms or notice any redness or swelling, check with your doctor; you might have a serious condition.

Coricidin Cold & Flu Tablets may cause drowsiness. Be especially cautious when driving and when operating machinery. They can also cause excitability, especially in children.

Possible food and drug interactions
when taking this medication
If you are taking a tranquilizer such as **Valium** or **Xanax**, or a sleep aid such as **Halcion** or **Seconal**, do not take Coricidin Cold & Flu Tablets without your doctor's approval; the combination could cause extreme drowsiness. For the same reason, avoid alcohol while taking this product.

Brand name:

Coricidin Cough & Cold Tablets

Pronounced: kor-i-SEE-din
Generic ingredients: Chlorpheniramine maleate, Dextromethorphan
hydrobromide

What this drug is used for

Coricidin Cough & Cold Tablets provide temporary relief from coughs. They also contain an antihistamine to relieve the sneezing, runny nose, and itchy, watery eyes that accompany colds and allergies such as hay fever. They do not contain a pain reliever or an ingredient to combat stuffy nose. Because they lack a decongestant, they are safe for people with high blood pressure.

How should you take this medication?

For adults and children 12 years and over, the usual dose is 1 tablet every 6 hours. Do not take more than 4 tablets each 24 hours.

■ STORAGE
Store at room temperature.

Do not take this medication if...

Unless your doctor approves, do not take Coricidin Cough & Cold Tablets if you have high pressure within the eye (glaucoma), an enlarged prostate gland, or a breathing problem such as emphysema or chronic bronchitis.

Also check with your doctor before using this product for the type of chronic cough that results from smoking or asthma, or for a cough that brings up lots of phlegm.

Not for children under 12.

Special warnings about this medication

If your cough doesn't improve within 7 days or tends to come back— or if you also have a fever, rash, or lasting headache—check with your doctor. A lingering cough could signal a serious condition.

The antihistamine in Coricidin Cough & Cold Tablets may cause marked drowsiness; use caution when driving and when operating machinery. This product may also cause excitability, especially in children.

Possible food and drug interactions when taking this medication

Do not use Coricidin Cough & Cold Tablets within 2 weeks of taking a drug classified as an MAO inhibitor, such as the antidepressants **Nardil** and **Parnate**.

If you are taking a tranquilizer such as **Valium** or **Xanax**, or a sleep aid such as **Halcion** or **Seconal**, do not take Coricidin Cough & Cold Tablets without your doctor's approval; the combination could cause extreme drowsiness. For the same reason, avoid alcohol while taking this product.

Brand name:

Coricidin Nighttime Cold & Cough Liquid

Pronounced: kor-i-SEE-din
Generic ingredients: Acetaminophen, Diphenhydramine hydrochloride

What this drug is used for

Coricidin Nighttime Cold & Cough Liquid temporarily relieves the minor aches, pains, headache, cough, sore throat, and fever that often accompany colds and flu. It also contains an antihistamine to relieve runny nose, sneezing, and itchy, watery eyes due to allergies such as hay fever. Because it does not contain an ingredient to combat stuffy nose, it is safe for people who cannot take such medications, like those with high blood pressure.

How should you take this medication?

■ ADULTS

For adults and children 12 years and over, the usual dosage is 2 tablespoonfuls every 4 hours. Do not take more than 6 doses each 24 hours.

■ CHILDREN

For children 6 to 12, the usual dose is 1 tablespoonful every 4 hours. Do not give more than 5 doses each 24 hours. For children under 6, consult your doctor.

■ STORAGE

Store at room temperature.

Do not take this medication if...

Unless your doctor approves, do not take Coricidin Nighttime Cold & Cough Liquid if you have high pressure within the eye (glaucoma), an enlarged prostate gland, or a breathing problem such as emphysema or chronic bronchitis.

Also check with your doctor before using this product for the type of chronic cough that results from smoking or asthma, or for a cough that brings up lots of phlegm.

Special warnings about this medication

Do not take this product for more than 10 days for pain (5-day limit for children) or 3 days for fever without your doctor's approval. If your pain or fever won't go away or gets worse, or if you develop new symptoms or notice any redness or swelling, check with your doctor; you might have a serious condition.

You should also check with your doctor immediately if you have a severe sore throat that lasts for more than 2 days, or if your sore throat is accompanied or followed by fever, headache, rash, nausea, or vomiting.

Coricidin Nighttime Cold & Cough Liquid may cause marked drowsiness; use caution when driving and when operating machinery. The product can also cause excitability, especially in children.

Possible food and drug interactions
when taking this medication

If you are taking a tranquilizer such as **Valium** or **Xanax**, or a sleep aid such as **Halcion** or **Seconal**, do not take Coricidin Nighttime Cold & Cough Liquid without your doctor's approval; the combination could cause extreme drowsiness. For the same reason, avoid alcohol while taking this product.

Brand name:

Correctol

Pronounced: koh-REK-tall
Generic name: Bisacodyl
Other brand name: Dulcolax

What this drug is used for

Correctol and Dulcolax are laxatives. They produce a bowel movement, providing relief from occasional constipation and irregularity.

Correctol is available in tablet and caplet form. Dulcolax comes in tablets and suppositories.

How should you take this medication?

Do not chew tablets or caplets, and do not take these products within 1 hour of taking an antacid or drinking milk.

To use the suppositories, remove the foil wrapper, then lie on your side and, with pointed end first, insert the suppository high enough in the rectum so that it does not feel as though it will come out immediately. Retain it for 15 to 20 minutes.

■ ADULTS AND CHILDREN 12 YEARS AND OVER
Tablets and caplets: 1 to 3 pills once a day
Suppositories: 1 a day

■ CHILDREN 6 TO 12
Tablets and caplets: 1 a day
Suppositories: Half a suppository once a day

■ CHILDREN UNDER 6
Consult a physician.

■ STORAGE
Store all formulations at room temperature. Keep dry.

Do not take this medication if...

Unless your doctor approves, do not use either of these products if you have nausea, vomiting, or abdominal pain, or if you've noticed a sudden change in bowel habits lasting 2 weeks or more.

Special warnings about this medication

In the process of restoring normal bowel function, these products may cause faintness and abdominal discomfort, including cramps.

If you begin to bleed from the rectum or fail to have a bowel movement after taking one of these products, stop using it and call your doctor.

Do not use a laxative for more than a week without your doctor's approval.

Brand name:

Correctol Herbal Tea

See Senokot

Brand name:

Correctol Stool Softener

See Colace

Brand name:

Delsym Cough Formula

See Benylin Adult Formula Cough Suppressant

Brand name:

Dexatrim

See Acutrim

Brand name:

Di-Gel

Pronounced: DYE-jell
Generic ingredients: Magnesium hydroxide, Simethicone, Aluminum
  hydroxide (liquid only), Calcium carbonate (tablets only)

What this drug is used for

Di-Gel temporarily relieves acid indigestion, heartburn, sour stomach, and gas.

How should you take this medication?

The usual dose is 2 to 4 tablets or teaspoonfuls every 2 hours, or as directed by your doctor. Chew the tablets. Shake the liquid well before using and take with a spoon.

Do not take more than 20 teaspoonfuls or 24 tablets each 24 hours, or use the maximum dosage of this product for more than 2 weeks, without first checking with your doctor.

Do not take this medication if...

If you have kidney disease, do not take Di-Gel unless your doctor approves.

Special warnings about this medication

Di-Gel tablets may cause either constipation or loose bowels.

**Possible food and drug interactions
when taking this medication**

Antacids interact with a variety of prescription drugs when taken at the same time. An interaction is unlikely, however, if you keep doses of the two at least 2 or 3 hours apart. Drugs that may interact include the following:

Alendronate (**Fosamax**)
Allopurinol (**Zyloprim**)
Antibiotics classified as quinolones, such as **Cipro**, **Floxin**, and **Noroxin**
Aspirin
Atenolol (**Tenormin**)
Captopril (**Capoten**)
Chlordiazepoxide (**Librium**)
Cimetidine (**Tagamet**)
Digoxin (**Lanoxin**)
Doxycycline (**Vibramycin**)
Fosfomycin (**Monurol**)
Gabapentin (**Neurontin**)
Glipizide (**Glucotrol**)
Glyburide (**Micronase, DiaBeta**)
Isoniazid (**Rifamate**)
Ketoconazole (**Nizoral**)
Levothyroxine (**Synthroid**)
Methenamine (**Urised**)
Metronidazole (**Flagyl**)
Misoprostol (**Cytotec**)
Mycophenolate mofetil (**CellCept**)
Nonsteroidal anti-inflammatory drugs such as **Dolobid, Motrin, Naprosyn**, and **Voltaren**
Penicillamine (**Cuprimine**)
Phenytoin (**Dilantin**)
Quinidine (**Quinidex**)

Sodium polystyrene sulfonate (**Kayexalate**)
Sucralfate (**Carafate**)
Tetracycline antibiotics such as **Achromycin V** and **Minocin**
Tilodronate (**Skelid**)
Ursodiol (**Actigall**)

Prolonged and heavy use of calcium-containing antacids such as the tablet form of Di-Gel, combined with a high intake of calcium-rich foods such as milk, can lead to an overload of calcium in the system. Early symptoms are constipation, weakness, nausea, and vomiting; and a severe overload can cause kidney damage. If you need a high-calcium diet, check with your doctor about a substitute for Di-Gel tablets.

A high-protein meal, such as a steak dinner, can reduce the effectiveness of aluminum-containing antacids such as the liquid form of Di-Gel.

Brand name:

Diabe-Tuss DM

See Benylin Adult Formula Cough Suppressant

Brand name:

Dialose

See Colace

Brand name:

Dialose Plus

Pronounced: DYE-uh-lohs
Generic ingredients: Docusate sodium, Yellow phenolphthalein

What this drug is used for
Like regular Dialose tablets, Dialose Plus contains a stool softener. However, Dialose Plus also includes a stimulant laxative. The stool softener makes bowel movements easier, thus easing constipation and painful straining. The laxative provokes the bowel into action.

How should you take this medication?
Take each dose with a full glass of water. Use only as needed.

■ ADULTS

For adults and children 12 and over, the usual daily dose is 1 or 2 tablets at bedtime or after waking up.

■ CHILDREN

For children 6 to 12, the usual dose is 1 tablet daily. For children under 6, consult your doctor.

Do not take this medication if...

Unless your doctor approves, do not use Dialose Plus if you have abdominal pain, nausea, or vomiting.

Special warnings about this medication

If you develop a rash, stop taking this product and avoid any other product containing phenolphthalein.

Do not use this product for more than 1 week. Prolonged or frequent use can lead to dependence.

Possible food and drug interactions
when taking this medication

Do not take Dialose Plus if you are also using mineral oil or taking a prescription drug.

Brand name:

Diarrid

See Imodium A-D

Brand name:

Dimetapp

Pronounced: DYE-meh-tap
Generic ingredients: Brompheniramine maleate, Phenylpropanol-
amine hydrochloride

What this drug is used for

This basic Dimetapp formulation relieves the stuffy nose that accompanies colds, inflamed sinuses, hay fever, and similar allergies. It is also a temporary remedy for such hay fever symptoms as runny nose, sneezing, itchy nose or throat, and itchy, watery eyes.

Dimetapp comes in tablets, softgels, and elixir. For children, a reduced dose of the medication is available in the form of Dimetapp Cold & Allergy Chewable Tablets. For adults, timed-release Extentabs are also available.

How should you take this medication?

■ TABLETS, LIQUIGELS, AND ELIXIR
Do not take more than 6 doses each 24 hours.

Adults and children 12 years and over
The usual dose is 1 pill or 2 teaspoonfuls every 4 hours.

Children 6 to 12
The usual dose is half a tablet or 1 teaspoonful every 4 hours.

■ COLD & ALLERGY CHEWABLE TABLETS

Children 6 to 12
The usual dose is 2 chewable tablets every 4 hours. Do not give more than 6 doses each 24 hours.

■ EXTENTABS

Adults and children 12 years and over
The usual dose is 1 pill every 12 hours. Allow a full 12 hours between pills; do not take more than 2 pills each 24 hours. Not for children under 12 without your doctor's approval.

■ STORAGE
All forms may be stored at room temperature.

Do not take this medication if...

Unless your doctor approves, do not take Dimetapp if you have heart disease, high blood pressure, thyroid disease, diabetes, high pressure within the eye (glaucoma), an enlarged prostate gland, or a breathing problem such as emphysema or chronic bronchitis. Also avoid Dimetapp if any of the ingredients have ever given you an allergic reaction.

Special warnings about this medication

If you become dizzy or nervous, or you have trouble sleeping, stop taking Dimetapp and check with your doctor.

Dimetapp may cause drowsiness. Be especially cautious when driving and when operating machinery. This medication can also cause excitability, especially in children.

If your symptoms do not improve within 7 days or you develop a fever, call your doctor.

Possible food or drug interactions when taking this medication

Do not use Dimetapp within 2 weeks of taking a drug classified as an MAO inhibitor, such as the antidepressants **Nardil** and **Parnate**.

If you are taking a tranquilizer such as **Valium** or **Xanax**, or a sleep aid such as **Halcion** or **Seconal**, do not take Dimetapp without your doctor's approval; the combination could cause extreme drowsiness. For the same reason, avoid alcohol while taking this product.

Brand name:

Dimetapp Allergy

Pronounced: DYE-meh-tap
Generic name: Brompheniramine maleate

What this drug is used for

Unlike other Dimetapp products, Dimetapp Allergy does NOT relieve stuffiness due to a cold or inflamed sinuses. Its single ingredient fights only those symptoms usually associated with hay fever and similar allergies, including runny nose, sneezing, itchy nose or throat, and itchy, watery eyes.

Dimetapp Allergy is available as a dye-free elixir.

How should you take this medication?
■ ADULTS

For adults and children 12 years and over, the usual dose is 2 teaspoonfuls every 4 to 6 hours. Do not take more than 12 teaspoonfuls each 24 hours.

■ CHILDREN

For children 6 to 12, the usual dose is 1 teaspoonful every 4 to 6 hours, up to a maximum of 6 teaspoonfuls each 24 hours. For children under 6, consult a doctor.

■ STORAGE

Store at room temperature.

Do not take this medication if...

Unless your doctor approves, do not take Dimetapp Allergy if you have an enlarged prostate gland, high pressure within the eye (glaucoma), or a breathing problem such as emphysema or chronic bronchitis.

Special warnings about this medication

Dimetapp Allergy may cause drowsiness. Be especially cautious when driving and when operating machinery.

The product could also cause excitability, especially in a child.

Possible food and drug interactions when taking this medication

If you are taking a tranquilizer such as **Valium** or **Xanax**, or a sleep aid such as **Halcion** or **Seconal**, do not take Dimetapp Allergy without your doctor's approval; the combination could cause extreme drowsiness. For the same reason, avoid alcohol while taking this product.

Brand name:

Dimetapp Allergy Sinus

Pronounced: DYE-meh-tap
Generic ingredients: Acetaminophen, Brompheniramine maleate,
  Phenylpropanolamine hydrochloride

What this drug is used for

Like most other Dimetapp products, Dimetapp Allergy Sinus relieves stuffiness due to a cold or sinus inflammation, and fights hay fever symptoms such as runny nose, sneezing, itchy nose or throat, and itchy, watery eyes. In addition, the acetaminophen in this product relieves minor aches and pains, eases headache, and reduces fever. The product comes in caplet form.

How should you take this medication?

For adults and children 12 years and over, the usual dose is 2 caplets every 6 hours. Do not take more than 8 caplets each 24 hours. For children under 12, consult a doctor.

■ STORAGE
Store at room temperature.

Do not take this medication if...

Unless your doctor approves, do not take Dimetapp Allergy Sinus if you have heart disease, high blood pressure, thyroid disease, diabetes, high pressure within the eye (glaucoma), an enlarged prostate gland, or a breathing problem such as emphysema or chronic bronchitis.

Special warnings about this medication

If you become dizzy or nervous, or have trouble sleeping, stop taking Dimetapp Allergy Sinus and check with your doctor.

Dimetapp Allergy Sinus may cause drowsiness. Be especially cautious when driving and when operating machinery. This medication can also cause excitability, especially in children.

Do not take this product for more than 7 days. (The limit is 3 days for fever.) If your pain or fever won't go away or gets worse, if you develop new symptoms, or if you notice any redness or swelling, check with your doctor; you might have a serious condition.

Possible food and drug interactions when taking this medication

Do not use Dimetapp Allergy Sinus within 2 weeks of taking a drug classified as an MAO inhibitor, such as the antidepressants **Nardil** and **Parnate**.

If you are taking a tranquilizer such as **Valium** or **Xanax**, or a sleep aid such as **Halcion** or **Seconal**, do not take Dimetapp Allergy Sinus without your doctor's approval; the combination could cause extreme drowsiness. For the same reason, avoid alcohol while taking this product.

Brand name:

Dimetapp Cold & Allergy

Pronounced: DYE-meh-tap
Generic ingredients: Brompheniramine maleate,
    Phenylpropanolamine hydrochloride

What this drug is used for

Dimetapp Cold & Allergy is formulated specifically for children. It temporarily relieves the stuffy nose that often accompanies a cold, inflamed sinuses, or allergies such as hay fever. It also relieves other hay fever symptoms, including runny nose, sneezing, and itchy, watery eyes. It comes as a quick-dissolving grape-flavored tablet.

How should you take this medication?

Do not give more than 6 doses each 24 hours.

■ CHILDREN

Age 6 to 12
The usual dose is 2 tablets every 4 hours.

Under 6
Consult a physician.

■ STORAGE
Store at room temperature.

Do not take this medication if...

Unless your doctor approves, do not give Dimetapp Cold & Allergy to children who have a breathing problem such as chronic bronchitis, or to a child with heart disease, high blood pressure, thyroid disease, diabetes, or high pressure within the eye (glaucoma).

Special warnings about this medication

Dimetapp Cold & Allergy may cause excitability. If the child becomes dizzy or nervous, or has trouble sleeping, stop using this product and check with your doctor. Call your doctor, too, if the child's symptoms do not improve within 7 days or are accompanied by fever.

Dimetapp Cold & Allergy contains an antihistamine that may cause drowsiness. It also contains phenylalanine. If your child must avoid this chemical, do not use Dimetapp Cold & Allergy.

Possible food and drug interactions
when taking this medication

If a child is taking a tranquilizer such as **Valium** or **Xanax**, or a sleep aid such as **Halcion** or **Seconal**, do not give Dimetapp Cold & Allergy without your doctor's approval; the combination could cause extreme drowsiness.

Do not use Dimetapp Cold & Allergy within 2 weeks of giving the child a drug classified as an MAO inhibitor, such as the antidepressants **Nardil** and **Parnate**.

Brand name:

Dimetapp Cold and Cough Products

Pronounced: DYE-meh-tap
Generic ingredients: Brompheniramine maleate, Dextromethorphan
hydrobromide, Phenylpropanolamine hydrochloride

What this-drug is used for

Two Dimetapp products—Dimetapp Cold and Cough and Dimetapp
DM Elixir— share the same set of ingredients. Dimetapp Cold and
Cough delivers them in softgel form; Dimetapp DM provides them as
a liquid.

Both products relieve the stuffiness due to a cold, inflamed sinuses, or
allergies such as hay fever. They also relieve cough due to the minor
throat and bronchial irritation that occurs with a cold; and they combat hay fever symptoms such as runny nose, sneezing, itchy nose or
throat, and itchy, watery eyes.

How should you take this medication?

Do not take more than 6 doses each 24 hours.

■ ADULTS

For adults and children 12 years and over, the usual dose is 1 softgel
or 2 teaspoonfuls every 4 hours.

■ CHILDREN

For children 6 to 12, the usual dose is 1 teaspoonful of elixir every 4
hours. For children under 6, consult your doctor.

■ STORAGE

Both products may be stored at room temperature.

Do not take this medication if...

Unless your doctor approves, do not take either of these products if
you have heart disease, high blood pressure, thyroid disease, diabetes,
high pressure within the eye (glaucoma), an enlarged prostate gland,
or a breathing problem such as emphysema or chronic bronchitis.

Also check with your doctor before using these products for the type
of chronic cough that results from smoking or asthma, or a cough that
brings up lots of phlegm.

Special warnings about this medication

These products may cause drowsiness. Be especially cautious when driving and when operating machinery.

They can also cause excitability, especially in children. If you become dizzy or nervous, or have trouble sleeping, stop taking the product and check with your doctor.

If cough and other symptoms don't improve within 7 days or tend to come back—or if you also have a fever, rash, or lasting headache—check with your doctor. A lingering cough could signal a serious condition.

Possible food and drug interactions when taking this medication

Do not use either of these products within 2 weeks of taking a drug classified as an MAO inhibitor, such as the antidepressants **Nardil** and **Parnate**.

If you are taking a tranquilizer such as **Valium** or **Xanax**, or a sleep aid such as **Halcion** or **Seconal**, do not take Dimetapp Cold and Cough Products without your doctor's approval; the combination could cause extreme drowsiness. For the same reason, avoid alcohol while taking either of these products.

Brand name:

Dimetapp Cold and Fever

Pronounced: DYE-meh-tap
Generic ingredients: Acetaminophen, Brompheniramine maleate,
   Pseudoephedrine hydrochloride

What this drug is used for

This children's formulation fights much the same symptoms as Dimetapp Allergy Sinus. It relieves stuffiness due to a cold or sinus inflammation, and fights hay fever symptoms such as runny nose, sneezing, itchy nose or throat, and itchy, watery eyes. In addition, it reduces fever and relieves minor aches, pains, headache, and sore throat.

Dimetapp Cold and Fever comes in liquid form.

How should you take this medication?

Shake well before using.

■ CHILDREN 6 TO 12
The usual dose is 2 teaspoonfuls every 4 hours. Do not give more than 4 doses each 24 hours.

■ CHILDREN UNDER 6
Consult a doctor.

■ STORAGE
Store at room temperature.

Do not take this medication if...

Unless your doctor approves, do not use this product for children with high blood pressure, heart disease, diabetes, thyroid disease, high pressure within the eye (glaucoma), or breathing problems such as chronic bronchitis.

Special warnings about this medication

Unless your doctor approves, do not give this product for pain for more than 5 days. (For fever, the limit is 3 days.) If pain or fever won't go away or gets worse, if the child develops new symptoms, or if you notice any redness or swelling, check with your doctor; there might be a serious problem. If the child has a severe sore throat for more than 2 days, along with (or followed by) fever, headache, rash, nausea, or vomiting, call your doctor immediately.

Dimetapp Cold and Fever can cause excitability. If the child becomes nervous or dizzy, or can't get to sleep, stop giving the product and call your doctor. In some children, the product may cause drowsiness instead.

Possible food and drug interactions
when taking this medication

Do not use Dimetapp Cold and Fever within 2 weeks of giving the child a drug classified as an MAO inhibitor, such as the antidepressants **Nardil** and **Parnate**.

If the child is taking a tranquilizer such as **Valium** or **Xanax**, or a sleep aid such as **Halcion** or **Seconal,** do not use this product without your doctor's approval; the combination could cause extreme drowsiness.

Brand name:

Dimetapp Decongestant Pediatric Drops

See Sudafed

Brand name:

Dimetapp DM Elixir

See Dimetapp Cold and Cough Products

Brand name:

Doan's

Pronounced: DOHNZ
Generic name: Magnesium salicylate tetrahydrate
Other brand name: Backache Caplets

What this drug is used for

Doan's Analgesic Caplets and the similar product, Backache Caplets, provide temporary relief from minor backache pain.

Doan's Caplets are available in regular and extra strengths. Backache Caplets are equivalent to the extra-strength variety of Doan's.

How should you take this medication?

Drink a full glass of water with each dose. For children under 12, consult your doctor.

■ REGULAR STRENGTH DOAN'S
The usual dose is 2 caplets every 4 hours. Do not take more than 12 caplets in 24 hours.

■ EXTRA STRENGTH DOAN'S AND BACKACHE CAPLETS
The usual dose is 2 caplets every 6 hours. Do not take more than 8 caplets in 24 hours.

■ STORAGE
Store at room temperature. Keep the product dry.

Do not take this medication if...

Unless your doctor approves, do not take Doan's if you are allergic to aspirin and other salicylates, or if you have asthma, ulcers, bleeding problems, or stomach complaints—heartburn, upset stomach, or stomach pain—that fail to get better or keep coming back.

Special warnings about this medication

Salicylates such as the active ingredient in these products have been known to trigger a serious illness called Reye's syndrome in children and teenagers who catch a virus. If your child gets chickenpox or flu, do not treat the symptoms with Doan's.

If you develop ringing in the ears or notice a loss of hearing, stop taking this medicine and call your doctor.

Do not take either of these products for more than 10 days for pain or 3 days for fever, unless your doctor recommends. Call your doctor if you develop new symptoms, your pain or fever continues or gets worse, or you notice redness and swelling. These could be signs of a serious condition.

Possible food and drug interactions when taking this medication

Check with your doctor before combining these products with any of the following:

Anti-gout drugs such as **Anturane, Benemid,** and **Zyloprim**
Arthritis preparations such as **Aleve, Anaprox, Ecotrin, Indocin, Motrin, Naprosyn,** and **Orudis**
Blood-thinning drugs such as **Coumadin**
Diabetes medications, including **DiaBeta, Diabinese, Micronase,** and **Glucotrol**

Brand name:

Doan's P.M.

Pronounced: DOHNZ
Generic ingredients: Diphenhydramine, Magnesium salicylate tetrahydrate

What this drug is used for

Doan's P.M. combines the pain reliever in regular Doan's with an antihistamine that causes drowsiness. The product provides temporary relief from minor back pain and helps overcome sleeplessness.

How should you take this medication?

The usual dose for adults and children 12 years and over is 2 caplets at bedtime. Drink a full glass of water with each dose.

■ STORAGE
Store at room temperature in a dry place.

Do not take this medication if...

Unless your doctor approves, do not take Doan's P.M. if you are allergic to aspirin and other salicylates, or if you have ulcers, bleeding problems, or stomach complaints—heartburn, upset stomach, or stomach pain—that fail to get better or keep coming back. Also avoid Doan's P.M. if you have a breathing problem such as emphysema or chronic bronchitis, high pressure within the eye (glaucoma), or an enlarged prostate gland.

Not for children under 12.

Special warnings about this medication

Salicylates such as the pain reliever in Doan's P.M. have been known to trigger a serious illness called Reye's syndrome in children and teenagers who catch a virus. If your child gets chickenpox or flu, do not treat the symptoms with Doan's P.M.

If you develop ringing in the ears or notice a loss of hearing, stop taking this product and call your doctor.

Do not take Doan's P.M. for more than 10 days for pain or 3 days for fever, unless your doctor recommends. Call your doctor if you develop new symptoms, your pain or fever continues or gets worse, or you notice any redness or swelling. These symptoms could signal a serious problem. Also check with your doctor if your sleep problems last for more than 2 weeks.

Possible food and drug interactions when taking this medication

The salicylate in Doan's P.M. can interact with a number of prescription drugs. Check with your doctor before combining this product with any of the following:

Anti-gout drugs such as **Anturane, Benemid,** and **Zyloprim**
Arthritis preparations such as **Aleve, Anaprox, Ecotrin, Indocin, Motrin, Naprosyn,** and **Orudis**
Blood-thinning drugs such as **Coumadin**
Diabetes medications, including **DiaBeta, Diabinese, Micronase,** and **Glucotrol**

Also, if you are taking a tranquilizer such as **Valium** or **Xanax,** or a sleep aid such as **Halcion** or **Seconal,** do not take Doan's P.M. without your doctor's approval; the antihistamine it contains can interact with such drugs and cause extreme drowsiness. For the same reason, avoid alcohol while taking this product.

Brand name:

Donnagel

See Kaopectate

Brand name:

Doxidan

Pronounced: DOCKS-i-dan
Generic ingredients: Casanthranol, Docusate sodium
Other brand names: Fleet Sof-Lax Overnight, Peri-Colace

What this drug is used for

Doxidan and similar products combine a laxative to relieve constipation and a stool softener to ease bowel movements.

Doxidan and Fleet Sof-Lax Overnight come in gelcap form. Peri-Colace is available in capsules and syrup.

How should you take this medication?

■ DOXIDAN

Adults
The usual dose for adults and children 12 years and over is 1 to 3 pills in a single dose, once a day.

Children
For children 2 to 12, the usual dose is 1 pill a day. For children under 2, consult your doctor.

■ FLEET SOF-LAX OVERNIGHT

Adults
The usual dose for adults and children 12 years and over is 1 or 2 pills daily at bedtime.

Children
For children 6 to 12, the usual dose is 1 pill a day.

■ PERI-COLACE

Adults
The usual dose is 1 or 2 capsules or tablespoonfuls of syrup at bed time. For severe constipation, you can take 2 capsules or tablespoon fuls twice a day, or take 3 capsules at bedtime.

Children

The usual dose is 1 to 3 teaspoonfuls of syrup at bedtime. To avoid throat irritation, mix the syrup into 6 to 8 ounces of milk or fruit juice, or add it to infant formula.

■ STORAGE

May be stored at room temperature.

Do not take this medication if...

Unless your doctor approves, do not use this medicine if you have abdominal pain, nausea, or vomiting. If you have noticed a sudden change in bowel habits lasting for 2 weeks or longer, check with your doctor before using any laxative.

Special warnings about this medication

Stop using this medicine and call your doctor if you develop rectal bleeding or fail to have a bowel movement after taking the medicine. You might have a serious condition.

Side effects of this medicine are rare, but may include nausea, abdominal discomfort, diarrhea, and rash.

Used too often or too long, laxatives can become habit-forming. Do not use any laxative for more than a week without your doctor's approval.

Possible food and drug interactions
when taking this medication

Unless your doctor directs, do not use these products if you are taking mineral oil.

Brand name:

Dramamine

Pronounced: DRAM-uh-meen
Generic name: Dimenhydrinate

What this drug is used for

Dramamine prevents motion sickness. It can also be used to relieve the nausea, vomiting, and dizziness once it begins.

Dramamine is available in tablets and chewable tablets. A liquid form is available for children.

How should you take this medication?

To prevent motion sickness, take the first dose one-half to 1 hou
before traveling.

■ TABLETS AND CHEWABLE TABLETS

Adults

The usual dose is 1 or 2 tablets every 4 to 6 hours. Do not take mor
than 8 tablets each 24 hours.

Children 6 to 12

The usual dose is one-half to 1 tablet every 6 to 8 hours. Do not giv
more than 3 tablets in 24 hours.

Children 2 to 6

The usual dose is one-quarter to one-half tablet every 6 to 8 hours. D
not give more than 1½ tablets in 24 hours.

■ DRAMAMINE CHILDREN'S LIQUID

Children 12 and over

The usual dose is 4 to 8 teaspoonfuls every 4 to 6 hours. Do not giv
more than 32 teaspoonfuls in 24 hours.

Children 6 to 12

The usual dose is 2 to 4 teaspoonfuls every 6 to 8 hours. Do not giv
more than 12 teaspoonfuls in 24 hours.

Children 2 to 6

The usual dose is 1 or 2 teaspoonfuls every 6 to 8 hours. Do not giv
more than 6 teaspoonfuls in 24 hours.

Do not take this medication if...

Unless your doctor approves, do not use Dramamine if you have hig
pressure within the eye (glaucoma), an enlarged prostate gland, o
breathing problems such as emphysema or chronic bronchitis.

Not for children under 2 without your doctor's approval.

Special warnings about this medication

Dramamine may cause drowsiness. Be especially cautious when driv
ing and when operating machinery.

Use only when motion sickness is likely. You should not use this prod
uct frequently or regularly.

**Possible food and drug interactions
when taking this medication**

If you are taking a tranquilizer such as **Valium** or **Xanax**, or a sleep aid such as **Halcion** or **Seconal**, do not take Dramamine without your doctor's approval; the combination could cause extreme drowsiness. For the same reason, avoid alcohol while taking this product.

Brand name:

Dramamine II

See Bonine

Brand name:

Drixoral Allergy/Sinus

See Drixoral Cold & Flu

Brand name:

Drixoral Cold & Allergy

Pronounced: dricks-OR-al
*Generic ingredients: Dexbrompheniramine maleate, Pseudo-
  ephedrine sulfate*

What this drug is used for

Drixoral Cold & Allergy Sustained-Action Tablets temporarily relieve many of the symptoms of the common cold, inflamed sinuses, and allergies such as hay fever. They unclog stuffy nose and sinuses, and relieve runny nose, sneezing, itchy nose or throat, and itchy, watery eyes.

Unlike other Drixoral products, this formulation contains no acetaminophen.

How should you take this medication?

For adults and children 12 years and over, the usual dosage is 1 tablet every 12 hours. Do not take more than 2 tablets each 24 hours.

■ STORAGE
Store at room temperature in a dry place.

Do not take this medication if...

Unless your doctor approves, do not take Drixoral Cold & Allergy if you have heart disease, high blood pressure, thyroid disease, diabetes, high pressure within the eye (glaucoma), an enlarged prostate gland, or a breathing problem such as emphysema or chronic bronchitis.

Not for children under 12 without your doctor's approval.

Special warnings about this medication

If you become dizzy or nervous, or have trouble sleeping, stop taking Drixoral Cold & Allergy and check with your doctor.

You should also check with your doctor if your symptoms do not improve within 7 days or you have a fever.

This product may cause excitability, especially in children. It can also make you sleepy. Use caution when driving and when operating machinery.

Possible food and drug interactions when taking this medication

Do not use Drixoral Cold & Allergy within 2 weeks of taking a drug classified as an MAO inhibitor, such as the antidepressants **Nardil** and **Parnate**.

If you are taking a tranquilizer such as **Valium** or **Xanax**, or a sleep aid such as **Halcion** or **Seconal**, do not take Drixoral Cold & Allergy without your doctor's approval; the combination could cause extreme drowsiness. For the same reason, avoid alcohol while taking this product.

Brand name:

Drixoral Cold & Flu

Pronounced: dricks-OR-al
Generic ingredients: Acetaminophen, Dexbrompheniramine maleate,
*   Pseudoephedrine sulfate*
Other brand name: Drixoral Allergy/Sinus

What this drug is used for

Two products in the Drixoral line—Drixoral Cold & Flu and Drixoral Allergy/Sinus—share the same set of ingredients. The acetaminophen in these products temporarily relieves headache, fever, and minor aches and pains. The dexbrompheniramine component relieves sneezing, runny nose, itchy nose or throat, and itchy, watery eyes. The pseudoephedrine unclogs stuffy nose and sinuses.

Both products are 12-hour timed-release formulations.

How should you take this medication?

For adults and children 12 years and over, the usual dosage is 2 tablets every 12 hours. Do not use more than 4 tablets each 24 hours. For children under 12, consult your doctor.

■ STORAGE

Store at room temperature in a dry place.

Do not take this medication if...

Unless your doctor approves, do not take these products if you have heart disease, high blood pressure, thyroid disease, diabetes, high pressure within the eye (glaucoma), an enlarged prostate gland, or a breathing problem such as emphysema or chronic bronchitis.

Special warnings about this medication

If you become dizzy or nervous, or have trouble sleeping, stop taking Drixoral and check with your doctor.

Also check with your doctor if your symptoms do not improve within 7 days or you have a fever that lasts for more than 3 days or goes away and comes back.

If your pain or fever gets worse, if you have redness or swelling, or if you develop new symptoms, you could have a serious condition and should go to a doctor.

These products can cause excitability, especially in children. They can also make you drowsy. Use caution when driving and when operating machinery.

Possible food and drug interactions when taking this medication

Do not use these products within 2 weeks of taking a drug classified as an MAO inhibitor, such as the antidepressants **Nardil** and **Parnate**.

If you are taking a tranquilizer such as **Valium** or **Xanax**, or a sleep aid such as **Halcion** or **Seconal**, do not take these products without your doctor's approval; the combination could cause extreme drowsiness. For the same reason, avoid alcohol while taking this medication.

Brand name:

Drixoral Nasal Decongestant

See Sudafed

Brand name:

Dulcolax

See Correctol

Brand name:

Duration 12 Hour

See Afrin 12 Hour

Brand name:

Ecotrin

See Aspirin

Brand name:

Ex-Lax

Pronounced: EKS-laks
Generic ingredient: Sennosides

What this drug is used for

Ex-Lax relieves occasional constipation or irregular bowel movements, generally in 6 to 12 hours.

Ex-Lax comes in regular- and maximum-strength formulas, and in chocolated form.

How should you take this medication?

Take once or twice daily with a glass of water.

■ ADULTS

For adults and children 12 and over, each dose is 2 pills or chocolated pieces.

■ CHILDREN 6 TO 12

Each dose is 1 pill or chocolated piece.

■ CHILDREN UNDER 6

Consult your doctor.

Do not take this medication if...

Do not take a laxative when you have stomach pain, nausea, or vomiting. If you have noticed a sudden change in bowel habits lasting for 2 weeks or longer, check with your doctor before using any laxative.

Special warnings about this medication

Stop using this medicine and call your doctor if you develop rectal bleeding or fail to have a bowel movement after taking the medicine. You might have a serious condition.

Used too often or too long, laxatives can become habit-forming. Do not use any laxative for more than a week without your doctor's approval.

Brand name:

Ex-Lax Gentle Nature Laxative Pills

See Senokot

Brand name:

Ex-Lax Stool Softener

See Colace

Brand name:

Excedrin

Pronounced: ek-SED-rin
Generic ingredients: Acetaminophen, Aspirin, Caffeine

What this drug is used for

Excedrin provides temporary relief of headache, muscle aches, menstrual discomfort, toothache, and minor arthritis pain. It can also be used for the pain of colds and inflamed sinuses. It is available in tablets, caplets, and geltabs.

How should you take this medication?

For adults and children 12 years and over, the usual dose is 2 pills with water every 6 hours. Do not take more than 8 pills in 24 hours. For children under 12, consult your doctor.

Do not take this medication if...

Unless your doctor approves, do not use Excedrin if you are allergic to aspirin, or if you have asthma, ulcers, bleeding problems, or stomach problems—heartburn, upset stomach, or stomach pain—that do not get better or that go away and come back again.

Special warnings about this medication

The aspirin in Excedrin has been known to trigger a serious illness called Reye's syndrome in children and teenagers who catch a virus. If your child gets chickenpox or flu, do not treat the symptoms with Excedrin.

Do not take Excedrin for more than 10 days for pain or 3 days for fever, unless your doctor recommends. Call your doctor if you develop new symptoms, your pain or fever continues or gets worse, or you notice redness or swelling.

Do not take this product during the last 3 months of pregnancy. It could harm the baby or cause complications during delivery. Earlier during pregnancy, and while nursing a baby, check with your doctor before taking Excedrin.

If you develop ringing in the ears or a loss of hearing, stop taking this medicine and consult your doctor.

Possible food and drug interactions
when taking this medication

The aspirin and acetaminophen in Excedrin can interact with a number of prescription drugs. Check with your doctor before combining Excedrin with any of the following:

Acetazolamide (**Diamox**)
ACE-inhibitor-type blood pressure medications such as **Capoten**
Anti-gout drugs such as **Anturane, Benemid,** and **Zyloprim**
Arthritis preparations such as **Aleve, Anaprox, Ecotrin, Indocin, Motrin, Naprosyn,** and **Orudis**
Blood-thinning drugs such as **Coumadin**
Certain diuretics (water pills), including **Lasix**
Cholestyramine (**Questran**)
Diabetes medications, including **DiaBeta, Diabinese, Micronase,** and **Glucotrol**
Diltiazem (**Cardizem**)
Dipyridamole (**Persantine**)
Isoniazid (**Nydrazid**)
Oral contraceptives
Seizure medications such as **Depakene** and **Dilantin**
Steroids such as prednisone (**Deltasone, Orasone**)
Zidovudine (**Retrovir**)

Heavy drinking plus large doses of the acetaminophen in this product can lead to liver problems. If you drink more than 3 alcoholic beverages a day, check with your doctor before taking Excedrin.

Overdosage
Symptoms of Excedrin overdose include sweating, a generally uneasy feeling, nausea, and vomiting. If you suspect an overdose, seek medical help immediately.

Brand name:

Excedrin P.M.

Pronounced: Ek-SED-rin
Generic ingredients: Acetaminophen, Diphenhydramine citrate

What this drug is used for
Excedrin P.M. can be used for temporary relief of occasional headaches and minor aches and pains accompanied by sleeplessness.

The product is available in tablet, caplet, or geltab form.

How should you take this medication?

The usual dose for adults and children 12 and over is 2 pills at bedtime.

■ STORAGE

Store at room temperature.

Do not take this medication if...

Unless your doctor approves, do not take this medication if you have high pressure within the eye (glaucoma), an enlarged prostate gland, or a breathing problem such as emphysema or chronic bronchitis.

Do not give to children under 12 without your doctor's approval.

Special warnings about this medication

Do not take Excedrin P.M. for more than 10 days unless your doctor approves. If symptoms continue or get worse, if new ones crop up, or if you have trouble sleeping every night for more than 2 weeks, call your doctor. Sleeplessness sometimes signals a serious illness.

Possible food and drug interactions
when taking this medication

Check with your doctor before combining Excedrin P.M. with other sleep aids such as **Ambien** and **Halcion**, or with tranquilizers such as **Valium** and **Xanax**. You should also avoid alcoholic beverages while taking this product.

Overdosage

Massive doses of the acetaminophen in Excedrin P.M. can cause liver damage. Early signs of acetaminophen overdose include nausea, vomiting, sweating, and general discomfort.

If you suspect an overdose, seek immediate medical attention *even if you don't have symptoms*. To prevent liver damage, the drug must be cleared from your system quickly.

Brand name:

Excedrin, Aspirin Free

Pronounced: ek-SED-rin
Generic ingredients: Acetaminophen, Caffeine

What this drug is used for

This type of Excedrin contains acetaminophen instead of aspirin. It provides temporary relief from the minor pain of headache, toothache, inflamed sinuses, colds, muscular aches, menstrual discomfort, and arthritis. It comes in caplets and geltabs.

How should you take this medication?

The usual dose is 2 pills every 6 hours. Do not take more than 8 pills each 24 hours. For children under 12, consult a doctor.

■ STORAGE
Store at room temperature.

Special warnings about this medication

Do not take this product for more than 10 days for pain, or 3 days for fever without your doctor's approval. If your pain or fever won't go away or gets worse, if you develop new symptoms, or if you notice any redness or swelling, check with your doctor; you might have a serious condition.

Possible food and drug interactions when taking this medication

Combined with heavy drinking, the acetaminophen in this product could conceivably cause liver damage. Check with your doctor before taking this product if you generally have more than 3 alcoholic beverages a day.

Overdosage

A massive overdose of acetaminophen can harm the liver. Early symptoms of a potentially harmful overdose may include nausea and vomiting, sweating, and a generally uneasy feeling. If you suspect an overdose, seek medical attention immediately.

Brand name:

Femstat 3

Pronounced: FEM-stat
Generic name: Butoconazole nitrate

What this drug is used for

Femstat 3 cures most vaginal yeast infections in 3 days.

How should you take this medication?

■ DISPOSABLE CARDBOARD APPLICATOR
First familiarize yourself with the applicator: Pull the ends apart until you see an arrow pointing to the "full" line (see Step 3 below), then push the applicator back together.

Now follow these steps:

1. Open the tube of cream by removing the cap, turning it upside down, and using its point to puncture the protective seal on the tube.

2. Push the white end of the applicator over the opening of the tube until secure.

3. Slowly squeeze the tube until you see the "full" line on the applicator appear.

4. Remove the applicator from the tube of cream and use immediately.

5. Lie down with your knees bent. Hold the applicator with your thumb and forefinger, and, beginning with the white end, gently insert the applicator into your vagina as far as it will comfortably go.

6. Slowly push the blue end of the applicator in as far as it will go.

7. Remove the cardboard applicator and throw it away. (Do not flush it down the toilet). Some cream may be left in the applicator; but if you pushed the blue end until it stopped, you will have gotten the proper dosage.

Repeat for the next 2 days, preferably at bedtime.

■ PRE-FILLED APPLICATOR

1. Tear open the foil wrapper and remove 1 applicator. Do not take off the special tip on the end and do not use the applicator if the tip has been removed. Do not warm the applicator before using.

2. While holding the applicator firmly, pull the ring back to fully extend the plunger.

3. Lie down with your knees bent. Holding the applicator by the outer cylinder with your thumb and forefinger, insert the applicator into your vagina as far as it will comfortably go.

4. Push the plunger to release the cream.

5. Remove the applicator and throw it away. Some cream may be left in the applicator, but if you pushed the plunger until it stopped, you will have gotten the proper dosage.

Repeat for the next 2 days, preferably at bedtime.

■ STORAGE

Protect from excessive heat (above 86 degrees) and from freezing.

Do not take this medication if...

Do not use Femstat 3 if you have stomach pain, fever, or a foul-smelling discharge. Instead, see your doctor.

If you even think you may be pregnant, avoid using Femstat. Likewise, avoid this product if you have diabetes or have tested positive for HIV, the virus that causes AIDS.

If you are sensitive to any Femstat product, do not use Femstat 3 without first checking with your doctor. Also check with your doctor if you've never had vaginal itching and discomfort before.

Not for use by girls under 12.

Special warnings about this medication

Do not use tampons while using this product.

If your infection is not gone in 3 days, call your doctor. You may have a condition other than a yeast infection or you may need to use more medication. Also check with your doctor if your symptoms return within 2 months, or you think you may have been exposed to HIV. Repeated infections may be a sign of pregnancy or a serious condition such as AIDS or diabetes.

Femstat 3 can damage condoms and diaphragms and may cause them to fail. Use another form of birth control during treatment with Femstat 3.

Femstat 3 is for use only in the vagina; do not put it in your eyes or mouth.

Brand name:

FiberCon

Pronounced: FY-bur-con
Generic name: Calcium polycarbophil
Other brand name: Konsyl Fiber Tablets

What this drug is used for

Both FiberCon and Konsyl Fiber Tablets help restore and maintain regular bowel movements in people who are constipated.

Konsyl Tablets are also used to treat irritable bowel syndrome and, with other drugs, to relieve the constipation that sometimes accompanies diverticular disease (a pouch in the wall of the bowel), pregnancy, convalescence, and old age. Konsyl Tablets can also ease bowel movements in people suffering from hemorrhoids.

FiberCon is available in caplet form, Konsyl as tablets.

How should you take this medication?

Take these products with a full 8-ounce glass of water or other liquid. The dosage required will vary according to your diet, exercise, previous laxative use, and degree of constipation. You can expect results in 12 to 72 hours.

■ ADULTS

For adults and children over 12, the usual dosage is 2 pills taken 1 to 4 times a day.

■ CHILDREN

For children 6 to 12, the usual dosage is 1 pill taken 1 to 4 times a day (FiberCon) or 1 to 3 times a day (Konsyl). For children under 6, consult your doctor.

■ STORAGE

Store at room temperature. Protect from moisture.

Do not take this medication if...

Avoid these products if you have trouble swallowing. Also avoid them if you have an intestinal blockage or impacted stool. Check with your doctor *before* taking them if you have stomach pain, nausea, or vomiting, or have noticed a sudden change in bowel habits lasting 2 weeks or more.

Special warnings about this medication

Be sure to take each dose with a full glass of liquid. If you don't take enough liquid, the product could choke you.

If you have chest pain, vomiting, or difficulty swallowing or breathing after taking one of these products, see a doctor immediately.

If you don't have a bowel movement within 12 to 72 hours, or you notice bleeding from the rectum, stop taking the medication and call your doctor. Do not take either product for more than a week without your doctor's approval.

**Possible food and drug interactions
when taking this medication**

Take these products at least 1 hour before or 2 hours after taking a tetracycline antibiotic such as **Achromycin V** or **Sumycin**.

Brand name:

Fleet Sof-Lax

See Colace

Brand name:

Fleet Sof-Lax Overnight

See Doxidan

Brand name:

Fletcher's Castoria

See Senokot

Brand name:

4-Way Fast Acting Nasal Spray

*Generic ingredients: Naphazoline hydrochloride, Phenylephrine
hydrochloride, Pyrilamine maleate*

What this drug is used for

This product gives temporary relief of stuffy nose caused by colds, inflamed sinuses, hay fever, or other allergies.

How should you take this medication?

Metered Pump: Remove the cap and hold the bottle with your thumb at the base and the nozzle between your first and second fingers. With your head held upright, insert the nozzle into your nostril. Push the pump all the way down with a firm, even stroke and sniff deeply. Repeat in your other nostril. Do not tilt your head back while spraying. Wipe the tip clean after each use. Before using the first time, remove the cap and prime the pump by depressing it firmly several times.

Atomizer Spray: Hold your head in a normal upright position and place the atomizer tip in your nostril. Give the bottle a firm, quick squeeze while inhaling.

■ ADULTS
Spray twice into each nostril not more than every 6 hours.

■ SPECIAL STORAGE RECOMMENDATIONS
Store at room temperature.

Do not take this medication if...
Unless your doctor approves, do not use this product if you have diabetes, heart disease, high blood pressure, thyroid disease, or an enlarged prostate gland.

Do not give 4-Way Fast Acting Nasal Spray to children under 12.

Special warnings about this medication
Do not use more than the recommended dose; burning, stinging, sneezing, or increased runny nose could result. Do not use this product for more than 3 days. If your symptoms continue, contact your doctor. Do not share this medication, since this could spread infection.

Brand name:
4-Way 12 Hour

See Afrin 12 Hour

Brand name:
Gas-X

Generic name: Simethicone

What this drug is used for
Gas-X relieves the bloating, pressure, and fullness that result from gas. Similar products with the active ingredient simethicone include Maalox Anti-Gas, Mylanta Gas Relief, Phazyme, and Infants' Mylicon.

Regular-strength Gas-X comes in chewable tablet form. Extra-strength Gas-X is available in chewable tablets and softgel capsules.

How should you take this medication?

Take 1 or 2 pills as needed after meals and at bedtime. Chew tablets thoroughly. Swallow capsules whole with water. Unless directed by your doctor, do not take more than 6 regular-strength pills or 4 extra-strength pills each day.

Special warnings about this medication

If your condition does not clear up, contact your doctor.

Brand name:

Gaviscon

See Maalox

Brand name:

Goody's

Pronounced: GOOD-eez
Generic ingredients: Acetaminophen, Aspirin, Caffeine

What this drug is used for

The two Goody's products—Extra Strength Headache Powder and Extra Strength Pain Relief Tablets—share the same set of ingredients. (The Headache Powder is double the strength of the Pain Relief Tablets.)

The ingredients reduce fever and provide temporary relief from minor aches and pains such as headaches, arthritis pain, backaches, muscle strain, menstrual discomfort, toothaches, and the discomforts of colds and flu.

How should you take this medication?

Dosages are for adults and children 12 years and over. Do not take more than 4 doses each 24 hours. For children under 12, consult your doctor.

■ HEADACHE POWDER

Place 1 powder on your tongue and follow with liquid (or stir the powder into a glass of water or other liquid). You may repeat this dosage every 4 to 6 hours.

■ PAIN RELIEF TABLETS

Swallow 2 tablets with water or other liquid every 4 to 6 hours.

Do not take this medication if...

Avoid Goody's if you are allergic to aspirin.

Special warnings about this medication

When given to a child who has a virus, the aspirin in this product can trigger a rare but serious illness called Reye's Syndrome. Do not give Goody's to children or teenagers who have chickenpox or flu.

Avoid Goody's during the last 3 months of pregnancy. The aspirin it contains could harm the unborn child or cause problems during delivery. Earlier during pregnancy, and while nursing, check with your doctor before taking this product.

If your pain continues for more than 10 days, or if you develop redness, call your doctor immediately.

Possible food and drug interactions when taking this medication

Combined with heavy drinking, the acetaminophen in this product could conceivably cause liver damage. Check with your doctor before taking this product if you generally have more than 3 alcoholic beverages a day.

Brand name:

Halfprin

See Aspirin

Brand name:

Halls Cough Suppressant

Pronounced: Hawlz
Generic name: Menthol
Other brand names: Cepacol Sore Throat Lozenges, N'Ice, Vicks
  Cough Drops, Vicks Chloraseptic Cough & Throat Drops

What this drug is used for

These products relieve minor throat irritation, sore throat, and coughing due to colds or irritants. They come in a variety of strengths and flavors.

How should you take this medication?

Dissolve the lozenges slowly in your mouth.

■ HALLS

For most varieties, the usual dosage is 1 lozenge an hour. Give 2 Halls Juniors, one at a time, each hour. If you are taking Halls Plus for sore throat, take 1 or 2 lozenges every 2 hours. For children under 5, consult your doctor.

■ CEPACOL SORE THROAT LOZENGES

The usual dosage is 1 lozenge every 2 hours. Check with your doctor for children under 6.

■ N'ICE

The usual dosage is 1 lozenge an hour up to a maximum of 10 lozenges a day. For children under 6, check with your doctor.

■ VICKS COUGH DROPS

The usual dose is 2 menthol or 3 cherry lozenges. Repeat every hour for cough, or every 2 hours for sore throat. Check with your doctor for children under 5.

■ VICKS CHLORASEPTIC COUGH & THROAT DROPS

The usual dose is 1 lozenge. Repeat every hour for cough, or every 2 hours for sore throat. Check with your doctor for children under 5.

Do not take this medication if...

Unless your doctor approves, do not use these products for the type of chronic cough that results from smoking, asthma, or emphysema, or for a cough that brings up lots of phlegm.

Special warnings about this medication

You should check with your doctor immediately if you have a severe sore throat that lasts for more than 2 days, or if your sore throat is accompanied or followed by fever, headache, rash, nausea, or vomiting.

Likewise, call your doctor if you have a cough that lasts for more than 7 days or tends to come back, or a cough accompanied by rash, lasting headache, and fever. This could be a sign of a serious condition.

If you've been told to take N'Ice for a sore mouth, call your doctor or dentist immediately if there is no improvement in 7 days, or irritation, pain, or redness gets worse. Remember, too, that taking too many of these lozenges can have a laxative effect.

Brand name:

Imodium A-D

Pronounced: ih-MODE-ee-um
Generic name: Loperamide hydrochloride
Other brand names: Diarrid, Pepto Diarrhea Control

What this drug is used for:

These products control diarrhea. Imodium A-D is available in caplet and liquid form. Diarrid and Pepto Diarrhea Control come only in caplets.

How should you take this medication?

Diarrhea can quickly lead to dehydration. Drink plenty of water or other clear liquids until the problem clears up.

■ ADULTS
Caplets
The usual dosage is 2 caplets after your first loose bowel movement and 1 caplet after each loose movement thereafter. Do not take more than 4 caplets each 24 hours unless your doctor directs.

Liquid
The usual dose is 4 teaspoonfuls after your first loose bowel movement and 2 teaspoonfuls after each loose movement thereafter. Do not take more than 8 teaspoonfuls each 24 hours unless your doctor directs.

■ CHILDREN 6 TO 11 YEARS OLD
Caplets
The usual dose is 1 caplet after the first loose bowel movement and one-half caplet after each loose movement thereafter. Children 9 to 11 should not take more than 3 caplets a day; children aged 6 to 8 should take no more than 2 caplets.

Liquid
Give 2 teaspoonfuls after the first loose bowel movement and 1 teaspoonful after each loose movement that follows. The total daily dosage for children 9 to 11 should not be more than 6 teaspoonfuls; for children 6 to 8 the maximum is 4 teaspoonfuls.

■ CHILDREN 2 TO 5 YEARS OLD
Children this age should take only Imodium A-D liquid. The usual dose is 1 teaspoonful after the first loose bowel movement and 1 tea-

spoonful after each additional loose movement. Do not give a child this young more than 3 teaspoonfuls a day.

Do not take this medication if...
■ You have a fever higher than 101 degrees Fahrenheit.
■ You notice blood or mucus in your bowel movement.
■ Any other product containing loperamide hydrochloride has given you hives or a severe allergic reaction.

Special warnings about this medication
Do not use this medication for more than 2 days without your doctor's approval.

If you are taking antibiotics or have a history of liver disease, check with your doctor before taking any of these products.

Overdosage:
■ *Symptoms of overdose with one of these products may include:* Constipation, nausea, stupor

If you suspect an overdose, seek medical attention immediately.

Brand name:

Infants' Mylicon

Pronounced: MY-lick-on
Generic name: Simethicone

What this drug is used for
Infants' Mylicon relieves the bloating, pressure, and fullness that result from gas. Similar products with the active ingredient simethicone include Gas-X, Maalox Anti-Gas, Mylanta Gas Relief, and Phazyme.

How should you take this medication?
Do not exceed 12 doses a day unless your doctor directs.

■ ADULTS AND CHILDREN
Take 0.6 milliliters 4 times a day after meals and at bedtime.

■ INFANTS UNDER 2 YEARS OF AGE
Give 0.3 milliliters 4 times a day after meals and at bedtime. For easier administration, the dose may be mixed with 1 ounce of cool water, infant formula, or other liquid.

Special warnings about this medication

If the condition does not clear up, contact your doctor.

Brand name:

Kaopectate

Pronounced: KAY-oh-PECK-tayt
Generic name: Attapulgite
Other brand names: Donnagel, Rheaban

What this drug is used for

This medicine relieves diarrhea and cramping. Kaopectate is available in liquid and caplets, Donnagel in liquid and chewable tablets, Rheaban in caplets.

How should you take this medication?

For best results, take the full recommended dose at the first sign of diarrhea and after each subsequent bowel movement, up to a maximum of 6 doses each 24 hours (for Donnagel, 7 doses). Swallow caplets whole with water. Chew the chewable tablets thoroughly.

■ ADULTS AND CHILDREN 12 YEARS AND OVER
2 pills or tablespoonfuls.

■ CHILDREN 6 TO 12
1 pill or tablespoonful.

■ CHILDREN 3 TO 6
Half a chewable tablet or tablespoonful.

■ STORAGE
Store at room temperature.

Do not take this medication if...

Unless your doctor approves, do not give caplets to children under 6 or liquid or chewable tablets to children under 3. Do not use a product if it has caused an allergic reaction; and avoid these products if you have a high fever.

Special warnings about this medication

Limit use to 2 days. If diarrhea doesn't improve, call your doctor.

Brand name:

Kondremul

Pronounced: KON-druh-mul
Generic name: Mineral oil

What this drug is used for

Kondremul is used to relieve occasional constipation. It usually produces a bowel movement within 6 to 8 hours.

How should you take this medication?

Shake the bottle well. You can take the full dose all at once, or divide it into smaller doses; but do not take with meals.

■ ADULTS

For adults and children over 12, the usual dosage is 2 to 5 *table*spoonfuls.

■ CHILDREN

For children 6 to 12, the usual dosage is 2 to 5 *tea*spoonfuls.

■ STORAGE

Store at room temperature.

Do not take this medication if...

If you are pregnant, have trouble swallowing, or must remain in bed, do not take this product. If you have stomach pain, nausea, or vomiting, or you've noticed a sudden change in bowel habits lasting for 2 weeks or longer, check with your doctor before taking the product.

Not for children under 6.

Special warnings about this medication

Stop using Kondremul and call your doctor if you develop rectal bleeding or fail to have a bowel movement after taking the medicine. You might have a serious condition.

Used too often or too long, laxatives can become habit-forming. Do not use any laxative for more than a week without your doctor's approval.

Possible food and drug interactions
when taking this medication

Do not take this product if you are taking a stool softener laxative such as **Colace**, **Dialose**, or **Fleet Sof-Lax**.

Brand name:

Konsyl Fiber Tablets

See FiberCon

Brand name:

Konsyl Powder

See Metamucil

Brand name:

Legatrin PM

See Tylenol PM

Brand name:

Maalox

Pronounced: MAY-locks
Generic ingredients: Aluminum hydroxide, Magnesium
Other brand name: Gaviscon

What this drug is used for

Maalox and Gaviscon relieve acid indigestion, heartburn, and sour or upset stomach. The products come in a variety of strengths, including Maalox Suspension, Maalox Heartburn Relief Suspension (a weaker version), Gaviscon Liquid, Gaviscon Extra Strength Liquid, Gaviscon Tablets, Gaviscon-2 (double strength) Tablets, and Gaviscon Extra Strength Tablets.

How should you take this medication?

■ LIQUIDS

The usual dosage is 2 to 4 teaspoonfuls taken 4 times a day (for Gaviscon Liquid, 1 or 2 tablespoonfuls). Shake the bottle well and measure the dose with a spoon or other measuring device. Do not take more than 16 teaspoonfuls each 24 hours (for Gaviscon Liquid, 8 tablespoonfuls).

■ TABLETS

The usual dosage is 2 to 4 tablets taken 4 times a day. (For Gaviscon-2, the dose is 1 or 2 tablets.) Take the tablets after meals and at bedtime, or as needed. Chew the tablets; do not swallow them whole. Follow with half a glass of water or other liquid. Do not take more than 16 tablets each 24 hours. (For Gaviscon-2, the maximum is 8 tablets.)

■ STORAGE
Store at room temperature. Keep tightly closed. Protect liquids from freezing. Store tablets in a dry place.

Do not take this medication if...

Avoid these products if you have kidney disease. Do not use Gaviscon if you are on a salt-restricted diet.

Special warnings about this medication

Do not use the maximum dosage of either of these products for more than 2 weeks without your doctor's approval. Prolonged use of aluminum antacids can lead to loss of appetite, a general feeling of uneasiness, muscle weakness, and softened bones.

These products may have a laxative effect.

Possible food and drug interactions
when taking this medication

Antacids interact with a variety of prescription drugs when taken at the same time. However, an interaction is unlikely if you keep doses of the two at least 2 or 3 hours apart. Drugs that may interact include the following:

Alendronate (**Fosamax**)
Allopurinol (**Zyloprim**)
Antibiotics classified as quinolones, such as **Cipro**, **Floxin**, and
 Noroxin
Aspirin
Atenolol (**Tenormin**)
Captopril (**Capoten**)
Chlordiazepoxide (**Librium**)
Cimetidine (**Tagamet**)
Digoxin (**Lanoxin**)
Doxycycline (**Vibramycin**)
Fosfomycin (**Monurol**)
Gabapentin (**Neurontin**)
Glipizide (**Glucotrol**)
Glyburide (**Micronase**, **DiaBeta**)

Isoniazid (**Rifamate**)

Ketoconazole (**Nizoral**)

Levothyroxine (**Synthroid**)

Methenamine (**Urised**)

Metronidazole (**Flagyl**)

Misoprostol (**Cytotec**)

Mycophenolate mofetil (**CellCept**)

Nonsteroidal anti-inflammatory drugs such as **Dolobid, Motrin, Naprosyn**, and **Voltaren**

Penicillamine (**Cuprimine**)

Phenytoin (**Dilantin**)

Quinidine (**Quinidex**)

Sodium polystyrene sulfonate (**Kayexalate**)

Sucralfate (**Carafate**)

Tetracycline antibiotics such as **Achromycin V** and **Minocin**

Tilodronate (**Skelid**)

Ursodiol (**Actigall**)

A high-protein meal, such as a steak dinner, can reduce the effectiveness of aluminum-containing antacids such as Maalox and Gaviscon.

Brand name:

Maalox Antacid/Anti-Gas

Pronounced: MAY-locks
Generic ingredients: Aluminum hydroxide, Magnesium hydroxide, Simethicone

What this drug is used for

Maalox Antacid/Anti-Gas reduces the excess acid that accompanies such stomach problems as ulcer, inflammation, heartburn, and hiatal hernia (a weakening in the diaphragm above the stomach). It also relieves gas symptoms, including gas pain after surgery.

The product is available in regular and extra-strength tablets, and in extra-strength liquid.

How should you take this medication?

Chew tablets before swallowing.

■ REGULAR STRENGTH

The usual dose is 1 to 4 tablets 4 times a day. Do not take more than 16 tablets each 24 hours.

■ EXTRA STRENGTH

The usual dose is 1 to 3 tablets or 2 to 4 teaspoonfuls 4 times a day. Do not take more than 12 tablets or teaspoonfuls each 24 hours.

Do not take this medication if...

Unless your doctor approves, do not take this product if you have kidney disease.

Special warnings about this medication

Do not take the maximum dose for more than 2 weeks without your doctor's approval. Long-term use can cause a condition marked by loss of appetite, a generally uneasy feeling, muscle weakness, and weakened bones.

Possible food and drug interactions
when taking this medication

Antacids interact with a variety of prescription drugs when taken at the same time. An interaction is unlikely, however, if you keep doses of the two at least 2 or 3 hours apart. Drugs that may interact include the following:

Alendronate (**Fosamax**)

Allopurinol (**Zyloprim**)

Antibiotics classified as quinolones, such as **Cipro**, **Floxin**, and **Noroxin**

Aspirin

Atenolol (**Tenormin**)

Captopril (**Capoten**)

Chlordiazepoxide (**Librium**)

Cimetidine (**Tagamet**)

Digoxin (**Lanoxin**)

Doxycycline (**Vibramycin**)

Fosfomycin (**Monurol**)

Gabapentin (**Neurontin**)

Glipizide (**Glucotrol**)

Glyburide (**Micronase, DiaBeta**)

Isoniazid (**Rifamate**)

Ketoconazole (**Nizoral**)

Levothyroxine (**Synthroid**)

Methenamine (**Urised**)

Metronidazole (**Flagyl**)

Misoprostol (**Cytotec**)

Mycophenolate mofetil (**CellCept**)

Nonsteroidal anti-inflammatory drugs such as **Dolobid, Motrin, Naprosyn**, and **Voltaren**

Penicillamine (**Cuprimine**)

Phenytoin (**Dilantin**)

Quinidine (**Quinidex**)

Sodium polystyrene sulfonate (**Kayexalate**)

Sucralfate (**Carafate**)

Tetracycline antibiotics such as **Achromycin V** and **Minocin**

Tilodronate (**Skelid**)

Ursodiol (**Actigall**)

A high-protein meal, such as a steak dinner, can reduce the effectiveness of aluminum-containing antacids such as Maalox.

Brand name:

Maalox Anti-Gas

Pronounced: MAY-locks
Generic name: Simethicone

What this drug is used for

Maalox Anti-Gas tablets relieve the bloating, pressure, and fullness that result from gas. Similar products with the active ingredient simethicone include Gas-X, Mylanta Gas Relief, Phazyme, and Infants' Mylicon.

Maalox Anti-Gas tablets come in regular and extra strength.

How should you take this medication?

Chew tablets thoroughly. Dosage for both the regular- and extra-strength tablets is 1 or 2 tablets after meals or at bedtime, or as needed. Unless directed by your doctor, take no more than 3 extra-strength tablets or 6 regular-strength tablets each day.

Special warnings about this medication

If your condition does not clear up, contact your doctor.

Brand name:

Maltsupex

Pronounced: MALT-soup-ex
Generic name: Malt soup extract

What this drug is used for

Maltsupex relieves occasional constipation. It generally produces a bowel movement in 12 to 72 hours. The product is available in tablet, powder, and liquid forms.

How should you take this medication?

Maltsupex can be taken daily. Take the full dosage for 3 or 4 days until your constipation improves, then continue on a lower maintenance dosage as needed. Use the smallest dose that produces an effect, and lower the dosage as your condition clears up. Drink a full glass (8 ounces) of liquid with each dose.

■ ADULTS

The usual starting dose for adults and children 12 and over is up to 4 scoops of powder once or twice daily, 1 to 2 tablespoonfuls of liquid once or twice daily, or 4 tablets 4 times daily. Do not take more than 48 tablets a day.

■ CHILDREN

Age 6 to 12
The usual dose is up to 2 scoops of powder or 1 tablespoonful of liquid twice daily.

Age 2 to 6
The usual dose is 1 scoop of powder or half a tablespoonful of liquid twice daily.

Infants
The usual dose is 2 scoops of powder or 1 tablespoonful of liquid in water, fruit juice, or formula twice a day.

■ STORAGE

Store at room temperature. Protect the powder and tablets from moisture.

Do not take this medication if...

Unless your doctor approves, do not use Maltsupex if you have abdominal pain, nausea, or vomiting. Also check first with your doctor if you have noticed a sudden change in bowel habits lasting 2 weeks or longer.

If you are on a sodium-restricted diet, do not use the liquid form unless your doctor approves.

Special warnings about this medication

Laxative products should not be used for more than a week without your doctor's approval. If your constipation doesn't clear up, you should check with the doctor.

If you notice rectal bleeding or fail to have a bowel movement after using Maltsupex, stop taking it and call your doctor. These symptoms may signal a serious condition.

Brand name:

Maximum Strength Unisom

See Nytol

Brand name:

Metamucil

Pronounced: MET-uh-MEW-sil
Generic ingredients: Psyllium, Sennosides (Perdiem only)
Other brand names: Konsyl Powder, Perdiem

What this drug is used for

Metamucil, Konsyl Powder, and Perdiem, all of which are based on psyllium fiber, are used for constipation.

Metamucil and Konsyl Powder relieve chronic constipation and irritable bowel syndrome. Doctors also use them, along with other medications, to ease bowel movements in people with hemorrhoids and to treat the constipation that may accompany diverticular disease (a pouch in the wall of the bowel), occasional constipation during pregnancy, constipation during convalescence, and constipation in the very old. Metamucil is available in regular and smooth-texture powder form, as well as in wafers, in a variety of flavors. Konsyl Powder is sugar- and sugar substitute-free.

Perdiem products are used only for occasional constipation. Perdiem Fiber contains psyllium alone. Perdiem Plus Natural Vegetable Stimulant also contains sennosides. Both come in granule form.

How should you take this medication?

Take these products with at least 1 full glass (8 ounces) of water or other liquid. Expect results in 12 to 72 hours.

■ ADULTS AND CHILDREN 12 YEARS AND OVER

Metamucil

The usual dose is 2 wafers or 1 rounded tablespoonful of sugared Metamucil, 1 rounded teaspoonful of sugar-free Metamucil, or 1 packet mixed with 8 ounces of liquid. Start by taking 1 dose each day and gradually increase to 3 doses a day, if needed.

Konsyl

Place 1 rounded teaspoonful in a dry shaker cup or container that can be closed. Add 8 ounces of liquid and shake, don't stir, for 3 to 5 seconds. Drink promptly. If the mixture thickens, add more liquid and shake again. Follow with an 8-ounce glass of liquid. Take this dosage 1 to 3 times daily. To avoid bloating and to help your body adjust, you may wish to start with half-teaspoonful doses for several days, then increase the dose gradually over several more days.

Perdiem

Take 1 to 2 rounded teaspoonfuls in the evening and/or before breakfast. If your constipation is severe, you may take up to 2 rounded teaspoonfuls every 6 hours, but do not take more than 5 teaspoonfuls in 24 hours. Put the granules in your mouth and wash them down with a full glass of cool liquid. Do not chew them.

■ CHILDREN UNDER 12

Metamucil

Use half the adult dosage. For children under 6, consult your doctor.

Konsyl

Use half the adult dosage. For children under 6, consult your doctor.

Perdiem

The usual dosage is 1 rounded teaspoonful once or twice daily. For children under 7, consult your doctor.

■ STORAGE

Store at room temperature in a dry place.

Do not take this medication if...

Avoid these products if you have trouble swallowing, or have ever had an allergic reaction to psyllium. Also avoid them if you have an intestinal blockage or impacted stool. Check with your doctor *before* taking them if you have stomach pain, nausea, vomiting, or rectal bleeding, or have noticed a sudden change in bowel habits lasting 2 weeks or more.

Special warnings about this medication

Be sure to take each dose with at least 1 full glass of water. If you don't use enough liquid, the product could choke you.

If you have chest pain, vomiting, or difficulty in swallowing or breathing after taking one of these products, see your doctor immediately.

If you are still constipated after 1 week or notice rectal bleeding, stop taking the medication and call your doctor.

When handling Metamucil powder, spoon it into a glass according to the directions on the label in order to keep psyllium dust from escaping into the air.

Do not take one of these products less than 2 hours before or after taking a prescription drug. If you must avoid phenylalanine, do not use the smooth-texture, sugar-free, orange-flavored variety of Metamucil.

Brand name:

Midol Menstrual Formula

Pronounced: MY-dawl
Generic ingredients: Acetaminophen, Caffeine, Pyrilamine maleate

What this drug is used for

This type of Midol relieves menstrual symptoms such as cramps, bloating, headaches, backaches, muscle aches, fatigue, and weight gain caused by water retention. The product is available in caplet and gelcap form.

How should you take this medication?

Take 2 pills with water every 4 to 6 hours, as needed. Do not take more than 8 pills a day.

Do not take this medication if...

Unless your doctor approves, do not take this Midol formulation if you have high pressure within the eye (glaucoma) or a breathing problem such as emphysema or chronic bronchitis.

Midol is not intended for use by men or children.

Special warnings about this medication

Do not use Midol for more than 10 days. If pain lasts longer, call your doctor immediately.

The pyrilamine in this product can cause drowsiness. Until you know how the medication affects you, be careful when driving and when operating machinery.

This product may also cause excitability.

Possible food and drug interactions when taking this medication

If you are taking a tranquilizer such as Valium or Xanax, or a sleep aid such as Halcion or Seconal, do not take this type of Midol without your doctor's approval; the combination could cause extreme drowsiness. For the same reason, avoid alcohol while using this product.

A dose of Midol Menstrual Formula contains as much caffeine as a cup of coffee. To avoid the nervousness, irritability, sleeplessness, and rapid heartbeat that can come from too much caffeine, limit your use of caffeine-containing medicines, foods, and beverages while taking this product.

Brand name:

Midol PMS Formula

Pronounced: MY-dawl
Generic ingredients: Acetaminophen, Pamabrom, Pyrilamine maleate
Other brand name: Pamprin Multi-Symptom

What this drug is used for

Midol PMS and Multi-Symptom Pamprin relieve some of the problems commonly associated with premenstrual syndrome, including cramps, headaches, backaches, bloating, and weight gain caused by water retention.

Both products are available in caplets and gelcaps. Pamprin is also available in tablet form.

Another version of Pamprin—Maximum Pain Relief Pamprin—combats the same symptoms, but has a slightly different set of ingredients.

How should you take this medication?
The usual dosage is 2 pills with water every 4 to 6 hours as needed. Do not take more than 8 pills each 24 hours.

Do not take this medication if...
Unless your doctor approves, do not use these products if you have high pressure within the eye (glaucoma) or a breathing problem such as emphysema or chronic bronchitis.

These products are not intended for use by men or children.

Special warnings about this medication
Do not use these products for more than 10 days. If pain lasts longer, call your doctor immediately.

These products may make you sleepy. Be especially careful when driving and when operating machinery.

Both of these products may cause excitability.

Possible food and drug interactions
when taking this medication
If you are taking a tranquilizer such as **Valium** or **Xanax**, or a sleep aid such as **Halcion** or **Seconal**, do not take either of these products without your doctor's approval; the combination could cause extreme drowsiness. For the same reason, avoid alcohol.

Brand name:

Midol Teen Menstrual Formula

Pronounced: MY-dawl
Generic ingredients: Acetaminophen, Pamabrom

What this drug is used for
This type of Midol relieves menstrual symptoms such as cramps, headaches, backaches, muscle aches and pains, bloating, and weight gain caused by water retention. Unlike regular Midol Menstrual Formula, this

product contains no caffeine, which can cause nervousness, or pyrilamine, which can make you drowsy. It is available only in caplet form.

How should you take this medication?
The usual dosage is 2 caplets with water every 4 hours, as needed. Do not take more than 8 caplets a day.

Special warnings about this medication
Do not use Midol Teen Menstrual Formula for more than 10 days. If pain lasts longer, call your doctor immediately.

This product is not intended for men or children.

Brand name:
Motrin

See Advil

Brand name:
Mycelex-7

Pronounced: MY-sell-ex
Generic name: Clotrimazole

What this drug is used for
Mycelex-7 vaginal cream and inserts are used to treat vaginal yeast infections. Mycelex-7 external vulvar cream relieves yeast-related itching and irritation on the vaginal lips (the vulva). The vaginal cream is available with a reusable applicator, or a set of 7 disposable applicators. The vaginal inserts are available alone, or with the external vulvar cream.

How should you take this medication?
■ VAGINAL CREAM

Fill the applicator and insert one applicatorful of cream into the vagina, preferably at bedtime. Repeat this procedure daily for 7 consecutive days. If you are using a disposable applicator, throw it away after one use. (Do not flush it down the toilet.)

■ VAGINAL INSERTS

Unwrap one insert, put it in the applicator, and use the applicator to place the insert into the vagina, preferably at bedtime. Repeat daily for 7 consecutive days.

■ EXTERNAL VULVAR CREAM

Squeeze a small amount onto your finger and gently spread the cream over the irritated area of the vulva. Use 1 or 2 times a day for up to 7 days as needed.

■ STORAGE

Store at room temperature.

Do not take this medication if...

Do not use Mycelex-7 if you have stomach pain, fever, or a foul-smelling discharge. Instead, see your doctor.

Unless your doctor advises it, do not use Mycelex-7 during pregnancy. Also check with your doctor first if you've never had vaginal itching and discomfort before.

Not for use by girls under 12.

Special warnings about this medication

Do not use tampons while using this product.

If you do not improve in 3 days, or if you do not get well in 7 days, consult your doctor. You may have something other than a yeast infection.

Call your doctor if your symptoms return within 2 months, or if you have infections that do not clear up easily with proper treatment. You could be pregnant, or there might be a serious medical cause for your infections such as diabetes or damage to the immune system from HIV, the virus that causes AIDS.

Brand name:

Mylanta AR

See Pepcid AC

Brand name:

Mylanta Gas Relief

Pronounced: my-LAN-tuh
Generic name: Simethicone

What this drug is used for

Mylanta Gas Relief pills relieve the bloating, pressure, and fullness that result from gas. Similar products with the active ingredient simethicone include Gas-X, Maalox Anti-Gas, Phazyme, and Infants' Mylicon.

Mylanta Gas Relief chewable tablets come in regular and extra strengths. Regular-strength gelcaps are also available.

How should you take this medication?

■ TABLETS

Chew tablets thoroughly. Dosage for both the regular- and extra-strength tablets is 1 tablet 4 times a day after meals and at bedtime. Alternatively, you can take up to 6 regular-strength tablets as needed each day.

■ GELCAPS

Take 2 to 4 gelcaps as needed after meals and at bedtime. Unless directed by your doctor, do not take more than 8 gelcaps a day.

Special warnings about this medication

If your condition does not clear up, contact your doctor.

Brand name:

Mylanta Liquid

Pronounced: my-LAN-tuh
Generic ingredients: Aluminum hydroxide, Magnesium hydroxide,
  Simethicone

What this drug is used for

Mylanta liquid relieves acid indigestion, heartburn, and sour stomach, as well as gas from these conditions. You can also use Mylanta liquid to control excess acid associated with an ulcer, stomach inflammation, inflammation of the food canal (the esophagus), or a weakened stomach diaphragm (a hiatal hernia), and to relieve gas after surgery.

How should you take this medication?

Shake well before using. The usual dose is 2 to 4 teaspoonfuls between meals and at bedtime.

Do not take this medication if...

Avoid Mylanta liquid if you have kidney disease.

Special warnings about this medication

Unless directed by your doctor, do not take more than 24 teaspoonfuls of Mylanta liquid or 12 teaspoonfuls of Maximum-Strength Mylanta liquid each 24 hours. Do not use the maximum dose for more than 2 weeks.

Possible food and drug interactions
when taking this medication

Antacids interact with a variety of prescription drugs when taken at the same time. An interaction is unlikely, however, if you keep doses of the two at least 2 or 3 hours apart. Drugs that may interact include the following:

Alendronate (**Fosamax**)

Allopurinol (**Zyloprim**)

Antibiotics classified as quinolones, such as **Cipro**, **Floxin**, and **Noroxin**

Aspirin

Atenolol (**Tenormin**)

Captopril (**Capoten**)

Chlordiazepoxide (**Librium**)

Cimetidine (**Tagamet**)

Digoxin (**Lanoxin**)

Doxycycline (**Vibramycin**)

Fosfomycin (**Monurol**)

Gabapentin (**Neurontin**)

Glipizide (**Glucotrol**)

Glyburide (**Micronase, DiaBeta**)

Isoniazid (**Rifamate**)

Ketoconazole (**Nizoral**)

Levothyroxine (**Synthroid**)

Methenamine (**Urised**)

Metronidazole (**Flagyl**)

Misoprostol (**Cytotec**)

Mycophenolate mofetil (**CellCept**)

Nonsteroidal anti-inflammatory drugs such as **Dolobid**, **Motrin**, **Naprosyn**, and **Voltaren**

Penicillamine (**Cuprimine**)

Phenytoin (**Dilantin**)

Quinidine (**Quinidex**)

Sodium polystyrene sulfonate (**Kayexalate**)

Sucralfate (**Carafate**)

Tetracycline antibiotics such as **Achromycin V** and **Minocin**
Tilodronate (**Skelid**)
Ursodiol (**Actigall**)

A high-protein meal, such as a steak dinner, can reduce the effectiveness of aluminum-containing antacids such as Mylanta liquid.

Overdosage

Heavy long-term use of aluminum antacids can lead to symptoms such as loss of appetite, a general feeling of uneasiness, muscle weakness, and bone pain. If you suspect an overdose, call your doctor immediately.

Brand name:

Mylanta Soothing Lozenges

See Tums

Brand name:

Mylanta Tablets and Gelcaps

Pronounced: my-LAN-tuh
Generic ingredients: Calcium carbonate, Magnesium hydroxide

What this drug is used for

Mylanta tablets and gelcaps relieve heartburn, acid indigestion, and sour or upset stomach. You can also use them to control excess acid associated with an ulcer, stomach inflammation, inflammation of the food canal (the esophagus), or a weakened stomach diaphragm (a hiatal hernia).

Unlike Mylanta liquid, the tablets and gelcaps do not contain an anti-gas ingredient. If gas is also a problem, you may find the liquid preferable.

How should you take this medication?

Chew tablets thoroughly.

■ FAST-ACTING MYLANTA TABLETS
The usual dose is 2 to 4 tablets between meals and at bedtime. Do not take more than 20 tablets each 24 hours.

■ MAXIMUM STRENGTH FAST-ACTING MYLANTA TABLETS
The usual dose is 2 to 4 tablets between meals and at bedtime. Do not take more than 10 tablets each 24 hours.

■ MYLANTA GELCAPS
The usual dose is 2 to 4 gelcaps as needed. Do not take more than 24 gelcaps in a 24-hour period.

Do not take this medication if...
Unless your doctor directs, do not take Mylanta tablets or gelcaps if you have kidney disease.

Special warnings about this medication
Do not use the maximum dosage for more than 2 weeks.

Possible food and drug interactions
when taking this medication
Antacids interact with a variety of prescription drugs when taken at the same time. An interaction is unlikely, however, if you keep doses of the two at least 2 or 3 hours apart. Drugs that may interact include the following:

Alendronate (**Fosamax**)
Allopurinol (**Zyloprim**)
Antibiotics classified as quinolones, such as **Cipro**, **Floxin**, and
 Noroxin
Aspirin
Atenolol (**Tenormin**)
Captopril (**Capoten**)
Chlordiazepoxide (**Librium**)
Cimetidine (**Tagamet**)
Digoxin (**Lanoxin**)
Doxycycline (**Vibramycin**)
Fosfomycin (**Monurol**)
Gabapentin (**Neurontin**)
Glipizide (**Glucotrol**)
Glyburide (**Micronase, DiaBeta**)
Isoniazid (**Rifamate**)
Ketoconazole (**Nizoral**)
Levothyroxine (**Synthroid**)
Methenamine (**Urised**)

Metronidazole (**Flagyl**)

Misoprostol (**Cytotec**)

Mycophenolate mofetil (**CellCept**)

Nonsteroidal anti-inflammatory drugs such as **Dolobid, Motrin, Naprosyn,** and **Voltaren**

Penicillamine (**Cuprimine**)

Phenytoin (**Dilantin**)

Quinidine (**Quinidex**)

Sodium polystyrene sulfonate (**Kayexalate**)

Sucralfate (**Carafate**)

Tetracycline antibiotics such as **Achromycin V** and **Minocin**

Tilodronate (**Skelid**)

Ursodiol (**Actigall**)

Prolonged and heavy use of antacids such as Mylanta tablets or gel-caps, combined with a high intake of calcium-rich foods such as milk, can lead to an overload of calcium in the system. Early symptoms are constipation, weakness, nausea, and vomiting; a severe overload can cause kidney damage. If you need a high-calcium diet, check with your doctor about a substitute for this product.

Overdosage

An overdose of magnesium-containing antacids such as Mylanta tablets and gelcaps may be signaled by difficult or painful urination, dizziness or light-headedness, irregular heartbeat, mood shifts, and unusual fatigue. If you suspect an overdose, check with your doctor immediately.

Brand name:

Naphcon A

Pronounced: NAF-con
Generic ingredients: Naphazoline hydrochloride, Pheniramine maleate
Other brand name: OcuHist

What this drug is used for

Naphcon A and OcuHist eyedrops share the same pair of active ingredients. Both products temporarily relieve eye itchiness and redness caused by ragweed, pollen, grass, and animal hair and dander.

How should you use this medication?

Put 1 or 2 drops in the affected eye up to 4 times daily. Remove contact lenses before using. For children under 6, consult your doctor.

■ STORAGE

Store at room temperature away from light.

Do not use this medication if...

Unless your doctor approves, do not use these eyedrops if you have heart disease, high blood pressure, an enlarged prostate gland, or high pressure within the eye (glaucoma). Avoid these products if you've had a reaction to any of their ingredients.

Special warnings about this medication

If you experience eye pain, changes in vision, or continued redness or irritation—or if the condition gets worse or lasts more than 3 days—stop using the drops and call your doctor.

To avoid contaminating the eyedrops, do not touch the tip of the container to any surface. Replace the cap after using. If the solution becomes cloudy or changes color, do not use it.

Overdosage

Overuse of these products can make the redness worse. If an infant or child drinks the solution, it could lead to coma and a marked loss of body temperature.

Brand name:

Nasalcrom

Pronounced: NAY-zul-krohm
Generic name: Cromolyn sodium

What this drug is used for

Formerly available only by prescription, Nasalcrom both relieves and *prevents* symptoms of allergies such as hay fever. It works by blocking certain cells in the body from releasing substances that make the bronchial tubes tighten and constrict. It combats symptoms such as sneezing and runny, itchy, stuffy nose.

Unlike nonprescription antihistamines, this medication does not cause drowsiness. It comes in a nasal spray bottle.

How should you take this medication?

For adults and children 6 years and older, the usual dosage is 1 spray in each nostril every 4 to 6 hours, up to a maximum of 6 times a day.

Nasalcrom should be used daily as long as you are in contact with the cause of your allergy. It may be several days before you notice an effect, and 1 to 2 weeks before the effect reaches its peak. To *prevent* allergy symptoms, begin using the medication as much as a week before you expect to encounter the cause.

Use the pump spray as follows:

1. Blow your nose.
2. Remove the plastic cap and yellow safety clip.
3. Hold the pump with your thumb at the bottom and the nozzle between your fingers. (The first time you use the pump, or after not using it for 14 days, spray into the air until a fine mist appears.)
4. Insert the nozzle into a nostril and spray upward while breathing in through the nose.

■ STORAGE
Store at room temperature. Protect from light.

Do not take this medication if...

Nasalcrom is not for treatment of sinus infections, colds, or asthma. Check with your doctor before using the product if you have a fever, discolored nasal discharge, sinus pain, or wheezing.

Not for children under 6 unless your doctor recommends.

Special warnings about this medication

You may have a brief fit of sneezing or stinging immediately after using this drug.

Stop using this product and check with your doctor if your symptoms get worse or fail to improve after 2 weeks, or if any new symptoms develop.

Do not share the Nasalcrom bottle; this could spread germs.

Possible food and drug interactions
when taking this medication

Nasalcrom *can* be used with other medicines, including other allergy remedies.

Brand name:

Neo-Synephrine

Pronounced: NEE-oh-si-NEF-rin
Generic name: Phenylephrine hydrochloride
Other brand names: Afrin 4 Hour, Vicks Sinex

What this drug is used for

These products provide short-term relief of stuffy nose due to the common cold, inflamed sinuses, or allergies such as hay fever. All of these brands are also available in 12-hour formulations containing a different active ingredient. (*See Afrin 12 Hour.*)

All the products are available as nasal sprays. Neo-Synephrine is also available as nasal drops, and comes in three strengths: mild, regular, and extra. Vicks Sinex also offers an ultra-fine mist.

How should you take this medication?

The usual dose is 2 or 3 sprays or drops in each nostril every 4 hours. Neo-Synephrine Mild formula can be given to children 6 years and over. With all other formulations, consult a doctor for children under 12.

Spray quickly and firmly into the nostril and inhale deeply. Do not tilt the head backward while spraying. Wipe the nozzle clean after each use. Do not use more often than every 4 hours.

When using Vicks Sinex Ultra Fine Mist for the first time, you'll need to prime the pump by firmly depressing its rim several times. Then hold the container with your thumb at the base and the nozzle between your first and second fingers, insert the nozzle into your nostril, and spray.

■ STORAGE
Store at room temperature.

Do not take this medication if...

Unless your doctor approves, do not use these products if you have heart disease, high blood pressure, thyroid disease, diabetes, or an enlarged prostate gland.

Special warnings about this medication

These products may cause temporary burning, stinging, sneezing, or runny nose.

Do not use these products for more than 3 days. Frequent or prolonged use can make stuffy nose come back or get worse. If your symptoms do not clear up, call your doctor.

Do not share containers. This could spread infection.

Brand name:

Neo-Synephrine 12 Hour

See Afrin 12 Hour

Brand name:

Nephrox

Pronounced: NEF-rocks
Generic ingredients: Aluminum hydroxide, Mineral oil

What this drug is used for
Nephrox relieves symptoms caused by excess stomach acid, including heartburn, upset stomach, sour stomach, and acid indigestion. Because it is low in sodium and has no magnesium, Nephrox is especially recommended for kidney patients.

How should you take this medication?
The usual dose is 2 teaspoonfuls at bedtime.

Do not take this medication if...
Do not take while pregnant or nursing, or give to an infant, unless your doctor directs.

Special warnings about this medication
Take only at bedtime.

Possible food and drug interactions
when taking this medication
Antacids interact with a variety of prescription drugs when taken at the same time. An interaction is unlikely, however, if you keep doses of the two at least 2 or 3 hours apart. Drugs that may interact include the following:

Alendronate (**Fosamax**)
Allopurinol (**Zyloprim**)

Antibiotics classified as quinolones, such as **Cipro**, **Floxin**, and **Noroxin**

Aspirin

Atenolol (**Tenormin**)

Captopril (**Capoten**)

Chlordiazepoxide (**Librium**)

Cimetidine (**Tagamet**)

Digoxin (**Lanoxin**)

Doxycycline (**Vibramycin**)

Fosfomycin (**Monurol**)

Gabapentin (**Neurontin**)

Glipizide (**Glucotrol**)

Glyburide (**Micronase, DiaBeta**)

Isoniazid (**Rifamate**)

Ketoconazole (**Nizoral**)

Levothyroxine (**Synthroid**)

Methenamine (**Urised**)

Metronidazole (**Flagyl**)

Misoprostol (**Cytotec**)

Mycophenolate mofetil (**CellCept**)

Nonsteroidal anti-inflammatory drugs such as **Dolobid**, **Motrin**, **Naprosyn**, and **Voltaren**

Penicillamine (**Cuprimine**)

Phenytoin (**Dilantin**)

Quinidine (**Quinidex**)

Sodium polystyrene sulfonate (**Kayexalate**)

Sucralfate (**Carafate**)

Tetracycline antibiotics such as **Achromycin V** and **Minocin**

Tilodronate (**Skelid**)

Ursodiol (**Actigall**)

A high-protein meal, such as a steak dinner, can reduce the effectiveness of aluminum-containing antacids such as Nephrox.

Overdosage

Heavy long-term use of aluminum antacids can lead to symptoms such as loss of appetite, a general feeling of uneasiness, muscle weakness, and bone pain. If you suspect an overdose, call your doctor immediately.

Brand name:

N'Ice

See Halls Cough Suppressant

Brand name:

Nicoderm CQ

See Nicotine Patches

Brand name:

Nicorette

Pronounced: nick-oh-RET
Generic name: Nicotine polacrilex

What this drug is used for

Nicorette is a chewing gum that can help when you resolve to stop smoking. It reduces withdrawal symptoms such as a craving for nicotine. To increase your odds of success, use it together with a support program and the encouragement of friends and family.

How should you use this medication?

Stop smoking completely when you begin using Nicorette.

Do not eat or drink for 15 minutes before starting a piece of the gum, or while chewing it. To improve your chances of quitting, start off with at least 9 pieces of Nicorette a day. With each piece, follow these steps:

1. Chew the gum very slowly several times. Stop chewing when you notice a peppery taste or a slight tingling in your mouth. This usually happens after about 15 chews.
2. Park the piece of gum between your cheek and gum and leave it there.
3. When the peppery taste or tingle is almost gone (in about a minute), chew slowly a few more times. When the taste or tingle returns, stop again and park the gum in a different place in your mouth.
4. Repeat these steps until most of the nicotine is gone from the gum (the peppery taste or tingle will not return). This usually takes about half an hour. Then throw away the used gum.

Do not chew more than 24 pieces a day. Cut back gradually, following this 12-week schedule:

Weeks 1 through 6: Chew 1 piece every 1 to 2 hours.
Weeks 7 through 9: Chew 1 piece every 2 to 4 hours.
Weeks 10 through 12: Chew 1 piece every 4 to 8 hours.
End of Week 12: Stop using the product. If you still crave cigarettes and feel you need Nicorette to control this feeling, talk to your doctor.

■ STORAGE
Store below 86 degrees Fahrenheit. Keep away from light.

Do not take this medication if...
Unless your doctor approves, do not use this product if you have heart disease or an irregular heartbeat, or have recently had a heart attack. Nicotine can increase your heart rate.

Check with your doctor about using Nicorette if you have high blood pressure that is not being controlled with medication. Nicotine can raise blood pressure. Check, too, if you have a stomach ulcer. Nicotine can cause stomach problems.

Special warnings about this medication
Stop using this product and see your doctor if you develop an irregular or pounding heartbeat, or have symptoms of nicotine overdose such as nausea, vomiting, dizziness, weakness, and a rapid heartbeat. Also stop use and see your doctor if you have mouth, tooth, or jaw problems.

If you chew the gum too fast or don't chew correctly, it can cause hiccups, heartburn, and stomach problems. Other side effects of nicotine include headache, nausea, and dizziness.

Although Nicorette reduces nicotine withdrawal symptoms, you may still have brief episodes. The symptoms include edginess, trouble concentrating, upset stomach, headaches, muscle aches, constipation, fatigue, insomnia, and a worsened cough.

If you are under 18 and wish to stop smoking, talk to your doctor about using Nicorette gum. It can't be sold over the counter to those under 18.

If you are pregnant or nursing a baby, check with your doctor before using this product. Nicorette can increase the baby's heart rate.

Possible food and drug interactions
when taking these medications

Do not smoke and use Nicorette at the same time. Also avoid using chewing tobacco, snuff, nicotine patches, and other nicotine-containing products while using the gum.

If you take a prescription medicine for depression or asthma, make sure your doctor knows you are giving up smoking. Your medication dosage may need to be adjusted. Do not use Nicorette if you must take insulin for diabetes.

Coffee, juice, wine, and soft drinks can reduce Nicorette's effectiveness.

Overdosage

■ *Symptoms of Nicorette overdose may include:*
Weakness, diarrhea, vomiting

In a child, the product could even cause seizures. If you suspect an overdose, seek medical attention immediately.

Category:

Nicotine Patches

Brand names: Nicoderm CQ, Nicotrol

What this drug is used for

Nicotine patches are designed to help smokers give up the habit by reducing withdrawal symptoms such as nervousness, irritability, and the craving for tobacco.

While you wear the patch, a small amount of nicotine steadily travels out of the patch, through your skin, and into your bloodstream, keeping a constant low level of nicotine in your body. Although cigarettes deliver higher levels of nicotine in sudden bursts, the lower level maintained by the patch may be enough to eliminate your craving for cigarettes.

Two brands are available over the counter. Nicoderm CQ permits a stepwise reduction in nicotine levels by providing patches in 3 strengths: 21 milligrams (Step 1), 14 milligrams (Step 2), and 7 milligrams (Step 3). Nicotrol offers a simpler regimen with a single 15-milligram strength.

How should you take this medication?

Stop smoking completely when you begin using the patch.

Remove the backing from the patch and immediately press it onto your outer upper arm or any clean, dry, hairless skin on your trunk. (Do not apply it to broken, burned, or irritated areas.) Hold it in place with the heel of your hand for 10 seconds. If the patch won't stick, try using medical adhesive tape over it. When finished, wash your hands. Any nicotine sticking to your fingers could get into your eyes or nose, causing irritation.

Each day, apply a new patch to a different place on your skin. To reduce the chances of irritation, do not return to a previously used spot for at least a week. To prevent loss of nicotine, do not remove the patch from its sealed protective pouch until you are ready to apply it. If the pouch is unsealed, do not use the patch.

As a memory aid, pick a specific time of day and always apply a fresh patch at that time. You may change the schedule if you need to. Just remember not to wear any single patch for more than the recommended time. After that time, the patch will begin to lose strength and could start irritating your skin. If you miss a dose, apply the patch as soon as you remember. Never use 2 patches at once.

■ NICODERM CQ
Use 1 patch a day. Leave it on for 16 hours. If you crave cigarettes when you wake up, wear it for 24 hours.

Light smokers (10 cigarettes a day or less)
Use "Step 2" patches (14 milligrams) for 6 weeks and "Step 3" patches (7 milligrams) for 2 weeks; then stop.

Heavy smokers (more than 10 cigarettes a day)
Use "Step 1" patches (21 milligrams) for 6 weeks, "Step 2" patches (14 milligrams) for 2 weeks, and "Step 3" patches (7 milligrams) for 2 weeks; then stop.

■ NICOTROL
Use 1 patch a day for 6 weeks. Leave it on all day (16 hours); remove it at bedtime.

■ STORAGE
Store your supply of patches at temperatures no higher than 86 degrees Fahrenheit; remember that in warm weather the inside of a car can get much hotter than this.

Do not take this medication if...

Do not smoke, chew tobacco, take snuff, or use nicotine gum while using the patch.

Unless your doctor approves, do not use the patch if you have heart disease or an irregular heartbeat, or have recently had a heart attack. Nicotine can increase your heart rate.

Also check with your doctor if you have high blood pressure that is not being controlled with medication. Nicotine can raise blood pressure. Check, too, if you have a stomach ulcer. Nicotine can cause stomach problems.

If you are allergic to adhesive tape or bandages, or have any other skin problem, the patch may not be right for you. Ask your doctor before you proceed.

Special warnings about this medication

Stop using the patch and see your doctor if you develop:

■ Redness where a patch was applied that lasts for 4 days or more
■ Swelling or a rash on your skin
■ Irregular or pounding heartbeat
■ Nausea, vomiting, dizziness, weakness, or rapid heartbeat. These are symptoms of nicotine overdose.

If you begin to have vivid dreams or other disruptions of your sleep, be sure to remove the patch at bedtime.

Do not smoke after removing a patch. The nicotine from the patch will already be in your skin, and will continue to reach the bloodstream for several hours.

If you are taking prescription medicine for depression or asthma, make sure your doctor knows that you are giving up smoking. Your dosage may need to be adjusted.

If you are pregnant or nursing, remember that the nicotine from the patch can increase your baby's heart rate. When a baby is involved, it is best to quit smoking without taking nicotine in other forms. If this proves impossible, talk with your doctor.

If you are under 18 and wish to stop smoking, talk to your doctor about using the patch. It can't be sold over the counter to those under 18.

If you use soap containing lanolin or moisturizers, the patch may not stick well. Also, do not apply body creams, lotions, or sunscreens to the area where the patch will be applied.

Water will not harm a Nicoderm CQ patch; you can bathe, swim, shower or use a hot tub for short periods while wearing it. If your patch falls off, apply a new one on a clean, dry, non-hairy, non-irritated area of skin.

You may feel some mild itching, burning, or tingling when you first put on the patch. This is normal and should disappear within 1 hour. You may also notice redness on the skin under the patch after it's removed. The redness should disappear within a day.

For safety, dispose of used patches by folding them in half and throwing them into a trash container that cannot be reached by children or pets. If you are using Nicoderm CQ, insert the used patch in the disposal tray provided in the box.

Nicotine, from any source, can be poisonous and addictive. Do not use the patches for longer than the recommended period. If you still feel the need for a patch after you have finished your program, talk with your doctor.

Possible food and drug interactions when taking this medication
Ask your doctor before using nicotine patches if you are taking:

Acetaminophen-containing drugs such as **Tylenol** and **Panadol**
Caffeine-containing drugs such as **No Doz**
Certain airway-opening drugs such as **Isuprel**, **Dristan**, and **Neo-Synephrine**
Certain blood pressure medicines such as **Minipress**, **Trandate**, and **Normodyne**
Cimetidine (**Tagamet**)
Haloperidol (**Haldol**)
Imipramine (**Tofranil**)
Insulin
Lithium drugs including **Lithonate**
Oxazepam (**Serax**)
Pentazocine (**Talwin**)
Propranolol (**Inderal**)
Theophylline (**Theo-Dur**)

Overdosage

■ *Symptoms of nicotine overdose may include:*
Abdominal pain, diarrhea, dizziness, nausea, pounding or rapid heartbeat, sweating, vomiting, weakness

If you suspect an overdose, seek medical attention immediately.

Brand name:

Nicotrol

See Nicotine Patches

Brand name:

Nolahist

Pronounced: NO-luh-hist
Generic name: Phenindamine tartrate

What this drug is used for

Nolahist temporarily relieves the runny nose, sneezing, itchy nose or throat, and itchy, watery eyes caused by allergies such as hay fever.

How should you take this medication?

■ ADULTS

For adults and children 12 years and over, the usual dosage is 1 tablet every 4 to 6 hours. Do not take more than 6 tablets each 24 hours.

■ CHILDREN

For children 6 to 12, the usual dosage is half a tablet every 4 to 6 hours. Do not give more than 3 tablets each 24 hours. For children under 6, consult your doctor.

■ STORAGE

Keep the bottle tightly closed. Store at room temperature, away from light.

Do not take this medication if...

Unless your doctor approves, do not take Nolahist if you have high pressure within the eye (glaucoma), an enlarged prostate gland, or a breathing problem such as emphysema or chronic bronchitis.

Special warnings about this medication

This product may cause overexcitement, especially in children. You may also find that it makes you nervous or interferes with sleep.

On the other hand, antihistamines such as Nolahist often cause drowsiness. Be especially careful when driving, and when operating machinery.

Possible food and drug interactions
when taking this medication

If you are taking a tranquilizer such as **Valium** or **Xanax**, or a sleep aid such as **Halcion** or **Seconal**, do not take Nolahist without your doctor's approval; the combination could cause extreme drowsiness. For the same reason, avoid alcohol while taking this product.

Brand name:

12 Hour Nostrilla

See Afrin 12 Hour

Brand name:

Novahistine

Pronounced: nov-uh-HIST-een
Generic ingredients: Chlorpheniramine maleate, Phenylephrine
hydrochloride

What this drug is used for

Novahistine liquid temporarily relieves the stuffy or runny nose, sneezing, itchy nose or throat, and itchy, watery eyes that result from the common cold and allergies such as hay fever.

How should you take this medication?
■ ADULTS

For adults and children 12 years and over, the usual dose is 2 teaspoonfuls every 4 hours. Do not take more than 12 teaspoonfuls each 24 hours.

■ CHILDREN

For children 6 to 12, the usual dose is 1 teaspoonful every 4 hours, up to a maximum of 6 teaspoonfuls in 24 hours. For children under 6, consult your doctor.

■ STORAGE

Keep the bottle tightly closed and protect from excessive heat and light. Do not freeze.

Do not take this medication if...

Avoid Novahistine if you have any sort of breathing problem, including asthma, emphysema, chronic bronchitis, or shortness of breath. Also avoid the product if you have heart disease, high blood pressure, thyroid disease, diabetes, ulcers, high pressure within the eye (glaucoma), or an enlarged prostate gland.

Because of the phenylephrine in this product, do not take it while nursing a baby. Also avoid it if you are sensitive to stimulant drugs or antihistamines.

Special warnings about this medication

If you become dizzy or nervous, develop weakness or tremors, feel an irregular heartbeat, or have trouble sleeping, stop taking Novahistine and check with your doctor.

Novahistine may cause excitability, especially in children. The antihistamine in this product has been known to cause a variety of other side effects, including anxiety, convulsions, double vision, dry mouth, hallucinations, headache, heartburn, loss of appetite, nausea, and vomiting.

Novahistine can also make you drowsy. Be especially cautious when driving, and when operating machinery.

If you do not feel better in 7 days, or you develop a fever, call your doctor.

Possible food and drug interactions when taking this medication

Do not use Novahistine within 2 weeks of taking any drug classified as an MAO inhibitor, including the antidepressants **Nardil** and **Parnate**.

If you are taking a tranquilizer such as **Valium** or **Xanax**, or a sleep aid such as **Halcion** or **Seconal**, do not take Novahistine without your doctor's approval; the combination could cause extreme drowsiness. For the same reason, avoid alcohol while taking this product.

Brand name:

Novahistine DMX

Pronounced: nov-uh-HIST-een
Generic ingredients: Dextromethorphan hydrobromide, Guaifenesin,
  Pseudoephedrine hydrochloride

What this drug is used for

Novahistine DMX liquid has a completely different set of ingredients than regular Novahistine. It does not include an antihistamine for fighting the symptoms of allergy, and therefore is unlikely to make you drowsy. It is used for temporary relief from the cough and stuffy nose that often accompany a cold. It also helps rid the bronchial passageways of mucus, and helps relieve feelings of pressure and stuffiness in the sinuses.

How should you take this medication?

■ ADULTS

For adults and children 12 years and over, the usual dose is 2 teaspoonfuls every 4 hours. Do not take more than 8 teaspoonfuls each 24 hours.

■ CHILDREN

For children 6 to 12, the usual dose is 1 teaspoonful every 4 hours, up to a maximum of 4 teaspoonfuls in 24 hours. For children under 6, consult your doctor.

■ STORAGE

Keep the bottle tightly closed and protect from excessive heat and light. Do not freeze.

Do not take this medication if...

Never take Novahistine DMX if you have severely high blood pressure or clogged coronary arteries. Also avoid it if any of the ingredients has ever given you an allergic reaction. Get your doctor's approval before taking it if you have any kind of heart disease, high blood pressure, thyroid disease, diabetes, or an enlarged prostate gland.

Also check with your doctor before using Novahistine DMX for the type of chronic cough that accompanies smoking, asthma, chronic bronchitis, or emphysema, or for a cough that brings up lots of phlegm.

Do not take Novahistine DMX while nursing a baby. Infants are especially sensitive to the pseudoephedrine in this product.

Special warnings about this medication

If you become dizzy or nervous, develop weakness or tremors, feel an irregular heartbeat, or have trouble sleeping, stop taking Novahistine DMX and check with your doctor.

If cough and other symptoms don't improve within 7 days or tend to come back—or if you also have a fever, rash, or lasting headache—check with your doctor. A lingering cough could signal a serious condition.

Novahistine DMX occasionally may cause stomach upset and nausea. If you are sensitive to the pseudoephedrine in the product, there is also a possibility of such side effects as anxiety, convulsions, hallucinations, headache, difficulty breathing, and problems with urination.

Possible food and drug interactions when taking this medication

Avoid using Novahistine within 2 weeks of taking any drug classified as an MAO inhibitor, including the antidepressants **Nardil** and **Parnate**.

Brand name:

Nuprin

See Advil

Brand name:

Nytol

Pronounced: NIGHT-all
Generic name: Diphenhydramine hydrochloride
Other brand names: Sleepinal, Maximum Strength Unisom

What this drug is used for

Nytol, Sleepinal, and Maximum Strength Unisom all contain an antihistamine that tends to make you drowsy. They can be used to relieve occasional sleeplessness. Another variety of Unisom, not labeled "maximum strength," is also available. It contains a different antihistamine, but is subject to the same precautions as these products.

Nytol is available in caplets and double-strength softgels. Sleepinal comes in softgels and capsules. Maximum Strength Unisom is available only in softgels.

How should you take this medication?
■ NYTOL

The usual dosage is 2 caplets or 1 softgel at bedtime as needed.

■ SLEEPINAL AND UNISOM

The usual dosage is 1 capsule or softgel at bedtime as needed.

■ STORAGE

Store at room temperature in a dry place. Protect softgels from light.

Do not take this medication if...
Do not take these products while pregnant or nursing a baby; and do not give them to children under 12 years of age.

Unless your doctor approves, do not take these products if you have high pressure within the eye (glaucoma), an enlarged prostate gland, or a breathing problem such as asthma, emphysema, or chronic bronchitis.

Special warnings about this medication
These products are for occasional use. If you have problems sleeping for more than 2 weeks, talk to your doctor. There may be a serious underlying problem.

Possible food and drug interactions
when taking this medication
If you are taking a tranquilizer such as **Valium** or **Xanax**, or a sleep aid such as **Halcion** or **Seconal**, do not take any of these products without your doctor's approval; the combination could cause extreme drowsiness. For the same reason, avoid alcohol while using one of these sleep aids.

Also avoid taking these products if you are taking any drug classified as an MAO inhibitor, including the antidepressants **Nardil** and **Parnate**. Such drugs increase the effects of the antihistamine in these products.

Overdosage
An overdose of these products will cause severe problems. If you suspect an overdose, seek medical help immediately.

■ *Symptoms of overdose may include:*
Coma, convulsions, delirium, difficulty breathing, dilated pupils, dry mouth, flushed skin, loss of appetite, low blood pressure, nausea, tremor, vomiting

In a child, initial sleepiness may be followed by overexcitement.

Brand name:

OcuHist

See Naphcon A

Brand name:

Orudis KT

Pronounced: oh-REW-dis
Generic name: Ketoprofen
Other brand name: Actron

What this drug is used for

Orudis and Actron are over-the-counter versions of the prescription drug ketoprofen. They provide temporary relief from headache, toothache, muscle ache, backache, arthritis, menstrual cramps, and the minor aches and pains of a cold. They also reduce fever.

Both products come in tablet and caplet form.

How should you take this medication?

The usual dose is 1 pill with a full glass of liquid every 4 to 6 hours. If your pain or fever does not get better in 1 hour, you may take 1 more pill. Some people find they need 2 pills for the first dose.

Do not take more than 2 pills in a 4- to 6-hour period, or more than 6 pills each 24 hours.

■ STORAGE
Store at room temperature. Avoid too much heat.

Do not take this medication if...

Avoid these products if any other pain reliever has given you asthma, hives, or any other allergic reaction. Ketoprofen could cause a similar reaction.

Check with your doctor before using these products if the painful area is red or swollen, if you take other drugs on a regular basis, or if you are being treated for any continuing medical condition.

Not for children under 16 without your doctor's approval.

Special warnings about this medication

Do not use either product for more than 3 days for fever or 10 days for pain.

Avoid these products during the last 3 months of pregnancy; they could cause problems in your unborn child or complications during delivery. Earlier in pregnancy, and when nursing a baby, check with your doctor before taking these products.

Call your doctor if your symptoms continue or get worse, you develop new or unexpected symptoms, or you get stomach pain after using the product.

Possible food and drug interactions when taking this medication

Do not take Orudis or Actron if you are using another ketoprofen product such as **Oruvail**, or any other pain reliever such as **Aspirin**, **Aleve**, **Motrin**, or **Tylenol**.

Also, make sure to check with your doctor before combining either product with the following:

Blood-thinners such as **Coumadin**
Water pills (diuretics) such as **HydroDIURIL**
Lithium (**Lithonate**)
Methotrexate
Probenecid (the gout medication **Benemid**)

Brand name

Otrivin

Pronounced: OH-trih-vin
Generic name: Xylometazoline hydrochloride

What this drug is used for

Otrivin gives temporary relief from stuffy nose brought on by a cold, inflamed sinuses, and allergies such as hay fever. The product is available as a nasal spray, nasal drops, and pediatric nasal drops.

How should you take this medication?

The usual dosage is 2 or 3 sprays or drops in each nostril no more often than every 8 to 10 hours. For children under 12, give only the pediatric drops, using the dropper provided. For children under 2, consult your doctor.

■ STORAGE

Store at room temperature.

Do not take this medication if...

Unless your doctor approves, avoid Otrivin if you have heart disease, high blood pressure, thyroid disease, diabetes, or an enlarged prostate gland.

Special warnings about this medication

Otrivin may cause temporary burning, stinging, or sneezing, and may worsen a runny nose.

Do not use this product for more than 3 days. If you use it longer or more frequently than recommended, your stuffy nose may return or get worse. If you feel no improvement, call your doctor.

Do not use a container of this product for more than 1 person. Sharing a container could spread infection.

Overdosage

In a young child, an overdose can cause abnormal calmness (sedation). If you suspect an overdose, seek medical attention immediately.

Brand name:

Pamprin Maximum Pain Relief

Pronounced: PAM-prin
Generic ingredients: Acetaminophen, Magnesium salicylate, Pamabrom

What this drug is used for

Pamprin Maximum Pain Relief eases menstrual cramps and other pains associated with your period, such as backache and headache. It also contains a diuretic to get rid of the retained water that leads to temporary weight gain.

Another form of Pamprin—Multi-Symptom Pamprin—combats the same symptoms, but has a slightly different mix of ingredients.

How should you take this medication?

The usual dose is 2 caplets with a full glass of water every 4 to 6 hours, as needed. Do not take more than 8 caplets each 24 hours.

Do not take this medication if...

Unless your doctor approves, avoid this product if you are allergic to salicylates such as aspirin. Never give this medication to a child under 3 years of age.

Special warnings about this medication

Do not use this product for more than 10 days for menstrual problems—or, if you are using it for a fever, for more than 3 days—without your doctor's approval.

If you develop ringing in the ears or have trouble hearing, check with your doctor before taking any more of this product. Also call your doctor if your pain or fever continues or gets worse, if you develop new symptoms, or if you have any redness or swelling.

Do not use products such as Pamprin during the last 3 months of pregnancy; they could cause problems in your unborn child or complications during delivery. Earlier in pregnancy, and when nursing a baby, check with your doctor before using such products.

Salicylates such as the one in Pamprin have been known to trigger a serious illness called Reye's syndrome in children and teenagers who catch a virus. If your child gets chickenpox or flu, do not treat the symptoms with Pamprin.

Possible food and drug interactions when taking this medication

Unless directed by a doctor, do not take Pamprin if you are using any of the following:

Blood-thinning medications such as **Coumadin**
Diabetes drugs such as **DiaBeta**, **Orinase**, and **Tolinase**
Gout medicines such as **Anturane**, **Benemid**, and **Zyloprim**
Arthritis medications such as **Anaprox, Daypro, Ecotrin, Indocin, Motrin,** and **Naprosyn**

Brand name:

Pamprin Multi-Symptom

See Midol PMS Formula

Brand name:

Panadol

See Tylenol

Brand name:

PediaCare Cough-Cold

Pronounced: PEE-dee-uh-care
Generic ingredients: Chlorpheniramine maleate, Dextromethorphan
hydrobromide, Pseudoephedrine hydrochloride

What this drug is used for

PediaCare Cough-Cold products temporarily relieve a child's cough, stuffy or runny nose, and sneezing due to a cold or allergies such as hay fever.

Liquids and chewable tablets are available. The NightRest variety contains more of the cough reliever dextromethorphan than do the other PediaCare Cough-Cold products, but can be given either day or night.

How should you take this medication?

When giving one of the liquids, use the measuring cup that comes with the product to be sure the dosage is correct.

PediaCare Cough-Cold liquid and chewable tablets can be given every 4 to 6 hours. Give PediaCare NightRest liquid every 6 to 8 hours. Do not give more than 4 doses of any product each day.

Check with your doctor before giving these products to children under 6. The usual dosages are as follows:

Children 11 years old: 3 teaspoonfuls or tablets
Children 9 to 10: 2¹/₂ teaspoonfuls or tablets
Children 6 to 8: 2 teaspoonfuls or tablets
Children 4 to 5: 1¹/₂ teaspoonfuls or tablets
Children 2 to 3: 1 teaspoonful or tablet

Do not take this medication if...

Unless your doctor approves, do not use these products for the frequent, long-lasting coughing that marks conditions such as asthma, or for coughs that bring up lots of phlegm. Also check first with your doctor if the child has heart disease, high blood pressure, thyroid disease, diabetes, high pressure within the eye (glaucoma), or a breathing problem such as chronic bronchitis.

Special warnings about this medication

If the child becomes dizzy or nervous, or has trouble sleeping, stop giving PediaCare and check with your doctor.

If cough and other symptoms don't improve within 7 days or tend to come back—or if the child also has a fever, rash, or lasting headache—check with your doctor. A lingering cough could signal a serious condition.

These products can cause either overexcitement or drowsiness.

If the child must avoid phenylalanine, do not use the chewable tablets.

Possible food and drug interactions when taking this medication

Do not give any of these products within 2 weeks of a drug classified as an MAO inhibitor, such as the antidepressants **Nardil** and **Parnate**.

If the child is taking a tranquilizer such as **Valium** or **Xanax**, or a sleep aid such as **Halcion** or **Seconal**, do not give a PediaCare Cough-Cold product without your doctor's approval; the combination could cause extreme drowsiness.

Overdosage

■ *Symptoms of PediaCare overdose may include:*
Anxiety, rapid heartbeat, mild high blood pressure, nervous system problems, visual disturbances, failure to urinate, nausea, vomiting

If you suspect an overdose, get medical help immediately.

Brand name:

PediaCare Infants' Drops

Pronounced: PEE-dee-uh-care
Generic ingredients: Pseudoephedrine hydrochloride, Dextro-
methorphan hydrobromide (Decongestant Plus Cough only)

What this drug is used for

Two varieties of these drops are available: Decongestant and

Decongestant Plus Cough. Both temporarily relieve a stuffy nose caused by the common cold or allergies such as hay fever. The Decongestant Plus Cough product also relieves coughing brought on by colds and allergies.

How should you take this medication?

Use the dropper that comes with these products to measure the dosage accurately. Give only by mouth.

Doses may be repeated every 4 to 6 hours. Do not give more than 4 doses a day. Dosage is the same for both products:

Children 2 to 3 years old: 2 dropperfuls
Children 12 to 23 months old: 1½ dropperfuls
Infants 4 to 11 months old: 1 dropperful
Birth to 3 months old: ½ dropperful

Do not take this medication if...

Unless your doctor approves, do not give either variety of these drops to a child with heart disease, high blood pressure, thyroid disease, or diabetes.

In addition, get your doctor's approval before using the Decongestant Plus Cough formula for the type of frequent, long-lasting coughing that marks conditions such as asthma, or for coughs that bring up lots of phlegm.

Special warnings about this medication

If the child becomes dizzy or nervous, or has trouble sleeping, stop giving the drops and check with your doctor.

If cough and other symptoms don't improve within 7 days or tend to come back—or if the child also has a fever, rash, or lasting headache—check with your doctor. A lingering cough could signal a serious condition.

Possible food and drug interactions when taking this medication

Do not give these drops within 2 weeks of a drug classified as an MAO inhibitor, such as the antidepressants **Nardil** and **Parnate**.

Overdosage

■ *Symptoms of an overdose of PediaCare Decongestant Drops may include:*
Anxiety, rapid heartbeat, mild high blood pressure

■ *In addition, a massive overdose of the Decongestant Plus Cough formula may cause:*
Nervous system problems, visual disturbances, failure to urinate, nausea, vomiting

If you suspect an overdose, check with your doctor.

Brand name:
Pediatric Vicks 44E

See Robitussin-DM

Brand name:
Pediatric Vicks 44M

See Vicks NyQuil, Children's

Brand name:
Pepcid AC

Pronounced: PEP-sid
Generic name: Famotidine
Other brand name: Mylanta AR

What this drug is used for
Taken before a meal, Pepcid AC and Mylanta AR prevent heartburn and acid indigestion. They can also be used for relief after the problem develops.

These products are part of a family of acid-blocking prescription drugs recently released in over-the-counter formulations. Other members of the family are Axid AR, Tagamet HB, and Zantac 75.

How should you take this medication?
■ FOR PREVENTION
Swallow 1 tablet with water 1 hour before eating a meal that could cause trouble. Take no more than 2 tablets a day.

■ FOR RELIEF
Swallow 1 tablet with water.

■ STORAGE
Store at room temperature in a dry place.

Do not take this medication if...

Not for children under 12, unless your doctor approves.

Special warnings about this medication

Do not take 2 tablets of Pepcid AC or Mylanta AR every day for more than 2 weeks without your doctor's approval.

If you have trouble swallowing, or if you have stomach pain that does not go away, see your doctor promptly. You may have a serious condition that needs different treatment.

Possible food and drug interactions
when taking this medication

Unless your doctor approves, do not combine Pepcid AC or Mylanta AR with the following:

Itraconazole (**Sporanox**)
Ketoconazole (**Nizoral**)

Brand name:

Pepto Diarrhea Control

See Imodium A-D

Brand name:

Pepto-Bismol

Pronounced: PEP-toe BIZ-mahl
Generic name: Bismuth subsalicylate

What this drug is used for

Pepto-Bismol relieves upset stomach symptoms and diarrhea. It can be used for:

Heartburn and indigestion
Abdominal cramps from diarrhea
Nausea
Fullness caused by overeating

Pepto-Bismol is available in liquid, tablet, and caplet form.

How should you take this medication?

Tablets may be chewed or dissolved in the mouth. Swallow caplets with water—do not chew. Doses can be repeated every one-half to 1 hour if needed, up to a maximum of 8 doses in a 24-hour period (once an hour, up to a maximum of 4 doses if using the maximum strength liquid). Shake the liquid well before using. Drink plenty of clear fluids to help prevent the dehydration that may accompany diarrhea.

■ ADULTS

The usual dose is 2 pills or tablespoonfuls.

■ CHILDREN

Age 9 to 12

The usual dose is 1 pill or tablespoonful (half a dose cup, or 15 milliliters).

Age 6 to 9

The usual dose is two-thirds of a pill, or 2 teaspoonfuls (one-third of a dose cup, or 10 milliliters).

Age 3 to 6

The usual dose is one-third of a pill, or 1 teaspoonful (one-sixth of a dose cup, or 5 milliliters).

Under age 3

Consult a doctor.

Do not take this medication if...

Pepto-Bismol contains salicylates, which are chemically related to aspirin. If you are allergic to aspirin or non-aspirin salicylates, avoid Pepto-Bismol. Also, if you take Pepto-Bismol with aspirin and develop ringing in the ears, discontinue its use.

Special warnings about this medication

If diarrhea is accompanied by a high fever or continues for more than 2 days, consult a doctor.

Children or teenagers who have, or are recovering from, chickenpox or flu should not use Pepto-Bismol to treat nausea and vomiting. If these symptoms develop, consult a doctor. They could be early signs of Reye's syndrome, a rare but serious illness linked to certain viral infections.

Pepto-Bismol may cause a temporary and harmless darkening of the tongue and/or stool.

Possible food and drug interactions when taking this medication

Unless your doctor directs, do not combine Pepto-Bismol with the following:

Blood-thinning drugs such as **Coumadin**

Gout medications such as **ColBENEMID** and **Zyloprim**

Diabetes medications such as **DiaBeta** and **Micronase**

Brand name:

Perdiem

See Metamucil

Brand name:

Peri-Colace

See Doxidan

Brand name:

Pertussin CS

See Benylin Pediatric Cough Suppressant

Brand name:

Pertussin DM

See Benylin Adult Formula Cough Suppressant

Brand name:

Phazyme

Pronounced: FAY-zime
Generic name: Simethicone

What this drug is used for

Phazyme relieves the bloating, pressure, and fullness that result from gas. Similar products with the active ingredient simethicone include Gas-X, Maalox Anti-Gas, Mylanta Gas Relief, and Infants' Mylicon.

Phazyme is available in five forms: tablets, chewable tablets, capsules, liquid, and infant drops.

How should you take this medication?

Do not take more than the maximum recommended dosage unless directed by your doctor.

■ TABLETS

Take 1 tablet 4 times a day after meals and at bedtime. Do not take more than 5 tablets a day.

■ CHEWABLE TABLETS

Take 1 chewable tablet 4 times a day after meals and at bedtime. Chew thoroughly. Do not take more than 4 tablets a day.

■ SOFTGEL CAPSULES

Take 1 softgel capsule 4 times a day after meals and at bedtime. Do not take more than 4 capsules a day.

■ LIQUID

Shake well before using. Take 2 teaspoonfuls 4 times a day after meals and at bedtime. Do not take more than 8 teaspoonfuls a day.

■ INFANT DROPS

Shake well before using. If more convenient, drops may be mixed with other liquids.

Adults and children over 12

Take two 0.6-milliliter doses 4 times daily after meals and at bedtime. Do not take more than 6 times a day.

Children 2 to 12 years of age

Give 0.6 milliliters 4 times a day after meals and at bedtime.

Infants under 2 years of age

Give 0.3 milliliters 4 times a day after meals and at bedtime.

■ STORAGE

All forms may be stored at room temperature.

Special warnings about this medication

If your condition does not clear up, contact your doctor.

Brand name:

Phillips' Gelcaps

Pronounced: FIL-ips
Generic ingredients: Docusate sodium, Phenolphthalein

What this drug is used for

Phillips' Gelcaps combine a laxative (phenolphthalein) and a stool softener to relieve occasional constipation. The product generally produces a bowel movement in 6 to 12 hours.

How should you take this medication?

The usual dose for adults and children 12 years and over is 1 or 2 gelcaps daily with a full glass of liquid. For children under 12, consult your doctor.

Do not take this medication if...

Do not take any laxative if you have abdominal pain, nausea, or vomiting, unless directed by a doctor. Also check first with your doctor if you have noticed a sudden change in bowel habits lasting more than 2 weeks.

Special warnings about this medication

Rectal bleeding or failure to have a bowel movement after taking a laxative may signal a serious condition. Stop taking Phillips' Gelcaps and consult your doctor. In any event, do not use a laxative for more than 1 week without your doctor's approval.

The phenolphthalein in this product may cause a rash. If one appears, stop using the product and avoid other phenolphthalein-based laxatives.

Possible food and drug interactions
when taking this medication

Unless your doctor approves, do not use this medication while taking mineral oil.

Brand name:

Phillips' Milk of Magnesia

Pronounced: FIL-ips
Generic name: Magnesium hydroxide

What this drug is used for

Phillips' Milk of Magnesia can be used for occasional constipation, or for acid indigestion, sour stomach, and heartburn. It comes in original, mint, and cherry flavors.

How should you take this medication?

■ AS A LAXATIVE

Follow the dose with a full glass of liquid. You can expect results in as little as a half hour or as long as 6 hours later.

Adults and children 12 years of age and older
Take 2 to 4 tablespoonfuls.

Children 6 to 11 years of age
Give 1 to 2 tablespoonfuls.

Children 2 to 5 years of age
Give 1 to 3 teaspoonfuls.

Children under 2 years
Consult a physician.

■ AS AN ANTACID
Adults and children 12 years of age and older
The usual dosage is 1 to 3 teaspoonfuls with a little water up to 4 times a day.

Do not take this medication if...

Do not take any laxative if you have abdominal pain, nausea, or vomiting, unless directed by a doctor. Also check first with your doctor if you have noticed a sudden change in bowel habits lasting more than 2 weeks. Unless your doctor approves, do not use this product if you have kidney disease.

Special warnings about this medication

Rectal bleeding or failure to have a bowel movement after taking a laxative may signal a serious condition. Stop taking Phillips' and consult your doctor. In any event, do not use the product as a laxative for more than 1 week without your doctor's approval.

When taking this product as an antacid, do not take more than the maximum daily dosage in each 24-hour period, or use the maximum dosage continuously for more than 2 weeks, unless directed by a doctor.

Possible food and drug interactions when taking this medication

Antacids interact with a variety of prescription drugs when taken at the same time. An interaction is unlikely, however, if you keep doses of the two at least 2 or 3 hours apart. Drugs that may interact include the following:

Alendronate (**Fosamax**)

Allopurinol (**Zyloprim**)

Antibiotics classified as quinolones, such as **Cipro**, **Floxin**, and **Noroxin**

Aspirin

Atenolol (**Tenormin**)

Captopril (**Capoten**)

Chlordiazepoxide (**Librium**)

Cimetidine (**Tagamet**)

Digoxin (**Lanoxin**)

Doxycycline (**Vibramycin**)

Fosfomycin (**Monurol**)

Gabapentin (**Neurontin**)

Glipizide (**Glucotrol**)

Glyburide (**Micronase, DiaBeta**)

Isoniazid (**Rifamate**)

Ketoconazole (**Nizoral**)

Levothyroxine (**Synthroid**)

Methenamine (**Urised**)

Metronidazole (**Flagyl**)

Misoprostol (**Cytotec**)

Mycophenolate mofetil (**CellCept**)

Nonsteroidal anti-inflammatory drugs such as **Dolobid**, **Motrin**, **Naprosyn**, and **Voltaren**

Penicillamine (**Cuprimine**)

Phenytoin (**Dilantin**)

Quinidine (**Quinidex**)

Sodium polystyrene sulfonate (**Kayexalate**)

Sucralfate (**Carafate**)

Tetracycline antibiotics such as **Achromycin V** and **Minocin**

Tilodronate (**Skelid**)

Ursodiol (**Actigall**)

Brand name:

Pin-X

Generic name: Pyrantel pamoate

What this drug is used for

Pin-X is used to treat pinworm, the most common parasite among U.S. children. Pinworm eggs are easily spread in clothing, bedding, and toys. The main symptom is itching in the anal area. Often, however, there are no symptoms at all.

How should you take this medication?

Shake the bottle well before using. The usual dosage for adults and children over the age of 2 years is 5 milligrams for each pound of body weight, taken in a single dose. The package gives doses in teaspoonfuls.

■ STORAGE

Store at room temperature.

Do not take this medication if...

Unless your doctor approves, do not use this product if you are pregnant or have liver disease.

Special warnings about this medication

No matter what your weight, do not take a dose of more than 1,000 milligrams.

Brand name:

Primatene Mist

Pronounced: PRIME-uh-teen
Generic name: Epinephrine

What this drug is used for

Primatene Mist temporarily relieves the shortness of breath, chest tightness, and wheezing that mark an asthma attack. It works by reducing spasms in the muscles of the bronchial passages.

Primatene Mist is available in an aerosol inhaler that delivers a preset dose with each use.

How should you take this medication?

To use Primatene Mist:

1. Take the cap off the mouthpiece, then remove the mouthpiece, turn it upside down, and put it back on the bottle.

2. Turn the bottle upside down. Place your thumb over the circular button on the bottom of the mouthpiece, and put your forefinger on top of the vial. Exhale as much as possible.

3. Put the mouthpiece in your mouth and close your lips tightly around it. Inhale deeply while squeezing the mouthpiece and bottle together.

4. Release immediately and remove the unit from your mouth. Finish inhaling, then hold your breath as long as possible. Exhale slowly while keeping your lips nearly closed.

■ DOSAGE
Start with 1 inhalation, then wait at least 1 minute. If necessary, you can use the product one more time. After that, do not use Primatene Mist again for at least 3 hours.

For children under 4, consult a physician.

■ STORAGE
Wash the mouthpiece daily with soap and hot water. Rinse thoroughly and dry with a lint-free cloth. Store the unit at room temperature. Protect from excessive heat.

Do not take this medication if...
Do not use Primatene Mist unless you have been diagnosed with an actual case of asthma. Also, unless your doctor approves, do not use Primatene Mist if you have heart disease, high blood pressure, thyroid disease, diabetes, or an enlarged prostate gland, or if you have ever been hospitalized with asthma.

Special warnings about this medication
If your asthma symptoms do not improve within 20 minutes, or become worse, seek medical attention immediately.

**Possible food and drug interactions
when taking this medication**
Do not use Primatene Mist within 2 weeks of taking a drug classified as an MAO inhibitor, including the antidepressants **Nardil** and **Parnate**. Also, unless your doctor approves, do not use Primatene Mist while taking a prescription drug for asthma.

Overdosage

High doses of Primatene Mist can lead to symptoms such as nervousness and rapid heartbeat, and could be harmful to the heart. Never take more than the usual dose, and never use the product more often than recommended.

Brand name:

Primatene Tablets

Pronounced: PRIME-uh-teen
Generic ingredients: Ephedrine hydrochloride, Guaifenesin

What this drug is used for

Primatene tablets temporarily relieve the shortness of breath, chest tightness, and wheezing that mark an asthma attack. They work by reducing muscle spasms that tend to constrict the walls of the bronchial passages, and by loosening phlegm to keep the passageways clear.

How should you take this medication?

For adults and children 12 and over, the initial dosage is 2 tablets. You may take an additional 2 tablets every 2 to 4 hours if needed; but do not take more than 12 tablets in 24 hours. For children under 12, consult a doctor.

■ STORAGE
Store the tablets at room temperature.

Do not take this medication if...

Do not use Primatene tablets unless you have been diagnosed with an actual case of asthma. Also, unless your doctor approves, do not use Primatene tablets if you have heart disease, high blood pressure, thyroid disease, diabetes, or an enlarged prostate gland, or if you have ever been hospitalized with asthma.

Primatene tablets should be used only for asthma attacks. Do not take them for the chronic cough that sometimes accompanies smoking, asthma, bronchitis, or emphysema, and avoid them if your cough is already bringing up excessive phlegm. If you have a persistent cough or a cough accompanied by fever, rash, or headache, see your doctor.

Special warnings about this medication

If your asthma symptoms do not improve within 1 hour, or become worse, seek medical attention immediately.

Possible side effects of Primatene tablets include nervousness, sleeplessness, tremor, nausea, and loss of appetite. If these symptoms don't subside, or become worse, call your doctor.

Possible food and drug interactions when taking this medication

Do not use Primatene tablets within 2 weeks of taking a drug classified as an MAO inhibitor, including the antidepressants **Nardil** and **Parnate**. Also, unless your doctor approves, do not use Primatene tablets while taking a prescription drug for asthma.

Overdosage

Overuse of this product can be harmful or even fatal. If you suspect an overdose, seek medical help immediately.

Brand name:

Privine

Pronounced: pry-VEEN
Generic name: Naphazoline hydrochloride

What this drug is used for

Privine provides temporary relief of stuffy nose caused by colds, inflamed sinuses, hay fever, and other allergies. It is available as nasal drops and a nasal spray.

How should you take this medication?

The usual dose is 1 or 2 drops or sprays in each nostril. Do not use more often than every 6 hours.

■ STORAGE
Store at room temperature.

Do not take this medication if...

Unless your doctor approves, do not use Privine if you have diabetes, heart disease, high blood pressure, thyroid disease, or an enlarged prostate gland.

Not for use in children under 12 unless directed by your doctor.

Special warnings about this medication

Do not use Privine for more than 3 days. If you use it too often or for too long, your stuffy nose may come back or get worse. If your symptoms do not clear up, call your doctor.

Privine may cause temporary burning, stinging, sneezing, or increased runny nose.

Do not share this medication, since this could spread infection.

Brand name:

Prodium

Pronounced: PRO-dee-um
Generic name: Phenazopyridine hydrochloride

What this drug is used for

Prodium relieves the minor pain, urgency, frequency, and burning caused by an infection in the urinary tract. Prodium does not cure the infection itself. For that you need prescription antibiotics; so be sure to see your doctor.

How should you take this medication?

The usual dosage is 2 tablets 3 times a day after meals. You should use this product for no more than 2 days.

■ STORAGE
Store at room temperature.

Do not take this medication if...

Avoid Prodium if it has ever given you an allergic reaction. Also, unless your doctor approves, do not take Prodium if you have any liver or kidney problems.

Not for children under 12 unless directed by a doctor.

Special warnings about this medication

If your symptoms don't clear up, check with your doctor. Also call your doctor if your skin or eyes turn yellowish. This is a sign that the drug is building up in your system, and that you may need to stop taking it.

Prodium turns urine reddish orange, and could stain your clothes. The drug has also been known to stain contact lenses.

If Prodium upsets your stomach, you should stop taking it. Taking the drug with or following meals makes stomach upset less likely.

3M TITRALAC ANTACID

3M

Available in: Regular Strength 40, 100, 1000 Tablets and Extra Strength 100 Tablets only

3M TITRALAC PLUS ANTACID

3M

Antacid with Simethicone
Available in:
100 Tablets and 12 Fl. oz. liquid

4-WAY 12 HOUR NASAL SPRAY

Bristol-Myers Products

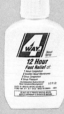

1/2 oz. Atomizers

4-WAY NASAL SPRAY

Bristol-Myers Products

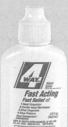

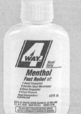

Regular available in:
1/2 oz. and 1 oz. Atomizers
Mentholated also available

ACTIFED ALLERGY DAYTIME/NIGHTTIME

Warner-Lambert Consumer Healthcare

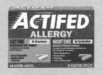

Available in 24 Daytime Caplets and 8 Nighttime Caplets

ACTIFED COLD & ALLERGY

Warner-Lambert Consumer Healthcare

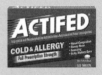

Available in 12, 24, 48 tablets and bottles of 100

ACTIFED COLD & SINUS

Warner-Lambert Consumer Healthcare

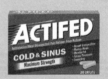

Available in 20 Tablets and Caplets

ACTIFED SINUS DAYTIME/NIGHTTIME

Warner-Lambert Consumer Healthcare

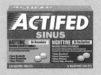

Available in 18 Daytime and 6 Nighttime Tablets or Caplets

ACTRON

**Bayer Corporation
Consumer Care Division**

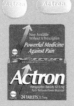

**Ketoprofen Tablets
and Caplets 12.5 mg**

ACUTRIM

Novartis Consumer Health, Inc.

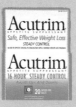

**Appetite Suppressants
Steady Control,
Maximum Strength,
Late Day Strength
Caffeine Free/Works all Day**

AFRIN EXTRA
MOISTURIZING NASAL
SPRAY

**Schering-Plough HealthCare
Products**

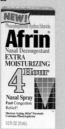

Extra-Moisturizing 4 Hour

AFRIN EXTRA
MOISTURIZING NASAL
SPRAY

**Schering-Plough HealthCare
Products**

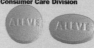

Extra-Moisturizing 12 Hour

AFRIN NASAL SPRAY

**Schering-Plough HealthCare
Products**

**Regular 12 Hour
Safety Sealed**

ALEVE

**Bayer Corporation
Consumer Care Division**

**Tablets and Caplets
available in 24, 50, 100
and 150 count. Caplets
also available in 200 count.**

ALKA-MINTS

**Bayer Corporation
Consumer Care Division**

**Spearmint, Cherry, Tropical
and Assorted Chewable
Antacid**

ALKA-SELTZER

**Bayer Corporation
Consumer Care Division**

**Original, Extra Strength,
Lemon Lime and Cherry
Effervescent Antacid and
Pain Reliever**

ALKA-SELTZER GOLD

**Bayer Corporation
Consumer Care Division**

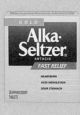

Effervescent Antacid

ALKA-SELTZER PLUS COLD MEDICINE

**Bayer Corporation
Consumer Care Division**

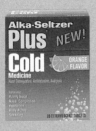

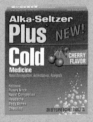

Orange and Cherry Flavors

ALKA-SELTZER PLUS COLD MEDICINE

**Bayer Corporation
Consumer Care Division**

**Cold, Cold & Cough,
Night-Time and Sinus
Effervescent Tablets**

ALKA-SELTZER PLUS COLD MEDICINE LIQUI-GELS

**Bayer Corporation
Consumer Care Division**

**Cold, Cold & Cough,
Flu & Body Aches
and Night-Time.**

ALKA-SELTZER PLUS FLU AND BODY ACHES

**Bayer Corporation
Consumer Care Division**

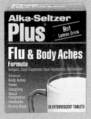

Effervescent Tablets

ALTERNAGEL

J&J-Merck Consumer

5 fl oz

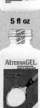

12 fl oz

**High potency aluminum
hydroxide antacid**

AMPHOJEL

Wyeth-Ayerst Laboratories

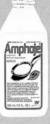

**0.6 gram (10 gr.)
Tablet shown above
12 Fl. oz. bottle and
100 tablets
Tablets and
Suspension Antacid**

ASCRIPTIN

Novartis Consumer Health, Inc.

**Regular Strength,
Maximum Strength and
Arthritis Pain**

ASCRIPTIN ENTERIC

Novartis Consumer Health, Inc.

**Adult Low Strength and
Regular Strength**

BASALJEL

Wyeth-Ayerst Laboratories

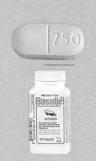

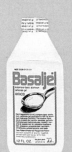

**Antacid Tablets, Capsules and
Suspension Antacid 12 Fl. oz.**

BAYER ASPIRIN

**Bayer Corporation
Consumer Care Division**

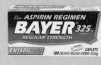

**Genuine Bayer, Aspirin
Regimen 81 mg,
Aspirin Regimen 325 mg**

ASPIRIN REGIMEN
BAYER CHILDREN'S

**Bayer Corporation
Consumer Care Division**

**Low Strength, Chewable
Aspirin
Orange and Cherry Flavors**

ASPIRIN REGIMEN BAYER 81 MG WITH CALCIUM

**Bayer Corporation
Consumer Care Division**

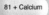

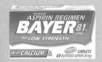

EXTENDED-RELEASE BAYER 8 HOUR

**Bayer Corporation
Consumer Care Division**

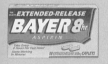

Only Extended-Release Aspirin

EXTRA STRENGTH BAYER ASPIRIN

**Bayer Corporation
Consumer Care Division**

Extra Strength, Plus,
Arthritis Pain Regimen
and PM

BENADRYL ALLERGY

**Warner-Lambert Consumer
Healthcare**

**Capsules and Tablets
Available in boxes of 24
and 48**

**Tablets also available in
bottles of 100**

BENADRYL ALLERGY CHEWABLES

**Warner-Lambert Consumer
Healthcare**

Available in boxes of 24
chewable Tablets

BENADRYL ALLERGY LIQUID MEDICATION

**Warner-Lambert Consumer
Healthcare**

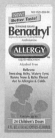

Available in 4 oz. and 8
oz. bottles

BENADRYL ALLERGY/COLD

**Warner-Lambert Consumer
Healthcare**

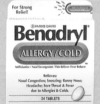

Available in boxes of
24 Tablets

BENADRYL ALLERGY DECONGESTANT

**Warner-Lambert Consumer
Healthcare**

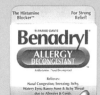

Available in boxes of
24 Tablets

BENADRYL ALLERGY DECONGESTANT LIQUID MEDICATION

Warner-Lambert Consumer Healthcare

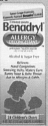

Available in 4 oz. bottles

BENADRYL ALLERGY SINUS HEADACHE

Warner-Lambert Consumer Healthcare

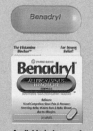

Available in boxes of 24 and 48 Caplets

BENYLIN MULTI-SYMPTOM

Warner-Lambert Consumer Healthcare

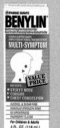

Available in 4 oz. bottles

BENADRYL DYE-FREE ALLERGY LIQUID MEDICATION

Warner-Lambert Consumer Healthcare

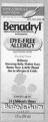

Available in 4 Fl. oz. bottles

BENYLIN ADULT COUGH SUPPRESSANT

Warner-Lambert Consumer Healthcare

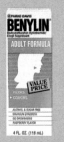

Available in 4 oz. bottles

BENYLIN PEDIATRIC COUGH SUPPRESSANT

Warner-Lambert Consumer Healthcare

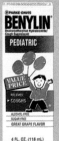

Available in 4 oz. bottles

BENADRYL DYE-FREE ALLERGY LIQUI-GELS SOFTGELS

Warner-Lambert Consumer Healthcare

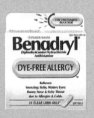

Available in Boxes of 24

BENYLIN COUGH SUPPRESSANT EXPECTORANT

Warner-Lambert Consumer Healthcare

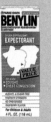

Available in 4 oz. bottles

BUFFERIN ARTHRITIS STRENGTH

Bristol-Myers Products

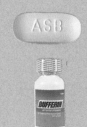

Bottles of 130 coated caplet

BUFFERIN COATED ANALGESIC

Bristol-Myers Products

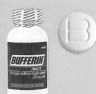

Bottles of 39, 65, 130
and 275 tablets

BUFFERIN EXTRA STRENGTH

Bristol-Myers Products

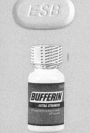

Bottles of 39, 65 and 130
coated tablets

CEPACOL

J.B. Williams Co.

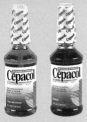

Maximum Strength
Sore Throat Spray

Cool Menthol and
Cherry Flavors.

4 Fl. oz. bottles

Cepacol

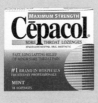

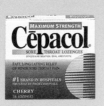

Maximum Strength
Sore Throat Lozenges
Mint and Cherry Flavors

Also Available in
Regular Strength.

18 lozenges per pack

CEPASTAT

**SmithKline Beecham
Consumer Healthcare, L.P.**

Sore Throat Lozenges
Extra Strength and Cherry
18 lozenges per package

CEROSE DM

Wyeth-Ayerst Laboratories

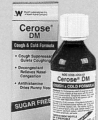

4 Fl. oz. Cough/Cold Formula
with Dextromethorphan
Also available in 1 pint
bottles

CHERACOL D

Roberts Pharmaceutical Corp.

4 oz., 6 oz. Cough Formula
Also available Cheracol Plus
Head Cold/Cough Formula
4 oz., 6 oz.

CHLOR-TRIMETON

Schering-Plough HealthCare
Products

4 Hour Allergy Tablets
8 Hour Allergy Tablets
12 Hour Allergy Tablets
4 Hour Allergy
Decongestant Tablets
12 Hour Allergy
Decongestant Tablets

CITRUCEL

SmithKline Beecham
Consumer Healthcare, L.P.

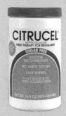

Fiber Therapy for Regularity

Sugar Free Orange available
in: 8.6 oz. and 16.9 oz.

Regular Orange available in:
16 oz. and 30 oz. containers

COLACE

Roberts Pharmaceutical Corp.

Stool softener - 50mg/100mg
100 mg available:
Two tone color 30, 60,
100, 250, 1000
50 mg available: 30, 60, 100
Available in Liquid and Syrup

PERI-COLACE

Roberts Pharmaceutical Corp.

Bottles of 30, 60, 100,
250, 1000
Laxative and Stool Softener
Available in Syrup

COMTREX ALLERGY-SINUS

Bristol-Myers Products

Available in blister packs of
24 and bottles of 50

COMTREX MULTI-SYMPTOM COLD & FLU RELIEF

Bristol-Myers Products

**Liqui-Gels in blister packs of 24 and 50
Coated caplets in blister packs of 24 and bottles of 50
Coated tablets in blister packs of 24 and bottles of 50**

COMTREX NON-DROWSY MULTI-SYMPTOM COLD & FLU RELIEF

Bristol-Myers Products

**Multi-Symptom Cold Reliever Caplets
Blister packs of 24 and bottles of 50**

CONTAC 12 HOUR

SmithKline Beecham Consumer Healthcare, L.P.

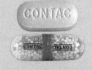

**Continuous Action
Nasal Decongestant
Antihistamine
Packages of 10 and 20
capsules and caplets**

CONTAC 12 HOUR ALLERGY

SmithKline Beecham Consumer Healthcare, L.P.

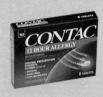

CONTAC DAY & NIGHT COLD & FLU AND ALLERGY/SINUS

SmithKline Beecham Consumer Healthcare, L.P.

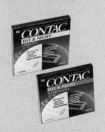

CONTAC SEVERE COLD & FLU

SmithKline Beecham Consumer Healthcare, L.P.

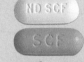

**Non-Drowsy Formula
Packages of 16 caplets**

CORICIDIN COLD & FLU

Schering-Plough HealthCare Products

For Relief Of Cold & Flu Symptoms

CORICIDIN COUGH & COLD

Schering-Plough HealthCare Products

For Relief Of Cold & Cough Symptoms

CORICIDIN NIGHTTIME COLD & COUGH

Schering-Plough HealthCare Products

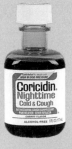

For Relief Of Cold and Cough Symptoms.

CORICIDIN-D

Schering-Plough HealthCare Products

For Relief Of Cold, Flu & Sinus Symptoms

CORRECTOL

Schering-Plough HealthCare Products

Laxative Tablets and Caplets and Stool Softener Soft Gels

CORRECTOL HERBAL TEA LAXATIVE

Schering-Plough HealthCare Products

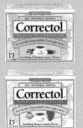

Cinnamon Spice and Honey Lemon Flavors

MAXIMUM STRENGTH DEXATRIM

Thompson Medical Co., Inc.

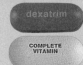

Available in 20 and 40 count package. Dexatrim Plus Vitamins available in 14 count

DIALOSE

J&J-Merck Consumer

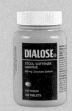

100 mg

Bottles of 100 tablets

DIALOSE PLUS

J&J-Merck Consumer

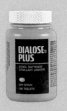

100 mg / 65 mg

Bottles of 100 tablets

DONNAGEL

Wyeth-Ayerst Laboratories

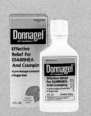

Available in bottles of 4 and
8 Fl. oz.
Chewable tablets
available in cartons of 18

DOXIDAN LIQUI-GELS

Pharmacia & Upjohn

Stimulant/Stool
Softener Laxative

Packages of 10, 30,
100, 1,000,
and 100 unit dose

DRAMAMINE

Pharmacia & Upjohn

Tablets, Chewables and
Children's Liquid

DRAMAMINE II

Pharmacia & Upjohn

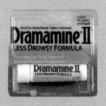

Tablets

DRIXORAL COLD & ALLERGY

**Schering-Plough HealthCare
Products**

12 Hour Sustained-Action
Tablets

DULCOLAX LAXATIVE

Novartis Consumer Health, Inc.

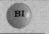

Tablets & Suppositories

ECOTRIN

**SmithKline Beecham
Consumer Healthcare, L.P.**

Adult Low Strength Tablets
in Bottles of 36

ECOTRIN

**SmithKline Beecham
Consumer Healthcare, L.P.**

Regular Strength Tablets
in bottles of 100, 250

ECOTRIN

**SmithKline Beecham
Consumer Healthcare, L.P.**

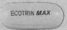

Maximum Strength Tablets
in bottles of 60, 150 and
Caplets in bottles of 60

EX-LAX

Novartis Consumer Health, Inc.

regular strength
ex·lax
laxative pills
gentle, dependable
overnight relief
30 pills

maximum relief formula
ex·lax
laxative pills
50% more
ex·lax medicine
24 pills

extra gentle
ex·lax
laxative pills
a mild laxative
dose plus softener
24 pills

gentle nature formula
ex·lax
gentle nature laxative pills
for natural-feeling
overnight relief
16 pills

Regular Strength 8's,
30's, 60's
Maximum Relief Formula 24's,
48's
Extra Gentle 24's
Gentle Nature 16's

EX-LAX CHOCOLATED

Novartis Consumer Health, Inc.

original regular strength
ex·lax
chocolated laxative
gentle, dependable
overnight relief
18 tablets

**Chocolated Laxative
Tablets 6's, 18's, 48's
and 72's**

EX-LAX STOOL SOFTENER

Novartis Consumer Health, Inc.

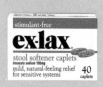

stimulant-free
ex·lax
stool softener caplets
docusate sodium 100mg
mild, natural-feeling relief
for sensitive systems
40 caplets

**Stimulant-Free Stool
Softener Caplets**

ASPIRIN FREE EXCEDRIN

Bristol-Myers Products

**Bottles of 24, 50 and
100 caplets**

EXTRA STRENGTH EXCEDRIN

Bristol-Myers Products

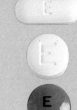

**Bottles of 12, 24, 50, 100,
175 and 275, metal tins of
12 tablets**

EXCEDRIN PM

Bristol-Myers Products

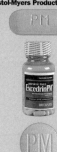

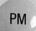

**Tablets and Caplets in Bottles
of 10, 24, 50 and 100
Geltabs in bottles of
24 and 50**

FEMSTAT 3

**Bayer Corporation
Consumer Care Division**

**3 - Day Treatment
Full Prescription Strength**

GAS-X

Novartis Consumer Health, Inc.

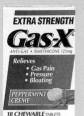

**Extra-Strength Cherry
18's, 48's
Extra-Strength Peppermint
18's, 48's**

Gas-X

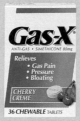

**Regular Strength
Cherry 12's, 36's
Peppermint 12's, 36's**

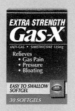

**Extra Strength Softgels
in packs of 10's and 30's**

GAVISCON ANTACID

**SmithKline Beecham
Consumer Healthcare, L.P.**

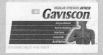

**100-Tablet bottles
30-Tablet box
(foil-wrapped 2s)**

GAVISCON LIQUID ANTACID

**SmithKline Beecham
Consumer Healthcare, L.P.**

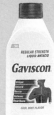

12 Fl. oz.

GAVISCON EXTRA STRENGTH ANTACID

SmithKline Beecham Consumer Healthcare, L.P.

Extra Strength Relief Formula 100-Tablet bottles

GAVISCON EXTRA STRENGTH LIQUID ANTACID

SmithKline Beecham Consumer Healthcare, L.P.

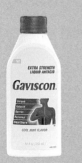

Extra Strength Relief Formula

HALLS JUNIORS SUGAR FREE

Warner-Lambert Co.

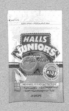

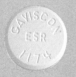

Sugar Free Cough Suppressant Drops Orange and Grape

HALLS MENTHO-LYPTUS

Warner-Lambert Co.

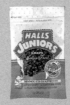

Cough Suppressant Drops Spearmint, Mentho-Lyptus, Ice Blue, Honey-Lemon and Cherry Flavors

HALLS SUGAR FREE MENTHO-LYPTUS

Warner-Lambert Co.

Black Cherry, Citrus Blend and Mountain Menthol

HALLS VITAMIN C DROPS

Warner-Lambert Co.

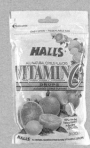

Assorted Citrus

MAXIMUM STRENGTH HALLS PLUS

Warner-Lambert Co.

Cough Suppressant Drops with Soothing Syrup Centers Honey-Lemon, Mentho-Lyptus and Cherry

IMODIUM A-D

McNeil Consumer Products

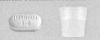

Available in 2 and 4 fl. oz. bottles with a convenient dosage cup, and caplets in 6's, 12's, 18's and 24's

KAOPECTATE ANTI-DIARRHEAL

Pharmacia & Upjohn

Regular, Peppermint, Children's Cherry Flavored Liquid and Maximum Strength Caplets

KONDREMUL

Novartis Consumer Health, Inc.

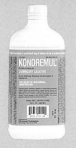

Plain (Mineral Oil) Lubricant Laxative

ADVANCED FORMULA LEGATRIN PM

Columbia

Pain Reliever / Sleep Aid Available in packages of 30 and 50 caplets.

MAALOX ANTACID

Novartis Consumer Health, Inc.

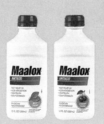

Cooling Mint and Smooth Cherry Also available in Refreshing Lemon Bottles of 5 (Mint Only), 12 & 26 oz.

MAALOX ANTACID/ANTI-GAS

Novartis Consumer Health, Inc.

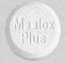

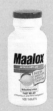

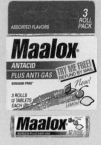

Refreshing Lemon, as well as Assorted & Smooth Cherry Flavors in Bottles of 50 & 100 Tablets Rollpacks in Assorted and Refreshing Lemon Flavors

EXTRA STRENGTH MAALOX ANTACID/ANTI-GAS

Novartis Consumer Health, Inc.

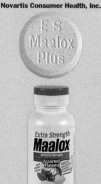

Assorted Flavors
(Mint, Cherry, Lemon)
Also available in Cooling Mint
Bottles of 38 and 75

EXTRA STRENGTH MAALOX ANTACID/ANTI-GAS

Novartis Consumer Health, Inc.

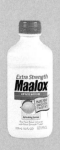

Refreshing Lemon
Also available in Cooling Mint
and Smooth Cherry
Bottles of 5 (Lemon only),
12 & 26 oz.

MAALOX ANTI-GAS

Novartis Consumer Health, Inc.

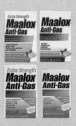

**Peppermint and Sweet
Lemon Flavor
Regular Strength 12's
Extra Strength 10's**

MALTSUPEX LIQUID

Wallace Laboratories

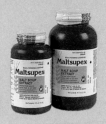

8 fl. oz. (1/2 pt) and
16 fl. oz. (1 pt)
(malt soup extract)

MALTSUPEX POWDER

Wallace Laboratories

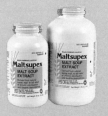

8 oz. (1/2 lb) and
16 oz. (1 lb)
(malt soup extract)

MALTSUPEX TABLETS

Wallace Laboratories

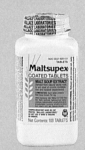

100 Tablets
(malt soup extract)

METAMUCIL

Procter & Gamble

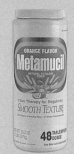

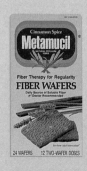

Available in 48, 72 and 114
dose canisters and 30
one-dose packets.
Also available in sugar free.

MIDOL MENSTRUAL

**Bayer Corporation
Consumer Care Division**

**Maximum Strength
Caplets and Gelcaps**

MIDOL PMS

**Bayer Corporation
Consumer Care Division**

**Maximum Strength
Gelcaps and Caplets**

MIDOL TEEN

**Bayer Corporation
Consumer Care Division**

Maximum Strength Caplets

MOTRIN IB

Pharmacia & Upjohn

**Tablets and Caplets: 24's,
50's, 100's, 130's
and 165's;
Gelcaps: 24's and 50's,
Convenience Pack (vial)
of 8 caplets**

CHILDREN'S MOTRIN IBUPROFEN ORAL SUSPENSION

McNeil Consumer Products

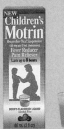

100 mg/5 mL

CHILDREN'S MOTRIN DROPS

McNeil Consumer Products

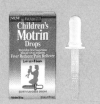

**50 mg/1.25 mL
Available in 1/2 fl. oz. bottle**

JUNIOR STRENGTH MOTRIN IBUPROFEN CAPLETS

McNeil Consumer Products

Available in blister packs of 24

MYCELEX-7

**Bayer Corporation
Consumer Care Division**

**Vaginal Cream 1%
Vaginal Cream with 7
disposable applicators
Vaginal Inserts and
external vulvar cream**

MYLANTA TABLETS

J&J-Merck Consumer

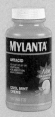

Available in Cool Mint Creme and Cherry Creme in bottles of 50 and 100 and rollpacks of 12

MAXIMUM STRENGTH MYLANTA GAS

J&J-Merck Consumer

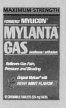

125 mg

12 & 24 tablet convenience packs

CHILDREN'S MYLANTA UPSET STOMACH RELIEF LIQUID

J&J-Merck Consumer

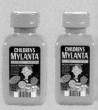

4 oz. Liquid

MYLANTA DOUBLE STRENGTH TABLETS

J&J-Merck Consumer

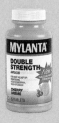

Tablets in bottles of 35, 70 and rollpacks of 8

MYLANTA GAS RELIEF GELCAPS

J&J-Merck Consumer

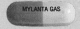

Boxes of 24 and 60 gelcaps

CHILDREN'S MYLANTA UPSET STOMACH RELIEF TABLETS

J&J-Merck Consumer

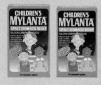

Boxes of 24 tablets.

MYLANTA GAS

J&J-Merck Consumer

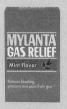

80 mg

12 & 30 tablet convenience packs, bottles of 60 and 100

MYLANTA GELCAPS ANTACID

J&J-Merck Consumer

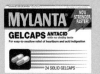

24 Solid Gelcaps

FAST-ACTING MYLANTA

J&J-Merck Consumer

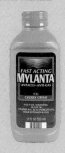

Bottles of 5, 12, 24 oz.

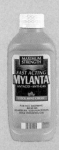
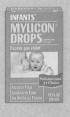
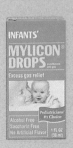

NOSTRILLA

Novartis Consumer Health, Inc.

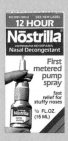

12 Hour Metered Pump Spray

NUPRIN

Bristol-Myers Products

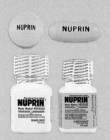

Bottles of 36, 75 and 150 tablets

OCUHIST

Pfizer Consumer Health Care

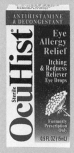

Itching and Redness Reliever Eye Drops

OTRIVIN

Novartis Consumer Health, Inc.

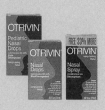

Nasal Decongestant Drops Pediatric Drops and Nasal Spray

PANADOL

SmithKline Beecham Consumer Healthcare, L.P.

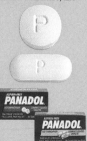

Aspirin-Free Tablets and Caplets

CHILDREN'S PANADOL

SmithKline Beecham Consumer Healthcare, L.P.

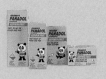

Chewable Tablets, Caplets, Liquid and Drops

PEDIACARE COUGH-COLD

McNeil Consumer Products

Blister Packs of 16 Chewable Tablets

Liquid available in 4 fl. oz. bottle with child-resistant safety cap and convenient dosage cup

PEDIACARE NIGHTREST COUGH-COLD LIQUID

McNeil Consumer Products

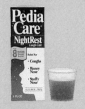

Available in 4 fl. oz. bottle with child-resistant safety cap and convenient dosage cup

PEDIACARE INFANTS' DECONGESTANT DROPS

Available in 1/2 fl. oz. bottle with child-resistant safety cap and calibrated dropper

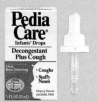

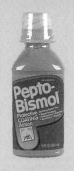
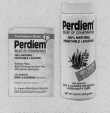
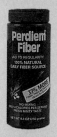
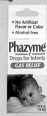

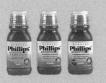
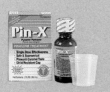

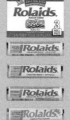
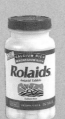
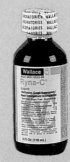
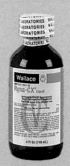

MAXIMUM STRENGTH SINE-AID

McNeil Consumer Products

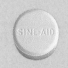

Tablets and Caplets in
blister packs
of 24 & bottles of 50

Gelcaps in blister packs
of 20 & bottles of 40

SINE-OFF

Hogil Pharmaceutical Corp.

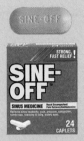

Packages of 24 and
100 caplets

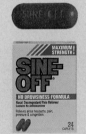

Maximum Strength
No Drowsiness Formula
Caplets

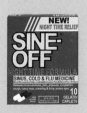

Night Time Formula Caplets

SINUTAB NON-DRYING LIQUID CAPS

Warner-Lambert Consumer Healthcare

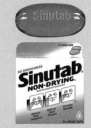

Available in Boxes of 24

SINUTAB SINUS

Warner-Lambert Consumer Healthcare

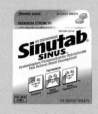

Maximum Strength
Without Drowsiness Formula
Available in 24 Caplets
or Tablets

SINUTAB SINUS ALLERGY

Warner-Lambert Consumer Healthcare

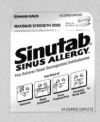

Maximum Strength Formula
Available in 24 Caplets
or Tablets

SLEEPINAL

Thompson Medical Co., Inc.

Available in 16 and 32
Capsule sizes
and 8 & 16 Softgel sizes

SUCRETS

**SmithKline Beecham
Consumer Healthcare, L.P.**

Sore Throat Lozenges
Available in: Regular Strength
(Wild Cherry, Original
Mint, Vapor Lemon
and Assorted)

Maximum Strength
(Wintergreen,
Vapor Black Cherry) and
Children's Cherry

SUCRETS 4-HOUR COUGH SUPPRESSANT

**SmithKline Beecham
Consumer Healthcare, L.P.**

Available in Wild Cherry and
Menthol-Eucalyptus

SUDAFED 12 HOUR

**Warner-Lambert Consumer
Healthcare**

12 Hour Caplets
Available in 10 and
20 caplets

SUDAFED COLD AND ALLERGY

**Warner-Lambert Consumer
Healthcare**

Available in boxes of 24
and 48 tablets.

SUDAFED COLD & COUGH

**Warner-Lambert Consumer
Healthcare**

Available in 10's or
20's Liquid Caps

SUDAFED COLD AND SINUS

**Warner-Lambert Consumer
Healthcare**

Available in boxes of
10 and 20 liquid caps

SUDAFED NASAL DECONGESTANT

**Warner-Lambert Consumer
Healthcare**

30 mg Tablets
Available in 24, 48 and 100

CHILDREN'S SUDAFED NASAL DECONGESTANT

Warner-Lambert Consumer Healthcare

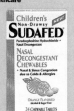

Available in boxes of 24 chewable tablets

CHILDREN'S SUDAFED NASAL DECONGESTANT LIQUID MEDICATION

Warner-Lambert Consumer Healthcare

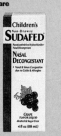

Available in 4 fl. oz. bottles

PEDIATRIC SUDAFED NASAL DECONGESTANT LIQUID ORAL DROPS

Warner-Lambert Consumer Healthcare

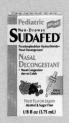

Available in 1/2 fl. oz. bottles

SUDAFED SEVERE COLD FORMULA

Warner-Lambert Consumer Healthcare

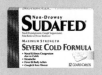

Available in 10 and 20 caplets and tablets

SUDAFED SINUS

Warner-Lambert Consumer Healthcare

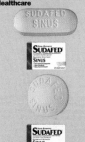

Available in 24 caplets and tablets

SUDAFED NON-DRYING SINUS LIQUID CAPS

Warner-Lambert Consumer Healthcare

Available in 24 Liquid Caps

SURFAK LIQUI-GELS STOOL SOFTENER

Pharmacia & Upjohn

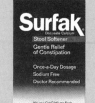

Packages of 10, 30, 100, 500 and 100 unit dose

TAGAMET HB 200

SmithKline Beecham Consumer Healthcare, L.P.

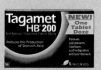

Acid Reducer Packages of 16, 32, 48 and 64

TAVIST-1

Novartis Consumer Health, Inc.

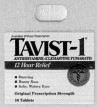

8's, 16's, 32's

TAVIST-D

Novartis Consumer Health, Inc.

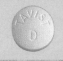

8's, 16's, 32's, 50's

TELDRIN

Hogil Pharmaceutical Corp.

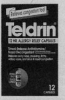

Timed-Release Capsules
Packages of 12, 24 and 48
capsules

THERAFLU

Novartis Consumer Health, Inc.

TheraFlu

Flu, Cold & Cough Medicine
Maximum Strength Nighttime
Flu, Cold & Cough Medicine
Maximum Strength, No
Drowsiness Flu, Cold &
Cough Medicine
In packs of 6 and 12 ct.

Flu and Cold Medicine
In packs of 6 and 12 ct.
Maximum Strength Flu and
Cold Medicine for Sore Throat
In packs of 6.

THERAFLU MAXIMUM STRENGTH

Novartis Consumer Health, Inc.

12's, 24's
Non-drowsy Flu, Cold
and Cough Caplets

THERAFLU MAXIMUM STRENGTH

Novartis Consumer Health, Inc.

12's, 24's
Flu, Cold & Cough Medicine
Nighttime Formula

THERAFLU SINUS

Novartis Consumer Health, Inc.

Maximum Strength Sinus
Non-Drowsy Formula in
packs of 24 caplets

TRIAMINIC AM COUGH & DECONGESTANT FORMULA

Novartis Consumer Health, Inc.

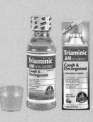

4 oz., 8 oz.

TRIAMINIC AM DECONGESTANT FORMULA

Novartis Consumer Health, Inc.

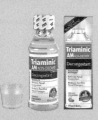

4 oz., 8 oz.

TRIAMINIC NIGHT TIME

Novartis Consumer Health, Inc.

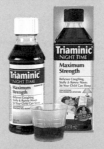

4 oz., 8 oz.

TRIAMINIC TRIAMINICOL

Novartis Consumer Health, Inc.

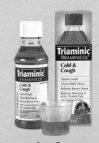

4 oz., 8 oz.

TRIAMINIC DM

Novartis Consumer Health, Inc.

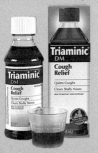

4 oz., 8 oz.

TRIAMINIC SORE THROAT

Novartis Consumer Health, Inc.

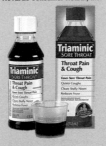

4 oz., 8 oz.

TRIAMINICIN

Novartis Consumer Health, Inc.

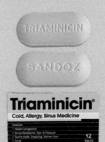

12's, 24's, 48's, 100's

TRIAMINIC EXPECTORANT

Novartis Consumer Health, Inc.

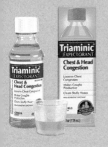

4 oz., 8 oz.

TRIAMINIC SYRUP

Novartis Consumer Health, Inc.

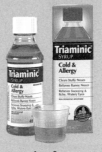

4 oz., 8 oz.

TUMS

SmithKline Beecham Consumer Healthcare, L.P.

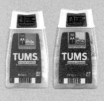

Peppermint and Assorted Flavors

TUMS E-X

**SmithKline Beecham
Consumer Healthcare, L.P.**

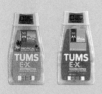

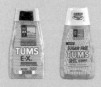

Tropical Fruit, Wintergreen,
Assorted Flavors and
SugarFree Orange Cream

TUMS ULTRA

**SmithKline Beecham
Consumer Healthcare, L.P.**

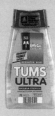

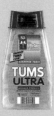

Assorted Mint and
Fruit Flavors

CHILDREN'S TYLENOL 80 MG CHEWABLE TABLETS

McNeil Consumer Products

Fruit Burst Flavor: bottles
of 30 with
child-resistant safety cap and
blister-packs of 60

Bubble Gum and Grape
Flavor Bottles of 30 with
child-resistant safety cap

CHILDREN'S TYLENOL ELIXIR

McNeil Consumer Products

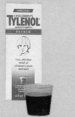

Available in cherry flavor
in 2 and 4 fl. oz. bottles with
child-resistant safety cap and
convenient dosage cup.
Alcohol Free, 80 mg.
per 1/2 teaspoon

CHILDREN'S TYLENOL FLU LIQUID

McNeil Consumer Products

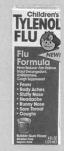

CHILDREN'S TYLENOL SUSPENSION LIQUID

McNeil Consumer Products

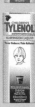

Available in Rich Cherry flavor
in 2 and 4 fl. oz. bottles.
Grape and Bubble
Gum Flavors in 4 fl. oz. with
child-resistant safety cap and
convenient dosage cup.
Alcohol Free, 80 mg
per 1/2 teaspoon

INFANT'S TYLENOL COLD DECONGESTANT AND FEVER REDUCER DROPS

McNeil Consumer Products

Available in 1/2 fl. oz. bottle with child-resistant safety cap and calibrated dropper. Bubble Gum Flavor, Alcohol-free.

INFANTS' TYLENOL SUSPENSION DROPS

McNeil Consumer Products

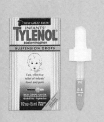

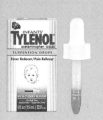

Available in rich cherry flavor and rich grape flavor 1/2 oz. bottle with child resistant safety cap and calibrated dropper. Rich Grape Flavor, Alcohol Free, 80 mg per 0.8 mL

JUNIOR STRENGTH TYLENOL

McNeil Consumer Products

Available in Fruit Burst and Grape Flavored Chewable tablets of 160 mg available in blister pack of 24

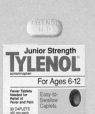

Swallowable Caplets: 160 mg blister packs of 30

CHILDREN'S TYLENOL COLD

McNeil Consumer Products

Available in bottles of 24 chewable tablets with child-resistant safety cap

CHILDREN'S TYLENOL COLD LIQUID

McNeil Consumer Products

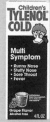

Multi-Symptom Formula

Available in 4 fl. oz. bottle with child-resistant safety cap and convenient dosage cup

CHILDREN'S TYLENOL COLD PLUS COUGH CHEWABLE

McNeil Consumer Products

Available in bottles of 24 chewable tablets with child-resistant safety cap

CHILDREN'S TYLENOL COLD PLUS COUGH LIQUID

McNeil Consumer Products

Multi-Symptom Plus Cough Formula

Available in 4 fl. oz. bottle with child-resistant safety cap and convenient dosage cup.

MAXIMUM STRENGTH TYLENOL ALLERGY SINUS NIGHTTIME

McNeil Consumer Products

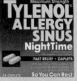

Caplets available in blister packs of 24's

TYLENOL COLD MEDICATION

McNeil Consumer Products

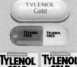

Gelcaps available in blister-packs of 24 and bottles of 40
Caplets available in blister-packs of 24 and bottles of 50
No Drowsiness Formula

MAXIMUM STRENGTH TYLENOL ALLERGY SINUS

McNeil Consumer Products

Caplets in blister packs of 24 & 48

Gelcaps in blister packs of 24 & 48

Geltabs in blister packs of 24 & 48

MAXIMUM STRENGTH TYLENOL SEVERE ALLERGY

McNeil Consumer Products

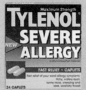

Caplets available in blister packs of 12's and 24's

TYLENOL COLD MEDICATION

McNeil Consumer Products

Caplets and Tablets available in blister-packs of 24 and bottles of 50

MULTI-SYMPTOM TYLENOL COLD

McNeil Consumer Products

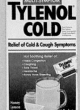

Available in cartons of 6 individual packets. Hot Liquid Medication

TYLENOL COLD SEVERE CONGESTION

McNeil Consumer Products

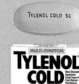

Available in blister packs of 12 and 24

MULTI-SYMPTOM TYLENOL COUGH

McNeil Consumer Products

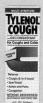

Available in 4 fl. oz. bottles

TYLENOL EXTENDED RELIEF

McNeil Consumer Products

Caplets available in 24's, 50's and 100's

MAXIMUM STRENGTH TYLENOL FLU

McNeil Consumer Products

Gelcaps available in blister-packs of 10's, and 20's No Drowsiness Formula

MAXIMUM STRENGTH TYLENOL FLU NIGHTTIME

McNeil Consumer Products

Gelcaps Available in Blister Packs of 10's and 20's

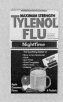

Hot Liquid Medication Available in cartons of 6 individual packets.

EXTRA STRENGTH TYLENOL

McNeil Consumer Products

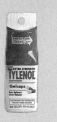

Gelcaps available in tamper-resistant bottles of 24's, 50's, 100's, 150's and 225's and FastCap™ bottle of 125's "for households without children"

Extra Strength TYLENOL

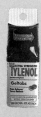

Geltabs available in tamper-resistant bottles of 24's, 50's and 100's and FastCap™ bottle of 125's "for households without children"

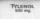

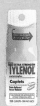

Caplets: tamper-resistant vials of 10 and bottles of 24's, 50's, 100's, 175's and 250's and FastCap™ bottle of 125's "for households without children"

Tablets: tamper-resistant vials of 10 and bottles of 30's, 60's, 100's and 200's Liquid: tamper-resistant bottles of 8 fl. oz.

TYLENOL PM

McNeil Consumer Products

Geltabs and Gelcaps available in tamper-resistant bottles of 24's and 50's. Caplets available in tamper-resistant bottles of 24's, 50's, 100's and 150's

REGULAR STRENGTH TYLENOL

McNeil Consumer Products

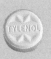

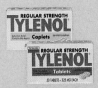

Tablets and Caplets available in: 24's, 50's, 100's and 200's and Tins of 12's

MAXIMUM STRENGTH TYLENOL SINUS

McNeil Consumer Products

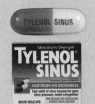

Maximum Strength TYLENOL Sinus

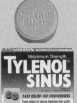

Caplets, Gelcaps, Geltabs and Tablets in blister packs of 24 & 48

VANQUISH

Bayer Corporation Consumer Care Division

Extra-Strength Pain Formula

Brand name:

Propagest

Pronounced: PROH-pah-jest
Generic name: Phenylpropanolamine hydrochloride

What this drug is used for

Propagest relieves the stuffy nose that accompanies the common cold, sinus inflammation, and allergies such as hay fever. Its active ingredient is responsible for the decongestant action of a number of other cold products. Here it's available without additional ingredients.

How should you take this medication?

■ ADULTS

For adults and children 12 years and over, the usual dose is 1 tablet every 4 hours. Do not take more than 6 tablets each 24 hours.

■ CHILDREN

For children 6 to 12, the usual dose is half a tablet every 4 hours. Do not give a total of more than 3 tablets each 24 hours. For children under 6, consult your doctor.

■ STORAGE

Keep tightly closed, away from light. Store at room temperature.

Do not take this medication if...

Unless your doctor approves, do not take Propagest if you have heart disease, high blood pressure, thyroid disease, diabetes, high pressure within the eye (glaucoma), or an enlarged prostate gland.

Special warnings about this medication

High doses of Propagest can cause dizziness, nervousness, sleeplessness, high blood pressure, and a rapid pulse. If you develop these symptoms, stop taking the drug and call your doctor.

Do not take this product for more than 7 days. If your symptoms do not improve or include a fever, check with your doctor.

Possible food and drug interactions
when taking this medication

Check with your doctor before combining Propagest with other medications, particularly high blood pressure drugs such as **Lopressor**, **Tenormin**, and **Zestril**, and drugs for depression, such as **Prozac**, **Tofranil**, and **Zoloft**.

Brand name:

Rheaban

See Kaopectate

Brand name:

Robitussin

Pronounced: ROW-bi-TUSS-in
Generic name: Guaifenesin

What this drug is used for

This basic form of Robitussin contains a single ingredient that helps loosen and thin bronchial mucus, making it easier to cough up.

Other products in the extensive Robitussin line have additional ingredients to combat other symptoms—but pose additional problems as well.

Robitussin comes as a liquid.

How should you take this medication?

A dosage cup is provided. Take a dose every 4 hours.

■ ADULTS

For adults and children 12 years and over, the usual dose is 2 to 4 teaspoonfuls.

■ CHILDREN

Age 6 to 12
The usual dose is 1 to 2 teaspoonfuls.

Age 2 to 6
The usual dose is ½ to 1 teaspoonful.

Under age 2
Consult a doctor.

■ STORAGE

Store at room temperature.

Do not take this medication if...

Unless your doctor approves, do not take Robitussin for the type of lasting cough that results from smoking, asthma, chronic bronchitis, or emphysema, or for coughs that bring up large amounts of mucus. Also avoid Robitussin if you've ever had a bad reaction to it.

Special warnings about this medication

If your cough doesn't improve within 7 days or tends to come back—or if you also have a fever, rash, or lasting headache—check with your doctor. A lingering cough could signal a serious condition.

Brand name:

Robitussin Cold & Cough

Pronounced: ROW-bi-TUSS-in
Generic ingredients: Dextromethorphan hydrobromide, Guaifenesin,
  Pseudoephedrine hydrochloride
Other brand name: Robitussin Pediatric Drops

What this drug is used for

Robitussin Cold & Cough provides temporary relief of the stuffy nose that often accompanies a common cold, inflamed sinuses, and allergies such as hay fever. It also relieves cough due to minor throat and bronchial irritation; and it thins and loosens bronchial mucus, making it easier to cough up.

For adults and older children, this formulation is available in liquigel form. For smaller children, the same ingredients are available in Robitussin Pediatric Drops.

How should you take this medication?

Doses can be repeated every 4 hours, but do not take more than 4 doses a day.

■ ADULTS

For adults and children 12 years and over, the usual dose is 2 liquigels.

■ CHILDREN
Age 6 to 12
The usual dose is 1 liquigel.

Age 2 to 6
The usual dose is 2.5 milliliters of the pediatric drops.

Under 2 years
Consult a doctor.

■ STORAGE

Both the liquigels and the drops can be stored at room temperature.

Do not take this medication if...

Unless your doctor approves, do not take Robitussin Cold & Cough for the type of lasting cough that results from smoking, asthma, chronic bronchitis, or emphysema, or for coughs that bring up large amounts of mucus. Also check with your doctor before using this product if you have heart disease, high blood pressure, thyroid disease, diabetes, or an enlarged prostate gland.

Special warnings about this medication

If you become dizzy or nervous, or have trouble sleeping, stop taking Robitussin Cold & Cough and check with your doctor.

If cough and other symptoms don't improve within 7 days or tend to come back—or if you also have a fever, rash, or lasting headache—check with your doctor. A lingering cough could signal a serious condition.

Possible food and drug interactions when taking this medication

Do not use Robitussin Cold & Cough within 2 weeks of taking a drug classified as an MAO inhibitor, such as the antidepressants **Nardil** and **Parnate**.

Brand name:

Robitussin Cold, Cough & Flu

Pronounced: ROW-bi-TUSS-in

Generic ingredients: Acetaminophen, Dextromethorphan hydrobromide, Guaifenesin, Pseudoephedrine hydrochloride

What this drug is used for

Robitussin Cold, Cough & Flu relieves the minor aches and pains, headache, muscular aches, and sore throat that often accompany a cold or the flu. It reduces fever and temporarily relieves cough and stuffy nose. It also helps loosen and thin bronchial mucus, making it easier to cough up.

This Robitussin formulation comes only in liquigel form.

How should you take this medication?

Doses may be repeated every 4 hours, but do not take more than 4 doses a day.

■ ADULTS

For adults and children 12 years and over, the usual dose is 2 Liquigels.

■ CHILDREN

For children 6 to 12, the usual dose is 1 Liquigel. Check with your doctor for children under 6.

■ STORAGE

Store at room temperature.

Do not take this medication if...

Unless your doctor approves, do not take this product for the type of lasting cough that results from smoking, asthma, chronic bronchitis, or emphysema, or for coughs that bring up large amounts of mucus. Also check with your doctor before using this product if you have heart disease, high blood pressure, thyroid disease, diabetes, or an enlarged prostate gland.

Special warnings about this medication

If you become dizzy or nervous, or have trouble sleeping, stop taking this product and check with your doctor.

If your pain or fever won't go away or gets worse, if you develop new symptoms, or if you notice any redness or swelling, check with your doctor; you might have a serious condition.

You should also check with your doctor immediately if you have a severe sore throat that lasts for more than 2 days, or if your sore throat is accompanied or followed by fever, headache, rash, nausea, or vomiting.

Likewise, call your doctor if you have a cough that lasts for more than 7 days or tends to come back, or have a cough accompanied by rash, lasting headache, and fever. A lingering cough may signal a serious problem.

In any event, do not take this product for more than 7 days (5 days maximum for children under 12) or use it for fever for more than 3 days unless directed by your doctor.

Possible food and drug interactions
when taking this medication

Do not use this product within 2 weeks of taking a drug classified as an MAO inhibitor, such as the antidepressants **Nardil** and **Parnate**.

Combined with heavy drinking, the acetaminophen in this product could conceivably cause liver damage. If you have more than 3 alcoholic beverages a day, you might want to check with your doctor about using this drug.

Generic name:

Robitussin Cough & Cold Products

Pronounced: ROW-bi-TUSS-in
Generic ingredients: Dextromethorphan hydrobromide,
Pseudoephedrine hydrochloride

What this drug is used for

Robitussin Cough & Cold products provide temporary relief from cough and stuffy nose. The "Maximum Strength" formulation is for adults and older children. The "Pediatric" formula is mainly for younger kids. Both varieties come only in liquid form.

How should you take this medication?

Doses may be repeated every 6 hours. Do not take more than 4 doses a day.

■ ROBITUSSIN MAXIMUM STRENGTH COUGH & COLD
The usual dose is 2 teaspoonfuls. For children under 12, check with your doctor.

■ ROBITUSSIN PEDIATRIC COUGH & COLD FORMULA
Age 12 and over
The usual dose is 4 teaspoonfuls.

Age 6 to 12
Give 2 teaspoonfuls.

Age 2 to 6
Give 1 teaspoonful.

Under age 2
Consult a doctor.

■ STORAGE
Store at room temperature.

Do not take this medication if...

Unless your doctor approves, do not take Robitussin Cough & Cold products for the type of lasting cough that results from smoking, asthma, chronic bronchitis, or emphysema, or for coughs that bring up large amounts of mucus. Also check with your doctor before using these products if you have heart disease, high blood pressure, thyroid disease, diabetes, or an enlarged prostate gland.

Special warnings about this medication

If you become dizzy or nervous, or have trouble sleeping, stop taking the product and check with your doctor.

If cough and other symptoms don't improve within 7 days or tend to come back—or if you also have a fever, rash, or lasting headache—check with your doctor. A lingering cough could signal a serious condition.

Possible food and drug interactions
when taking this medication

Do not use either of these products within 2 weeks of taking a drug classified as an MAO inhibitor, such as the antidepressants **Nardil** and **Parnate**.

Brand name:

Robitussin Cough Suppressant

See Benylin Adult Formula Cough Suppressant

Brand name:

Robitussin Night-Time Cold Formula

Pronounced: ROW-bi-TUSS-in
Generic ingredients: Acetaminophen, Dextromethorphan hydrobro-
*   mide, Doxylamine succinate, Pseudoephedrine hydrochloride*

What this drug is used for

Robitussin Night-Time Cold Formula temporarily relieves the minor aches and pains, headache, muscular aches, and sore throat that often accompany a cold or the flu. It reduces fever, relieves cough, and unclogs stuffy nose.

In addition, this Robitussin formulation contains an antihistamine that relieves symptoms of hay fever and similar allergies, including sneezing, runny nose, itchy nose or throat, and itchy, watery eyes. This ingredient can cause drowsiness, hence the "Night-Time" in the name.

Robitussin Night-Time Cold Formula is available in softgel form.

How should you take this medication?

The usual dose for adults and children 12 years and over is 2 softgels every 6 hours. Do not take more than 4 doses a day. The product is not recommended for children under 12.

■ STORAGE

Store at room temperature.

Do not take this medication if...

Unless your doctor approves, do not take Robitussin Night-Time Cold Formula for the type of lasting cough that results from smoking, asthma, chronic bronchitis, or emphysema, or for coughs that bring up large amounts of mucus. Also check with your doctor before using this product if you have heart disease, high blood pressure, thyroid disease, diabetes, or an enlarged prostate gland.

Special warnings about this medication

Robitussin Night-Time Cold Formula can cause excitability, especially in children. If you become dizzy or nervous, or have trouble sleeping, stop taking this product and check with your doctor.

Because this formula can also cause drowsiness, be especially cautious when driving, and when operating machinery.

If your pain or fever won't go away or gets worse, or if you develop new symptoms or notice any redness or swelling, check with your doctor; you might have a serious condition.

You should also check with your doctor immediately if you have a severe sore throat that lasts for more than 2 days, or if your sore throat is accompanied or followed by fever, headache, rash, nausea, or vomiting.

Likewise, call your doctor if you have a cough that lasts for more than 7 days or tends to come back, or a cough accompanied by rash, lasting headache, and fever.

In any event, do not take Robitussin Night-Time Cold Formula for more than 3 days for fever or 7 days in all unless directed by a doctor.

Possible food and drug interactions
when taking this medication

Do not use Robitussin Night-Time Cold Formula within 2 weeks of taking a drug classified as an MAO inhibitor, such as the antidepressants **Nardil** and **Parnate**.

If you are taking a tranquilizer such as **Valium** or **Xanax**, or a sleep aid such as **Halcion** or **Seconal**, do not take Robitussin Night-Time Cold Formula without your doctor's approval; the combination could cause extreme drowsiness. For the same reason, avoid alcohol while taking this product.

Brand name:

Robitussin Pediatric Cough & Cold Formula

See Robitussin Cough & Cold Products

Brand name:

Robitussin Pediatric Cough Suppressant

See Benylin Pediatric Cough Suppressant

Brand name:

Robitussin Pediatric Drops

See Robitussin Cold & Cough

Brand name:

Robitussin Severe Congestion Liqui-gels

See Robitussin-PE

Brand name:

Robitussin-CF

Pronounced: ROW-bi-TUSS-in
Generic ingredients: Dextromethorphan hydrobromide, Guaifenesin,
  Phenylpropanolamine hydrochloride

What this drug is used for

Robitussin-CF temporarily relieves cold symptoms such as stuffy nose and cough due to minor throat and bronchial irritation. It also helps loosen and thin bronchial mucus, making it easier to cough up.

Robitussin-CF comes as a liquid.

How should you take this medication?
Doses can be repeated every 4 hours. Do not take more than 6 doses each 24 hours.

■ ADULTS

For adults and children 12 years and over, the usual dose is 2 teaspoonfuls.

■ CHILDREN

Age 6 to 12

The usual dose is 1 teaspoonful.

Age 2 to 6

The usual dose is ½ teaspoonful.

Under 2

Consult a doctor.

Do not take this medication if...
Unless your doctor approves, do not take Robitussin-CF for the type of lasting cough that results from smoking, asthma, chronic bronchitis, or emphysema, or for coughs that bring up large amounts of mucus. Also get the doctor's approval before taking Robitussin-CF if you have heart disease, high blood pressure, thyroid disease, diabetes, or an enlarged prostate gland.

Special warnings about this medication
If you become dizzy or nervous, or have trouble sleeping, stop taking Robitussin-CF and check with your doctor.

If cough and other symptoms don't improve within 7 days or tend to come back—or if you also have a fever, rash, or lasting headache—check with your doctor. A lingering cough could signal a serious condition.

Possible food and drug interactions
when taking this medication
Do not use Robitussin-CF within 2 weeks of taking a drug classified as an MAO inhibitor, such as the antidepressants **Nardil** and **Parnate**.

Brand name:

Robitussin-DM

Pronounced: ROW-bi-TUSS-in
Generic ingredients: Dextromethorphan hydrobromide, Guaifenesin
Other brand names: Safe Tussin 30, Vicks 44E

What this drug is used for

Robitussin-DM, Safe Tussin 30, and Vicks 44E share the same pair of ingredients. All three relieve coughs due to the common cold and help loosen bronchial mucus, making it easier to cough up.

The products come in liquid form. Vicks 44E is available in regular and pediatric strengths.

How should you take this medication?

■ ROBITUSSIN-DM

Doses can be repeated every 4 hours, up to a maximum of 6 doses each 24 hours.

Adults

For adults and children 12 years and over, the usual dose is 2 teaspoonfuls.

Children

For children 6 to 12, the usual dose is 1 teaspoonful. For children 2 to 6, give ½ teaspoonful. For children under 2, consult your doctor.

■ SAFE TUSSIN 30

Doses can be repeated every 6 hours, up to a maximum of 4 doses each 24 hours.

Adults

For adults and children 12 years and over, the usual dose is 2 teaspoonfuls.

Children

For children 6 to 12, the usual dose is 1 teaspoonful. For children 2 to 6, give ½ teaspoonful. For children under 2, consult your doctor.

■ VICKS 44E

Doses can be repeated every 4 hours, up to a maximum of 6 doses each 24 hours.

Adults

For adults and children 12 years and over, the usual dose is 3 tea-spoonfuls.

Children

For children 6 to 12, the usual dose is 1½ teaspoonfuls. For children under 6, consult your doctor.

■ PEDIATRIC VICKS 44E

Doses can be repeated every 4 hours, up to a maximum of 6 doses each 24 hours.

For those 12 years and over, the usual dose is 2 tablespoonfuls. For children 6 to 12, give 1 tablespoonful; and for children 2 to 6, give ½ tablespoonful. Consult your doctor for children under 2.

■ STORAGE

Store at room temperature.

Do not take this medication if...

Unless your doctor approves, do not take these products for the type of lasting cough that results from smoking, asthma, chronic bronchitis, or emphysema, or for coughs that bring up large amounts of mucus. Also avoid these products if any has given you a bad reaction.

These products contain sodium. Check with your doctor if you are on a sodium-restricted diet.

Special warnings about this medication

If your cough doesn't improve within 7 days or tends to come back—or if you also have a fever, rash, or lasting headache—check with your doctor. A lingering cough could signal a serious condition.

**Possible food and drug interactions
when taking this medication**

Do not use any of these products within 2 weeks of taking a drug classified as an MAO inhibitor, such as the antidepressants **Nardil** and **Parnate**.

Brand name:

Robitussin-PE

Pronounced: ROW-bi-TUSS-in
Generic ingredients: Guaifenesin, Pseudoephedrine hydrochloride
Other brand name: Robitussin Severe Congestion Liqui-Gels

What this drug is used for

The ingredients in Robitussin-PE liquid are also available in pill form as Robitussin Severe Congestion Liqui-Gels. The guaifenesin in these products helps loosen bronchial mucus, making it easier to cough up. The pseudoephedrine relieves stuffy nose.

How should you take this medication?

Take a dose every 4 hours, but do not take more than 4 doses a day. A dosage cup is provided for Robitussin-PE.

■ ADULTS

The usual dose for adults and children 12 years and over is 2 tea-spoonfuls or Liqui-Gels.

■ CHILDREN

Age 6 to 12

The usual dose is 1 teaspoonful or Liqui-Gel.

Age 2 to 6

Give ½ teaspoonful of Robitussin-PE.

Under 2

Consult a doctor.

■ STORAGE

Store both products at room temperature.

Do not take this medication if...

Unless your doctor approves, do not take either of these products for the type of lasting cough that results from smoking, asthma, chronic bronchitis, or emphysema, or for coughs that bring up large amounts of mucus. Also check with your doctor before using these products if you have heart disease, high blood pressure, thyroid disease, diabetes, or an enlarged prostate gland.

Special warnings about this medication

If you become dizzy or nervous, or have trouble sleeping, stop taking this medication and check with your doctor.

If cough and other symptoms don't improve within 7 days or tend to come back—or if you also have a fever, rash, or lasting headache—check with your doctor. A lingering cough could signal a serious condition.

Possible food and drug interactions when taking this medication

Do not use either of these products within 2 weeks of taking a drug classified as an MAO inhibitor, such as the antidepressants **Nardil** and **Parnate**.

Brand name:

Rogaine

Pronounced: ROW-gane
Generic name: Minoxidil

What this drug is used for

Rogaine is a liquid scalp application that helps some men and women regrow hair in gradually thinning areas on the top of the head.

Rogaine's effect on each person is different, and can't be predicted. For some people, it doesn't work at all; and no one can expect 100 percent regrowth. Chances of success are best if you have been losing your hair for a short time or have little initial hair loss.

It generally takes at least 4 months for regrowth to begin. Women see best results in approximately 8 months; for men, up to a year is required. To keep the new hair, you must continue using the product. If you stop, you will probably lose the regrown hair within 3 to 4 months.

Rogaine comes in dropper and sprayer packages. The women's sprayer includes an extender. Each bottle includes enough liquid for 25 to 30 days.

How should you use this medication?

The usual dosage is 1 milliliter applied directly to the affected area of the scalp 2 times a day. There is no need to change your usual hair care routine when using Rogaine. However, you should apply it first and wait for it to dry before applying any styling aids. Use a mild shampoo if you wash your scalp before applying Rogaine.

If you miss one or two daily doses of Rogaine, do not try to make them up; just return to your regular schedule. Allow the product to remain on your scalp for about 4 hours before washing your hair. Using Rogaine more frequently or liberally than recommended will not improve results.

If you use your hands to apply Rogaine, wash them afterwards. Do not take the product by mouth.

■ DROPPER APPLICATION
While squeezing the rubber bulb, insert the dropper into the bottle.

Release the bulb, allowing the dropper to fill to the 1-milliliter line. If the level of the solution rises above the 1-milliliter line, squeeze the extra amount back into the bottle.

Place the tip of the dropper near the part of the scalp you are treating and gently squeeze the bulb to gradually release the solution. To keep the solution from running off the scalp, apply a small amount at a time.

■ SPRAYER APPLICATION
Insert the spray applicator into the bottle and twist it on firmly. (If you are using Rogaine for Women, continue by pulling off the small spray head from the plastic tube and replacing it with the extender spray. Push down firmly, then remove the cap from the end of the extender spray.)

Pump the spray 6 times to get one full dose (1 milliliter). Be careful not to inhale the mist.

Do not take this medication if...
If you have no family history of hair loss, or if hair loss is sudden, patchy, and unexplained, do not use Rogaine. Instead, see your doctor. An underlying disease or drug reaction may be at work.

You should also avoid Rogaine if the scalp is red, inflamed, infected, irritated, or painful, if you are using other prescription products on the scalp, or if you have ever had an allergic reaction to Rogaine.

Rogaine is not for the normal hair loss that may accompany childbirth, and is not for use in children under 18.

Special warnings about this medication

Stop using Rogaine and see your doctor if you have any of the following symptoms:

- Chest pain, rapid heartbeat, faintness, or dizziness
- Sudden, unexplained weight gain
- Swollen hands or feet
- Redness or irritation

The most common side effects of Rogaine are itching and other skin irritations on the treated area of the scalp. This product contains alcohol, which can cause burning or irritation of the eyes or sensitive skin areas. If Rogaine accidentally gets into those areas, rinse with large amounts of cold water. Contact your doctor if irritation continues.

Rogaine is not effective against the type of hair loss caused by medications, severe nutritional problems such as iron deficiency, or medical conditions such as hypothyroidism. The product is also ineffective for hair loss due to scarring or deep scalp burns from hair-care products, or hair loss due to grooming methods such as corn-rowing, which pull the hair tightly back from the scalp.

When you first start using Rogaine, hair loss may continue for up to 2 weeks. That hair loss is temporary. If you continue to lose hair after 2 weeks, see your doctor.

To prevent scalp irritation, make sure all of the Rogaine has been washed off your hair and scalp before using chemical products such as hair coloring or permanents.

Rogaine can cause unwanted hair growth elsewhere on the body. Be careful to limit use of the product to the scalp alone.

If you do not see hair regrowth after 8 to 12 months, stop using Rogaine and see your doctor.

Brand name:

Rolaids

Pronounced: ROLL-ayds
Generic ingredients: Calcium carbonate, Magnesium hydroxide

What this drug is used for

Rolaids neutralizes stomach acid. It can be taken for heartburn, sour stomach, acid indigestion, and upset stomach. Each Rolaids tablet also supplies 22 percent of the adult nutritional daily requirement for calcium and 11 percent of the requirement for magnesium.

Rolaids comes in chewable tablet form.

How should you take this medication?
Chew 1 to 4 tablets as symptoms occur. You can take additional doses each hour, but do not take more than 12 tablets a day.

Special warnings about this medication
Do not take the maximum dosage (12 tablets) every day for more than 2 weeks unless your doctor approves.

Possible food and drug interactions
when taking this medication
Antacids interact with a variety of prescription drugs when taken at the same time. An interaction is unlikely, however, if you keep doses of the two at least 2 or 3 hours apart. Drugs that may interact include the following:

Alendronate (**Fosamax**)
Allopurinol (**Zyloprim**)
Antibiotics classified as quinolones, such as **Cipro**, **Floxin**, and
  Noroxin
Aspirin
Atenolol (**Tenormin**)
Captopril (**Capoten**)
Chlordiazepoxide (**Librium**)
Cimetidine (**Tagamet**)
Digoxin (**Lanoxin**)
Doxycycline (**Vibramycin**)
Fosfomycin (**Monurol**)
Gabapentin (**Neurontin**)
Glipizide (**Glucotrol**)
Glyburide (**Micronase, DiaBeta**)
Isoniazid (**Rifamate**)
Ketoconazole (**Nizoral**)
Levothyroxine (**Synthroid**)
Methenamine (**Urised**)
Metronidazole (**Flagyl**)
Misoprostol (**Cytotec**)

Mycophenolate mofetil (**CellCept**)
Nonsteroidal anti-inflammatory drugs such as **Dolobid**, **Motrin**, **Naprosyn**, and **Voltaren**
Penicillamine (**Cuprimine**)
Phenytoin (**Dilantin**)
Quinidine (**Quinidex**)
Sodium polystyrene sulfonate (**Kayexalate**)
Sucralfate (**Carafate**)
Tetracycline antibiotics such as **Achromycin V** and **Minocin**
Tilodronate (**Skelid**)
Ursodiol (**Actigall**)

Prolonged and heavy use of antacids such as Rolaids, combined with a high intake of calcium-rich foods such as milk, can lead to an overload of calcium in the system. Early symptoms are constipation, weakness, nausea, and vomiting; a severe overload can cause kidney damage. If you need a high-calcium diet, check with your doctor about a substitute for Rolaids.

Brand name:

Ryna Liquid

Pronounced: RYE-nuh
Generic ingredients: Chlorpheniramine maleate, Pseudoephedrine hydrochloride

What this drug is used for

Ryna Liquid unclogs stuffy nose caused by colds and allergies such as hay fever. It also relieves allergy-related runny nose, sneezing, itchy nose or throat, and itchy, watery eyes.

How should you take this medication?

■ ADULTS

For adults and children 12 years and over, the usual dose is 2 teaspoonfuls every 4 to 6 hours, up to a maximum of 8 teaspoonfuls each 24 hours.

■ CHILDREN

For children 6 to 12, the usual dose is 1 teaspoonful every 4 to 6 hours, up to a maximum of 4 teaspoonfuls each 24 hours. For children under 6, consult your doctor.

■ STORAGE

Store at room temperature.

Do not take this medication if...

Unless your doctor approves, do not take Ryna Liquid if you have heart disease, high blood pressure, thyroid disease, diabetes, high pressure within the eye (glaucoma), an enlarged prostate gland, or a breathing problem such as emphysema or chronic bronchitis. Do not give the product to children taking other medication.

Special warnings about this medication

If you become dizzy or nervous, or have trouble sleeping, stop taking Ryna Liquid and check with your doctor.

If your symptoms do not improve within 7 days, or include a fever, check with your doctor.

Ryna Liquid may cause excitability, especially in children. It can also cause drowsiness. Be especially cautious when driving, and when operating machinery.

Possible food and drug interactions when taking this medication

Do not use Ryna Liquid within 2 weeks of taking a drug classified as an MAO inhibitor, such as the antidepressants **Nardil** and **Parnate**.

If you are taking a tranquilizer such as **Valium** or **Xanax**, or a sleep aid such as **Halcion** or **Seconal**, do not take Ryna Liquid without your doctor's approval; the combination could cause extreme drowsiness. For the same reason, avoid alcohol while taking this product.

Brand name:

Ryna-C Liquid

Pronounced: RYE-nuh
Generic ingredients: Chlorpheniramine maleate, Codeine phosphate, Pseudoephedrine hydrochloride

What this drug is used for

Like regular Ryna Liquid, Ryna-C unclogs stuffy nose caused by colds and allergies such as hay fever, and relieves allergy-related runny nose, sneezing, itchy nose or throat, and itchy, watery eyes. However, Ryna-C also includes codeine for relief of cough.

How should you take this medication?

■ ADULTS

For adults and children 12 years and over, the usual dose is 2 teaspoonfuls every 4 to 6 hours, up to a maximum of 8 teaspoonfuls each 24 hours.

■ CHILDREN

For children 6 to 12, the usual dose is 1 teaspoonful every 4 to 6 hours, up to a maximum of 4 teaspoonfuls each 24 hours. For children under 6, consult your doctor.

■ STORAGE

Store at room temperature, away from light. Keep the bottle tightly closed.

Do not take this medication if...

Unless your doctor approves, do not take Ryna-C if you have heart disease, high blood pressure, thyroid disease, diabetes, high pressure within the eye (glaucoma), an enlarged prostate gland, or a breathing problem such as emphysema or chronic bronchitis. Do not give the product to children taking other medication.

Also check with your doctor before using Ryna-C for the type of chronic cough that results from smoking or asthma, or for a cough that brings up lots of phlegm.

Special warnings about this medication

If you become dizzy or nervous, or have trouble sleeping, stop taking Ryna-C and check with your doctor.

If cough and other symptoms don't improve within 7 days or tend to come back—or if you also have a fever, rash, or lasting headache—check with your doctor. A lingering cough could signal a serious condition.

Ryna-C may cause excitability, especially in children. It can also cause drowsiness. Be especially cautious when driving, and when operating machinery.

Ryna-C may also cause constipation.

Possible food and drug interactions when taking this medication

Do not use Ryna-C within 2 weeks of taking a drug classified as an MAO inhibitor, such as the antidepressants **Nardil** and **Parnate**.

If you are taking a tranquilizer such as **Valium** or **Xanax**, or a sleep aid such as **Halcion** or **Seconal**, do not take Ryna-C without your doctor's approval; the combination could cause extreme drowsiness. For the same reason, avoid alcohol while taking this product.

Brand name:

Ryna-CX Liquid

Pronounced: RYE-nuh
Generic ingredients: Codeine phosphate, Guaifenesin, Pseudo-
  ephedrine hydrochloride

What this drug is used for

Like regular Ryna and Ryna-C, Ryna-CX unclogs stuffy nose caused by colds and allergies such as hay fever. Like Ryna-C, it contains codeine to quiet coughs. To all of this, the CX formulation adds guaifenesin, an ingredient that loosens phlegm, making it easier to cough up.

Unlike the two other Ryna products, Ryna-CX does *not* contain an antihistamine to relieve allergy symptoms such as sneezing and runny nose.

How should you take this medication?

■ ADULTS

For adults and children 12 years and over, the usual dose is 2 teaspoonfuls every 4 to 6 hours, up to a maximum of 8 teaspoonfuls each 24 hours.

■ CHILDREN

For children 6 to 12, the usual dose is 1 teaspoonful every 4 to 6 hours, up to a maximum of 4 teaspoonfuls each 24 hours. For children under 6, consult your doctor.

■ STORAGE

Store at room temperature, away from light. Keep bottle tightly closed.

Do not take this medication if...

Unless your doctor approves, do not take Ryna-CX if you have heart disease, high blood pressure, thyroid disease, diabetes, high pressure within the eye (glaucoma), an enlarged prostate gland, or a breathing problem such as shortness of breath, emphysema, or chronic bronchitis. Do not give the product to children taking other medication.

Also check with your doctor before using Ryna-CX for the type of chronic cough that results from smoking or asthma, or for a cough that brings up lots of phlegm.

Special warnings about this medication

If you become dizzy or nervous, or have trouble sleeping, stop taking Ryna-CX and check with your doctor.

If cough and other symptoms don't improve within 7 days or tend to come back—or if you also have a fever, rash, or lasting headache—check with your doctor. A lingering cough could signal a serious condition.

Ryna-CX may cause excitability, especially in children. It can also cause drowsiness. Be especially cautious when driving and when operating machinery.

Ryna-CX may also cause constipation.

Possible food and drug interactions
when taking this medication

Do not use Ryna-CX within 2 weeks of taking a drug classified as an MAO inhibitor, such as the antidepressants **Nardil** and **Parnate**.

If you are taking a tranquilizer such as **Valium** or **Xanax**, or a sleep aid such as **Halcion** or **Seconal**, do not take Ryna-CX without your doctor's approval; the combination could cause extreme drowsiness. For the same reason, avoid alcohol while taking this product.

Brand name:
Safe Tussin 30

See Robitussin-DM

Brand name:
Senokot

Pronounced: SEN-uh-cot
Generic ingredients: Senna, Docusate sodium (Senokot-S only)
Other brand names: Correctol Herbal Tea, Ex-Lax Gentle Nature Laxative Pills, Fletcher's Castoria

What this drug is used for

These products relieve constipation. All will usually produce a bowel movement within 6 to 12 hours. Fletcher's Castoria is marketed specifically for children.

Formulations range from pills and syrups to granules and tea bags. Note that Ex-Lax Gentle Nature is different from the rest of the Ex-Lax line, which contains another laxative ingredient called yellow phenolphthalein. The cherry flavor version of Fletcher's also contains this ingredient.

How should you take this medication?

■ ADULTS AND CHILDREN 12 YEARS AND OVER

Senokot

Take all forms of Senokot according to the instructions on the package or as directed by your doctor, preferably at bedtime.

Correctol Herbal Tea

Place 1 tea bag in a cup, add 6 ounces of boiling water, and let steep for 5 minutes. For iced tea, use 3 ounces of boiling water and add ice cubes after steeping. Remove the bag. You may sweeten to taste. Drink one 6-ounce cup of tea once a day. If you need a stronger laxative, make a second cup and drink as much as you feel you need, but do not take more than 3 cups a day. If you want a less powerful laxative, drink only two-thirds of a cup (4 ounces).

Ex-Lax Gentle Nature Laxative Pills

Take 1 or 2 pills with a glass of water, preferably at bedtime.

■ CHILDREN

Senokot

For children 6 to 12, the usual dosage is 1 to 1½ teaspoonfuls of Senokot Children's Syrup at bedtime. Do not give more than two 1½-teaspoonful doses a day. For children 2 to 6, the usual dosage is ½ to ¾ of a teaspoonful. Do not give more than two ¾-teaspoonful doses a day. For children under 2, consult your doctor.

Fletcher's Castoria

Shake the bottle well before using. For children 6 to 15, the usual dosage is 2 or 3 teaspoonfuls up to twice a day. For children 2 to 6, the usual dosage is 1 or 2 teaspoonfuls up to twice a day. For children under 2, consult your doctor.

Correctol Herbal Tea
Check with your doctor before giving this product to children under 12.

Ex-Lax Gentle Nature Laxative Pills
For children 6 to 12, the usual dosage is 1 pill with a glass of water at bedtime. For children under 6, consult your doctor.

■ OLDER ADULTS AND PREGNANT WOMEN
Your doctor may tell you to take half the starting dosage recommended on the package.

Do not take this medication if...
Unless your doctor approves, do not take a laxative when you have stomach pain, nausea, or vomiting. If you have noticed a sudden change in bowel habits lasting for 2 weeks or longer, check with your doctor before using a laxative.

Special warnings about this medication
Stop using this medicine and call your doctor if you develop rectal bleeding or fail to have a bowel movement after taking the medicine. You might have a serious condition.

Used too often or too long, laxatives can become habit-forming. Do not use any laxative for more than a week without your doctor's approval.

If you are using Correctol Herbal Tea, do not reuse individual tea bags; and do not take the tea while using other laxatives.

Brand name:
Sinarest

Pronounced: SIGN-uh-rest
Generic ingredients: Acetaminophen, Chlorpheniramine maleate, Pseudoephedrine hydrochloride

What this drug is used for
Sinarest temporarily unclogs stuffy nose and relieves the sneezing, runny nose, itchy nose or throat, and itchy, watery eyes that accompany inflamed sinuses and allergies such as hay fever. The acetaminophen in the product relieves headache and minor aches and pains.

Sinarest is available in regular-strength tablets and extra-strength caplets.

How should you take this medication?

■ ADULTS

For adults and children 12 years and over, the usual dose is 2 tablets. Regular-strength tablets can be taken every 4 to 6 hours; extra-strength caplets should be taken only every 6 hours. Do not take more than 8 pills each 24 hours.

■ CHILDREN

For children 6 to 12, the usual dose is 1 regular-strength tablet every 4 to 6 hours. Do not use the extra-strength caplets; and do not give more than 4 tablets a day. For children under 6, consult your doctor.

■ STORAGE

Store at room temperature.

Do not take this medication if...

Unless your doctor approves, do not take Sinarest if you have heart disease, high blood pressure, thyroid disease, diabetes, high pressure within the eye (glaucoma), an enlarged prostate gland, or a breathing problem such as emphysema or chronic bronchitis.

Special warnings about this medication

If you become dizzy or nervous, or have trouble sleeping, stop taking Sinarest and check with your doctor.

Sinarest may cause drowsiness. Be especially cautious when driving, and when operating machinery. This medication can also cause excitability, especially in children.

Do not take this product for more than 10 days (5-day limit for children). If your symptoms do not improve or include a fever that lasts more than 3 days—or if new symptoms appear—call your doctor.

Possible food and drug interactions
when taking this medication

Do not use Sinarest within 2 weeks of taking a drug classified as an MAO inhibitor, such as the antidepressants **Nardil** and **Parnate**.

If you are taking a tranquilizer such as **Valium** or **Xanax**, or a sleep aid such as **Halcion** or **Seconal**, do not take Sinarest without your doctor's approval; the combination could cause extreme drowsiness. For the same reason, avoid alcohol while taking this product.

Brand name:

Sine-Aid

Pronounced: SIGN-ade
Generic ingredients: Acetaminophen, Pseudoephedrine hydrochloride
Other brand names: Sudafed Sinus, Tylenol Sinus

What this drug is used for

These three sinus products all combine the decongestant pseudoephedrine with the pain reliever acetaminophen. The decongestant opens clogged sinuses and nasal passages. Acetaminophen relieves headache and other minor aches and pains.

Sine-Aid and Tylenol Sinus are available in caplets, tablets, and gels; Sudafed is available only in caplet and tablet form.

How should you take this medication?

The usual dose for adults and children 12 years and over is 2 pills every 4 to 6 hours. Do not take more than 8 pills each 24 hours.

■ STORAGE
Store at room temperature in a dry place. Protect from light.

Do not take this medication if...

Unless your doctor approves, do not take these products if you have heart disease, high blood pressure, thyroid disease, diabetes, or an enlarged prostate gland.

These products are not intended for children under 12.

Special warnings about this medication

If you become dizzy or nervous, or have trouble sleeping, stop taking the product and check with your doctor.

Generally speaking, you should not take any of these products for more than 7 days. If your symptoms do not improve or include a fever that lasts more than 3 days—or if new symptoms appear—call your doctor. Also check with your doctor if you notice any redness or swelling. These could be signs of a more serious condition.

Allergic reactions to these products are rare, but possible. Stop taking the drug immediately if a reaction develops.

Possible food and drug interactions
when taking this medication

Do not use any of these products within 2 weeks of taking a drug classified as an MAO inhibitor, such as the antidepressants **Nardil** and **Parnate**.

Do not combine any of these products with others that also contain acetaminophen. Large amounts of acetaminophen can conceivably cause liver damage, particularly if you are a heavy drinker. Check with your doctor before taking one of these products if you generally have more than 3 alcoholic beverages a day.

Overdosage

■ *Symptoms of overdose may include:*

Anxiety, a generally uneasy feeling, rapid heartbeat, sweating, nausea, vomiting

If you suspect an overdose, seek medical attention immediately.

Brand name:

Sine-Off

Pronounced: SIGN-off
Generic ingredients: Acetaminophen, Diphenhydramine hydrochloride, Pseudophedrine hydrochloride

What this drug is used for

The three ingredients in Sine-Off clear stuffy nose and sinuses, combat sneezing and runny nose due to a cold, flu, or hay fever, and relieve headache, fever, sore throat, and muscular aches and pains.

How should you take this medication?

The usual dosage is 2 gelatin caplets at bedtime. Doses can be repeated every 6 hours, up to a maximum of 8 caplets each 24 hours. Check with your doctor for children under 12.

■ STORAGE

Keep in a dry place. Protect from high temperatures.

Do not take this medication if...

Unless your doctor approves, do not take Sine-Off if you have heart disease, high blood pressure, thyroid disease, diabetes, high pressure within the eye (glaucoma), an enlarged prostate gland, or a breathing problem such as emphysema or chronic bronchitis.

Special warnings about this medication

Taking more than 8 caplets a day can lead to nervousness, dizziness, or trouble sleeping. The product can also cause overexcitement, especially in children.

On the other hand, Sine-Off makes some people drowsy. Be especially cautious when driving, and when operating machinery.

Do not take Sine-Off for more than 10 days. If your symptoms do not improve or include a fever that lasts more than 3 days—or if new symptoms appear—call your doctor.

You should also check with your doctor immediately if you have a severe sore throat that lasts for more than 2 days, or if your sore throat is accompanied or followed by fever, headache, rash, nausea, or vomiting.

Possible food and drug interactions
when taking this medication

Do not use Sine-Off within 2 weeks of taking a drug classified as an MAO inhibitor, such as the antidepressants **Nardil** and **Parnate**.

If you are taking a tranquilizer such as **Valium** or **Xanax**, or a sleep aid such as **Halcion** or **Seconal**, do not take Sine-Off without your doctor's approval; the combination could cause extreme drowsiness. For the same reason, avoid alcohol while taking this product.

Brand name:

Singlet

Pronounced: SING-let
Generic ingredients: Acetaminophen, Chlorpheniramine maleate,
   Pseudoephedrine hydrochloride

What this drug is used for

Singlet temporarily relieves stuffy nose, sinus pain, and headache due to a cold, inflamed sinuses, or an allergy such as hay fever. It reduces the fever that may accompany a cold; and it relieves allergy symptoms such as runny nose, sneezing, itchy nose or throat, and itchy, watery eyes.

How should you take this medication?

The usual dose for adults and children 12 years and over is 1 caplet every 4 to 6 hours. Do not take more than 4 caplets each 24 hours. For children under 12, consult your doctor.

■ STORAGE
Protect from excessive heat and moisture.

Do not take this medication if...

Unless your doctor approves, do not take Singlet if you have heart disease, high blood pressure, thyroid disease, diabetes, high pressure within the eye (glaucoma), an enlarged prostate gland, or a breathing problem such as emphysema or chronic bronchitis.

Special warnings about this medication

This product may cause excitability, especially in children. If you become dizzy or nervous, or have trouble sleeping, stop taking Singlet and check with your doctor. Singlet may also cause drowsiness. Be especially cautious when driving, and when operating machinery.

Do not take this product for more than 10 days. If your symptoms do not improve or include a fever that lasts more than 3 days—or if new symptoms appear—call your doctor.

Possible food and drug interactions when taking this medication

Do not use Singlet within 2 weeks of taking a drug classified as an MAO inhibitor, such as the antidepressants **Nardil** and **Parnate**.

If you are taking a tranquilizer such as **Valium** or **Xanax**, or a sleep aid such as **Halcion** or **Seconal**, do not take Singlet without your doctor's approval; the combination could cause extreme drowsiness. For the same reason, avoid alcohol while taking this product.

Brand name:

Sinulin

Pronounced: SIGN-you-lin
Generic ingredients: Acetaminophen, Chlorpheniramine maleate,
   Phenylpropanolamine hydrochloride

What this drug is used for

Sinulin gives temporary relief from many of the symptoms that accompany a cold, sinusitis, or an allergy such as hay fever. The product remedies headache, fever, stuffy nose and sinuses, runny nose, sneezing, itchy nose or throat, and itchy, watery eyes.

How should you take this medication?
■ ADULTS

The usual dose for adults and children 12 years and over is 1 tablet every 4 to 6 hours. Do not take more than 6 tablets each 24 hours.

■ CHILDREN

For children 6 to 12, the usual dose is half a tablet every 4 to 6 hours. Do not give a total of more than 3 tablets each 24 hours. For children under age 6, consult your doctor.

■ STORAGE

Store at room temperature.

Do not take this medication if...
Unless your doctor approves, do not take Sinulin if you have high blood pressure, heart disease, diabetes, thyroid disease, high pressure within the eye (glaucoma), an enlarged prostate gland, or a breathing problem such as emphysema, chronic bronchitis, or asthma.

Special warnings about this medication
High doses of this product can cause nervousness, dizziness, sleeplessness, rapid heartbeat, or high blood pressure.

The product can also make you drowsy. Be especially cautious when driving, and when operating machinery. Sinulin sometimes causes excitability, too, especially in children.

Allergic reactions to Sinulin are rare, but possible. If you develop any sort of reaction, stop taking the product and call your doctor.

Adults should not take Sinulin for more than 7 days. For children 6 to 12, the limit is 5 days. If your symptoms do not improve or include a fever that lasts more than 3 days or comes back—or if new symptoms appear—call your doctor.

Possible food and drug interactions
when taking this medication
Do not use Sinulin within 2 weeks of taking a drug classified as an MAO inhibitor, such as the antidepressants **Nardil** and **Parnate**.

Check with your doctor before combining Sinulin with any other anti-depressant, or with any medication for high blood pressure.

If you are taking a tranquilizer such as **Valium** or **Xanax**, or a sleep aid such as **Halcion** or **Seconal**, do not take Sinulin without your doctor's approval; the combination could cause extreme drowsiness. For the same reason, avoid alcohol while taking this product.

Overdosage
A massive overdose of the acetaminophen in Sinulin could conceivably cause liver damage. If you suspect an overdose, seek medical attention promptly.

Brand name:

Sinutab

Pronounced: SINE-you-tab
Generic ingredients: Guaifenesin, Pseudoephedrine hydrochloride

What this drug is used for
This is the basic Sinutab product. It relieves stuffiness due to inflamed sinuses and helps loosen and thin phlegm. It comes in a liquid-filled capsule (Liquid Cap).

How should you take this medication?
For adults and children 12 years and over, the usual dose is 2 capsules every 4 hours. Do not take more than 8 capsules each 24 hours. For children under 12, consult a doctor.

Do not take this medication if...
Unless your doctor approves, do not take Sinutab if you have heart disease, high blood pressure, thyroid disease, diabetes, or an enlarged prostate gland.

Also check with your doctor before using Sinutab for the type of nagging cough that results from smoking, asthma, emphysema, or chronic bronchitis, or for a cough that brings up lots of phlegm.

Special warnings about this medication
If you become dizzy or nervous, or have trouble sleeping, stop taking Sinutab and check with your doctor.

If cough and other symptoms don't improve within 7 days or tend to come back—or if you also have a fever, rash, or lasting headache—check with your doctor. A lingering cough could signal a serious condition.

Possible food and drug interactions when taking this medication

Do not use Sinutab within 2 weeks of taking a drug classified as an MAO inhibitor, such as the antidepressants **Nardil** and **Parnate**.

Brand name:

Sinutab Sinus Allergy

Pronounced: SINE-you-tab
Generic ingredients: Acetaminophen, Chlorpheniramine maleate,
  Pseudoephedrine hydrochloride

What this drug is used for

Like other Sinutab products, Sinutab Sinus Allergy temporarily relieves stuffiness due to inflamed sinuses. However, this formulation also eases minor aches, pains, and headache, and can be used for symptoms of hay fever and similar allergies, including runny nose, sneezing, itchy nose or throat, and itchy, watery eyes.

The product is available in tablet and caplet form.

How should you take this medication?

For adults and children 12 years and over, the usual dose is 2 pills every 6 hours. Do not take more than 8 pills each 24 hours. For children under 12, consult a doctor.

■ STORAGE
Store at room temperature.

Do not take this medication if...

Unless your doctor approves, do not take Sinutab Sinus Allergy if you have heart disease, high blood pressure, thyroid disease, diabetes, high pressure within the eye (glaucoma), an enlarged prostate gland, or a breathing problem such as emphysema or chronic bronchitis.

Special warnings about this medication

If you become dizzy or nervous, or have trouble sleeping, stop taking this product and check with your doctor.

Do not take Sinutab Sinus Allergy for more than 10 days. Check with your doctor if your symptoms don't improve or include a fever that lasts more than 3 days, or if new symptoms develop.

Sinutab Sinus Allergy may cause excitability, especially in children. This medication can also cause drowsiness. Be especially cautious when driving, and when operating machinery.

Possible food and drug interactions
when taking this medication
Do not use Sinutab Sinus Allergy within 2 weeks of taking a drug classified as an MAO inhibitor, such as the antidepressants **Nardil** and **Parnate**.

If you are taking a tranquilizer such as **Valium** or **Xanax**, or a sleep aid such as **Halcion** or **Seconal**, do not take Sinutab Sinus Allergy without your doctor's approval; the combination could cause extreme drowsiness. For the same reason, avoid alcohol while taking this product.

Brand name:

Sinutab Sinus Medication

Pronounced: SINE-you-tab
Generic ingredients: Acetaminophen, Pseudoephedrine hydrochloride

What this drug is used for
Like the other products in the Sinutab line, Sinutab Sinus Medication temporarily relieves stuffiness due to inflamed sinuses. This particular formulation also fights minor aches, pains, and headache. It is available in tablet or caplet form.

How should you take this medication?
For adults and children 12 years and over, the usual dose is 2 pills every 6 hours. Do not take more than 8 pills each 24 hours. For children under 12, consult a doctor.

Do not take this medication if...
Unless your doctor approves, do not take Sinutab Sinus Medication if you have heart disease, high blood pressure, thyroid disease, diabetes, or an enlarged prostate gland.

Special warnings about this medication
If you become dizzy or nervous, or have trouble sleeping, stop taking Sinutab Sinus Medication and check with your doctor.

Do not take Sinutab Sinus Medication for more than 10 days. Check with your doctor if your symptoms don't improve or include a fever that lasts more than 3 days, or if new symptoms develop.

**Possible food and drug interactions
when taking this medication**
Do not use Sinutab Sinus Medication within 2 weeks of taking a drug classified as an MAO inhibitor, such as the antidepressants **Nardil** and **Parnate**.

If you generally drink 3 or more alcoholic beverages a day, there is a remote possibility that the acetaminophen in this product could damage your liver. Ask your doctor whether you should be concerned.

Brand name:

Sleepinal

See Nytol

Brand name:

St. Joseph

See Aspirin

Brand name:

Sucrets

Pronounced: SOO-krets
Generic name: Dyclonine hydrochloride
Other brand name: Cepacol Sore Throat Spray

What this drug is used for
Both Sucrets lozenges and Cepacol Sore Throat Spray can be used for temporary relief of minor sore throat pain and sore mouth. In addition, the spray is marketed for relief of minor pain caused by canker sores and irritation from minor mouth injuries, dental procedures, dentures, and orthodontic appliances.

How should you take this medication?
■ SUCRETS
For adults and children 2 years and over, the usual dose is 1 lozenge slowly dissolved in the mouth. Doses may be repeated every 2 hours. For children under 2, consult your doctor.

■ CEPACOL SORE THROAT SPRAY

Spray this product in your mouth or throat, then swallow. Doses may be repeated up to 4 times a day.

Adults

For adults and children 12 years and over, the usual dose is 4 sprays.

Children

For children 2 to 12, the usual dose is 2 or 3 sprays under adult supervision. For children under 2, consult your doctor.

■ STORAGE

Store at room temperature. Protect the Cepacol spray from freezing.

Do not take this medication if...

Do not use these products for a severe sore throat, one that lasts more than 2 days, or a sore throat accompanied by a fever, headache, rash, swelling, nausea, or vomiting. Instead, see your doctor.

Special warnings about this medication

If symptoms don't improve in 7 days, or pain, irritation, or redness remains or gets worse, check with your doctor or dentist.

Overdosage

■ *Symptoms of overdose may include:*

Blurred vision, depression, dizziness, excitement, nervousness, tremors, slowed heartbeat, low blood pressure

If you suspect an overdose, seek medical attention immediately.

Brand name:

Sucrets 4 Hour Cough Suppressant

Pronounced: soo-KRETZ
Generic name: Dextromethorphan

What this drug is used for

These lozenges contain the same active ingredient found in a number of popular liquid cough suppressants (see Benylin Cough Suppressants). They provide temporary relief of cough due to sore throat or irritated bronchial tubes, as brought on by the common cold or an inhaled irritant.

How should you take this medication?

■ ADULTS AND CHILDREN 12 YEARS AND OVER

Take 1 cough lozenge every 4 hours as needed. Do not take more than 6 lozenges in any 24-hour period.

■ CHILDREN 6 TO 12

Give children this age 1 lozenge every 6 hours as needed. They should not take more than 4 lozenges in any 24-hour period.

■ STORAGE

Protect from high heat.

Do not take this medication if...

Unless your doctor tells you otherwise, do not use this product for cough due to smoking, asthma, or emphysema, or for coughs that bring up a lot of phlegm.

Do not give to children under 6 without your doctor's approval.

Special warnings about this medication

A persistent cough may be a sign of a serious illness. If you have a cough that lasts for more than 1 week, goes away and comes back, or is accompanied by a fever, rash, or long-lasting headache, call your doctor.

Possible food and drug interactions when taking this medication

Do not use this product within 2 weeks of taking a drug classified as an MAO inhibitor, including the antidepressants **Nardil** and **Parnate**.

Brand name:

Sudafed

Pronounced: SUE-da-fed
Generic name: Pseudoephedrine hydrochloride
Other brands: Dimetapp Decongestant Pediatric Drops, Drixoral
Nasal Decongestant, Triaminic Decongestant products

What this drug is used for

Sudafed 12 Hour Caplets, Sudafed Nasal Decongestant formulations, and several other products with "decongestant" in the name all share the single ingredient pseudoephedrine. This medication provides temporary relief of the stuffy nose that often accompanies a cold, sinus inflammation, or allergies such as hay fever.

How should you take these medications?

Here are the usual dosages for pseudoephedrine-based decongestant products.

■ SUDAFED NASAL DECONGESTANT

Take every 4 to 6 hours, up to 4 times each day.

Adults: 2 tablets.
Children 6 to 12: 1 tablet.
Children 2 to 6: Use a liquid product.

■ PEDIATRIC SUDAFED NASAL DECONGESTANT DROPS

Give by mouth only, using the supplied dropper. Give every 4 to 6 hours, up to 4 times each day.

Children 2 to 6: 2 dropperfuls.
Children under 2: Consult your doctor.

■ CHILDREN'S SUDAFED NASAL DECONGESTANT CHEWABLES

Give every 4 to 6 hours, up to 4 times each day.

Children 6 to 12: 2 tablets.
Children 2 to 6: 1 tablet.
Children under 2: Consult your doctor.

■ SUDAFED CHILDREN'S NASAL DECONGESTANT LIQUID / TRIAMINIC AM DECONGESTANT FORMULA

Take every 4 to 6 hours, up to 4 times each day.

Adults: 4 teaspoonfuls.
Children 6 to 12: 2 teaspoonfuls.
Children 2 to 6: 1 teaspoonful.
Children under 2: Consult your doctor.

■ DIMETAPP DECONGESTANT PEDIATRIC DROPS / TRIAMINIC INFANT ORAL DECONGESTANT DROPS

For administration by mouth only. Give every 4 to 6 hours, up to 4 times each day.

Children 2 to 3: 2 dropperfuls.
Children under 2: Consult your doctor.

■ SUDAFED 12 HOUR CAPLETS / DRIXORAL NASAL DECONGESTANT
Take 1 pill every 12 hours, up to twice each day. For children under 12, consult your doctor.

■ STORAGE
Store at room temperature. Protect tablets and caplets from excessive moisture. Store liquids away from light.

Do not take this medication if...
Unless your doctor approves, do not take any of these products if you have heart disease, high blood pressure, thyroid disease, diabetes, or an enlarged prostate gland.

Special warnings about this medication
If you become dizzy or nervous, or have trouble sleeping, stop taking this medication and check with your doctor. You should also call your doctor if symptoms do not improve within 7 days or you develop a fever.

If your child must avoid phenylalanine, do not give Children's Sudafed Nasal Decongestant Chewables, which contain the substance.

Possible food and drug interactions
when taking this medication
Do not use any of these products within 2 weeks of taking a drug classified as an MAO inhibitor, such as the antidepressants **Nardil** and **Parnate**.

Check with your doctor before combining Sudafed 12 Hour Caplets with any medication for depression or high blood pressure.

Brand name:

Sudafed Cold & Allergy

Pronounced: SUE-da-fed
Generic ingredients: Chlorpheniramine maleate, Pseudoephedrine
  hydrochloride

What this drug is used for
Like all Sudafed products, this one temporarily relieves the stuffy nose that comes with a cold. In addition, it contains an antihistamine

that combats allergy symptoms such as runny nose, sneezing, itchy nose or throat, and itchy, watery eyes.

How should you take this medication?

Doses may be repeated every 4 to 6 hours. Do not take more than 4 doses each 24 hours.

■ ADULTS

The usual dose for adults and children 12 years and over is 1 tablet.

■ CHILDREN

The usual dose for children 6 to 12 is half a tablet. For children under 6, consult your doctor.

■ STORAGE

Store at room temperature in a dry place. Protect from light.

Do not take this medication if...

Unless your doctor approves, do not take Sudafed Cold & Allergy if you have heart disease, high blood pressure, thyroid disease, diabetes, high pressure within the eye (glaucoma), an enlarged prostate gland, or a breathing problem such as emphysema or chronic bronchitis.

Special warnings about this medication

If you become dizzy or nervous, or have trouble sleeping, stop taking this product and check with your doctor.

The antihistamine in this product may cause drowsiness. Be especially cautious when driving and when operating machinery. This ingredient can also cause excitability, especially in children

If symptoms do not improve within 7 days or you develop a fever, call your doctor.

Possible food and drug interactions
when taking this medication

Do not use this product within 2 weeks of taking a drug classified as an MAO inhibitor, such as the antidepressants **Nardil** and **Parnate**.

If you are taking a tranquilizer such as **Valium** or **Xanax**, or a sleep aid such as **Halcion** or **Seconal**, do not take Sudafed Cold & Allergy without your doctor's approval; the combination could cause extreme drowsiness. For the same reason, avoid alcohol while taking this product.

Brand name:

Sudafed Cold & Cough

Pronounced: SUE-da-fed
Generic ingredients: Acetaminophen, Dextromethorphan hydrobro-
mide, Guaifenesin, Pseudoephedrine hydrochloride

What this drug is used for

Sudafed Cold & Cough, like other Sudafed products, relieves stuffy nose. In addition, the acetaminophen it contains will combat the minor aches and pains, headaches, muscle aches, sore throat, and fever that often accompany a common cold. Two other ingredients relieve cough and loosen bronchial mucus, making it easier to cough up.

How should you take this medication?

The usual dose for adults and children 12 years and over is 2 pills every 4 hours, up to a maximum of 8 pills each 24 hours. For children under 12, consult your doctor.

■ STORAGE

Store at room temperature in a dry place. Protect from light.

Do not take this medication if...

Unless your doctor approves, do not take Sudafed Cold & Cough if you have heart disease, high blood pressure, thyroid disease, diabetes, or an enlarged prostate gland.

Also check with your doctor before using this product for the type of chronic cough that results from smoking, asthma, chronic bronchitis, or emphysema, or for a cough that brings up lots of phlegm.

Special warnings about this medication

If you become dizzy or nervous, or have trouble sleeping, stop taking Sudafed Cold & Cough and check with your doctor.

Do not take this product for more than 10 days. If your symptoms do not improve or include a fever that lasts more than 3 days—or if new symptoms appear—call your doctor.

You should also check with your doctor immediately if you have a severe sore throat that lasts for more than 2 days, or if your sore throat is accompanied or followed by fever, headache, rash, nausea, or vomiting.

Likewise, call your doctor if you have a cough that lasts for more than 7 days or tends to come back, or your cough is accompanied by rash, lasting headache, and fever.

Possible food and drug interactions when taking this medication

Do not use Sudafed Cold & Cough within 2 weeks of taking a drug classified as an MAO inhibitor, such as the antidepressants **Nardil** and **Parnate**.

Combined with heavy drinking, the acetaminophen in this product could conceivably cause liver damage. Check with your doctor before taking this product if you generally have more than 3 alcoholic beverages a day.

Brand name:

Sudafed Cold & Sinus

Pronounced: SUE-da-fed
Generic ingredients: Acetaminophen, Pseudoephedrine hydrochloride

What this drug is used for

Sudafed Cold & Sinus temporarily relieves nasal congestion, allowing the sinuses to drain. In addition, the acetaminophen in this product relieves the minor aches, pains, headache, muscular aches, sore throat, and fever that often accompany a cold.

How should you take this medication?

The usual dose for adults and children 12 years and over is 2 pills every 4 to 6 hours, up to a maximum of 8 pills each 24 hours. For children under 12, consult your doctor.

■ STORAGE

Store at room temperature in a dry place. Protect from light.

Do not take this medication if...

Unless your doctor approves, do not take Sudafed Cold & Sinus if you have heart disease, high blood pressure, thyroid disease, diabetes, or an enlarged prostate gland.

Special warnings about this medication

If you become dizzy or nervous, or have trouble sleeping, stop taking Sudafed Cold & Sinus and check with your doctor.

Do not take this product for more than 10 days. If your symptoms do not improve or include a fever that lasts more than 3 days—or if new symptoms appear—call your doctor.

You should also check with your doctor immediately if you have a severe sore throat that lasts for more than 2 days, or if your sore throat is accompanied or followed by fever, headache, rash, nausea, or vomiting.

Possible food and drug interactions when taking this medication
Do not use Sudafed Cold & Sinus within 2 weeks of taking a drug classified as an MAO inhibitor, such as the antidepressants **Nardil** and **Parnate**.

Combined with heavy drinking, the acetaminophen in this product could conceivably cause liver damage. Check with your doctor before taking this product if you generally have more than 3 alcoholic beverages a day.

Brand name:

Sudafed Non-Drying Sinus

Pronounced: SUE-da-fed
Generic ingredients: Guaifenesin, Pseudoephedrine hydrochloride

What this drug is used for
Like all Sudafed products, Sudafed Non-Drying Sinus temporarily relieves nasal congestion. This helps the sinuses to drain, reducing sinus pressure. This variety of Sudafed also contains an ingredient that helps loosen and thin bronchial mucus, making it easier to cough up.

How should you take this medication?
The usual dose for adults and children 12 years and over is 2 pills every 4 hours, up to a maximum of 8 pills each 24 hours. For children under 12, consult your doctor.

■ STORAGE
Store at room temperature in a dry place. Protect from light.

Do not take this medication if...
Unless your doctor approves, do not take this product for the type of lasting cough that results from smoking, asthma, chronic bronchitis, or emphysema, or for coughs that bring up large amounts of mucus.

Also get your doctor's approval of this product if you have heart disease, high blood pressure, thyroid disease, diabetes, or an enlarged prostate gland.

Special warnings about this medication

If you become dizzy or nervous, or have trouble sleeping, stop taking Sudafed Non-Drying Sinus and check with your doctor.

If cough and other symptoms don't improve within 7 days or tend to come back—or if you also have a fever, rash, or lasting headache—check with your doctor. A lingering cough could signal a serious condition.

Possible food and drug interactions
when taking this medication

Do not use Sudafed Non-Drying Sinus within 2 weeks of taking a drug classified as an MAO inhibitor, such as the antidepressants **Nardil** and **Parnate**.

Brand name:

Sudafed Severe Cold Formula

Pronounced: SUE-da-fed
Generic ingredients: Acetaminophen, Dextromethorphan hydro-
*   bromide, Pseudoephedrine hydrochloride*

What this drug is used for

Like other Sudafed products, Sudafed Severe Cold Formula temporarily relieves stuffy nose. This variety also has an ingredient for cough, as well as acetaminophen to relieve the minor aches and pains, headache, muscle aches, sore throat, and fever that often accompany a cold.

This product is available in tablet and caplet forms.

How should you take this medication?

The usual dose for adults and children 12 years and over is 2 pills every 6 hours, up to a maximum of 8 pills a day. For children under 12, consult your doctor.

■ STORAGE

Store at room temperature in a dry place. Protect from light.

Do not take this medication if...

Unless your doctor approves, do not take Sudafed Severe Cold Formula if you have heart disease, high blood pressure, thyroid disease, diabetes, or an enlarged prostate gland.

Also check with your doctor before using Sudafed Severe Cold Formula for the type of chronic cough that results from smoking, emphysema, or asthma, or for a cough that brings up lots of phlegm.

Special warnings about this medication

If you become dizzy or nervous, or have trouble sleeping, stop taking this medication and check with your doctor.

Do not take this product for more than 10 days. If your symptoms do not improve or include a fever that lasts more than 3 days—or if new symptoms appear—call your doctor.

You should also check with your doctor immediately if you have a severe sore throat that lasts for more than 2 days, or if your sore throat is accompanied or followed by fever, headache, rash, nausea, or vomiting.

Likewise, call your doctor if you have a cough that lasts for more than 7 days or tends to come back, or your cough is accompanied by rash, lasting headache, and fever.

Possible food and drug interactions
when taking this medication

Do not use Sudafed Severe Cold Formula within 2 weeks of taking a drug classified as an MAO inhibitor, such as the antidepressants **Nardil** and **Parnate**.

Combined with heavy drinking, the acetaminophen in this product could conceivably cause liver damage. Check with your doctor before taking this product if you generally have more than 3 alcoholic beverages a day.

Brand name:

Sudafed Sinus

See Sine-Aid

Brand name:

Surfak

See Colace

Brand name:

Tagamet HB

Pronounced: TAG-uh-met
Generic name: Cimetidine

What this drug is used for

Taken before a meal, Tagamet HB prevents heartburn, acid indigestion, and sour stomach. It can also be used for relief after the problem develops.

Tagamet HB is part of a family of acid-blocking prescription drugs recently released in over-the-counter formulations. Others in the family are Axid AR, Mylanta AR, Pepcid AC, and Zantac 75.

How should you take this medication?

Do not take more than 2 tablets each 24 hours.

■ FOR PREVENTION
Swallow 1 tablet with water 30 minutes before eating a meal that could cause trouble.

■ FOR RELIEF
Swallow 1 tablet with water.

■ STORAGE
Store at room temperature.

Do not take this medication if...

Not for children under 12, unless your doctor approves.

Special warnings about this medication

Do not take 2 tablets of Tagamet HB every day for more than 2 weeks without your doctor's approval.

If you have trouble swallowing or constant stomach pain, see your doctor right away. You may have a serious problem that needs a different kind of medication.

Possible food and drug interactions when taking this medication

The prescription-strength version of Tagamet HB interacts with a number of medications. Check with your doctor before combining Tagamet HB with any of the following:

Aspirin

The antibiotic **Augmentin**

Blood-thinning drugs such as **Coumadin**

Chlorpromazine (**Thorazine**)

Cisapride (**Propulsid**)

Cyclosporine (**Sandimmune, Neoral**)

Digoxin (**Lanoxin**)

Drugs that clear up fungus infections such as **Diflucan** and **Nizoral**

Heart and blood pressure medications classified as calcium channel blockers, including **Cardizem**, **Calan**, and **Procardia**

Heart and blood pressure medications known as beta blockers, including **Inderal**, **Lopressor**, and **Tenormin**

Medications that control an irregular heartbeat, such as **Cordarone, Tonocard, Quinidex**, and **Procan**

Metoclopramide (**Reglan**)

Metronidazole (**Flagyl**)

Narcotic pain relievers such as **Demerol** and **morphine**

Nicotine (**Nicoderm, Nicorette**)

Oral diabetes drugs such as **Diabinese, Micronase**, and **Glucotrol**

Paroxetine (**Paxil**)

Pentoxifylline (**Trental**)

Phenytoin (the seizure medicine **Dilantin**)

Quinine

Sucralfate (**Carafate**)

Theophylline asthma medications such as **Theo-Dur**

Tranquilizers that contain benzodiazepine (**Valium** and **Librium**)

Brand name:

Tavist-1

Pronounced: TAV-ist
Generic name: Clemastine fumarate

What this drug is used for

Tavist-1 temporarily relieves the runny nose, sneezing, itchy nose or throat, and itchy, watery eyes that come from hay fever and similar allergies. Do not confuse this product with Tavist-D, which has an extra ingredient that fights stuffy nose.

How should you take this medication?

The usual dosage is 1 tablet every 12 hours. Do not exceed 2 tablets in 24 hours. For children under 12, consult a doctor.

Do not take this medication if...

Unless your doctor approves, do not take Tavist-1 if you have high pressure within the eye (glaucoma), an enlarged prostate gland, or a breathing problem such as emphysema or chronic bronchitis.

Special warnings about this medication

Since Tavist-1 may cause drowsiness, use caution when driving and when operating machinery. Tavist-1 may also cause excitability, especially in children.

Possible food and drug interactions
when taking this medication

If you are taking a tranquilizer such as **Valium** or **Xanax**, or a sleep aid such as **Halcion** or **Seconal**, do not take Tavist-1 without your doctor's approval; the combination could cause extreme drowsiness. For the same reason, avoid alcohol while taking this product.

Brand name:

Tavist-D

Pronounced: TA-vist
Generic ingredients: Clemastine fumarate, Phenylpropanolamine
  hydrochloride

What this drug is used for

Tavist-D temporarily relieves stuffy nose due to allergies or sinus inflammation.

How should you take this medication?

The usual dose for adults and children 12 years and older is 1 tablet swallowed whole every 12 hours. Do not take more than 2 tablets each 24 hours. For children under 12, consult your doctor.

Do not take this medication if...

Unless your doctor approves, do not take this drug if you have heart disease, high blood pressure, thyroid disease, diabetes, high pressure within the eye (glaucoma), a breathing problem such as emphysema or chronic bronchitis, or an enlarged prostate gland.

Special warnings about this medication

Tavist-D can make you sleepy. Use special caution when driving and when operating machinery.

Tavist-D also may cause excitability, especially in children. Do not take more than the recommended dosage; nervousness, dizziness, or sleeplessness could result.

Avoid taking Tavist-D for more than 7 days. If symptoms do not improve or are accompanied by fever, contact your doctor.

Possible food and drug interactions when taking this medication

Check with your doctor before combining Tavist-D with sleep aids such as **Ambien** and **Halcion** or tranquilizers such as **Valium** and **Xanax**; the combination can make you extra drowsy. For the same reason, do not drink alcoholic beverages while using Tavist-D.

Unless your doctor approves, you should also avoid Tavist-D if you are taking any of the following:

Antidepressant medications such as **Elavil**, **Sinequan**, and **Tofranil**
Decongestants such as **Entex**, **Rynatan**, and **Trinalin**
Drugs for high blood pressure, such as **Calan**, **Lotensin**, and **Tenormin**

Brand name:

Teldrin

Pronounced: TELL-drin
Generic ingredients: Chlorpheniramine maleate,
 • Phenylpropanolamine hydrochloride

What this drug is used for

Teldrin relieves the runny nose, sneezing, itchy nose or throat, and itchy, watery eyes that result from allergies such as hay fever. It also unclogs stuffy nose due to the common cold, hay fever, or sinus inflammation.

How should you take this medication?

For adults and children 12 years and over, the usual dose is 1 capsule every 12 hours. Do not take more than 2 capsules each 24 hours. For children under 12, consult your doctor.

■ STORAGE
Store in a dry place at room temperature.

Do not take this medication if...

Unless your doctor approves, do not take Teldrin if you have heart disease, high blood pressure, thyroid disease, diabetes, high pressure within the eye (glaucoma), an enlarged prostate gland, or a breathing problem such as emphysema or chronic bronchitis.

Special warnings about this medication

If you become dizzy or nervous, or have trouble sleeping, stop taking Teldrin and check with your doctor.

Teldrin may cause excitability, especially in children. In some people, it can also cause drowsiness. Be especially cautious when driving and when operating machinery.

If your symptoms do not improve within 7 days or include a fever, check with your doctor.

Possible food and drug interactions when taking this medication

Do not combine Teldrin with any other medication containing phenylpropanolamine, such as **Dimetane-DC, Ornade**, and **Triaminic**.

Also avoid using Teldrin within 2 weeks of taking a drug classified as an MAO inhibitor, such as the antidepressants **Nardil** and **Parnate**.

If you are taking a tranquilizer such as **Valium** or **Xanax**, or a sleep aid such as **Halcion** or **Seconal**, do not take Teldrin without your doctor's approval; the combination could cause extreme drowsiness. For the same reason, avoid alcohol while taking this product.

Brand name:

TheraFlu Flu and Cold Medicine

Pronounced: THAIR-uh-flew
Generic ingredients: Acetaminophen, Chlorpheniramine maleate,
  Pseudoephedrine hydrochloride

What this drug is used for

TheraFlu Flu and Cold Medicine relieves the headache, body aches, minor sore throat pain, and fever that accompany colds and flu. It also unclogs stuffy nose, and combats runny nose and sneezing. The product is available in regular and maximum strengths. It comes in powder form in foil packets.

How should you take this medication?

For adults and children 12 years and over, the usual dose is 1 packet. You can take the regular strength every 4 to 6 hours. The maximum strength should not be taken more often than every 6 hours. With either strength, take no more than 4 packets a day. Dissolve the powder in 6 ounces of hot water. For children under 12, consult your doctor.

Do not take this medication if...

Unless your doctor approves, do not take TheraFlu Flu and Cold Medicine if you have heart disease, high blood pressure, thyroid disease, diabetes, high pressure within the eye (glaucoma), an enlarged prostate gland, or a breathing problem such as emphysema or chronic bronchitis.

Special warnings about this medication

If you become dizzy or nervous, or have trouble sleeping, stop taking TheraFlu Flu and Cold Medicine and check with your doctor.

TheraFlu Flu and Cold Medicine may cause drowsiness. Be especially cautious when driving and when operating machinery. The product can also cause excitability, especially in children.

Do not take this product for more than 10 days for pain or 3 days for fever without your doctor's approval. If your pain or fever won't go away or gets worse, or if you develop new symptoms or notice any redness or swelling, check with your doctor; you might have a serious condition.

You should also check with your doctor immediately if you have a severe sore throat that lasts for more than 2 days, or if your sore throat is accompanied or followed by fever, headache, rash, nausea, or vomiting.

If you must avoid phenylalanine, do not use the maximum-strength version of this product.

Possible food and drug interactions when taking this medication

Do not use TheraFlu Flu and Cold Medicine within 2 weeks of taking a drug classified as an MAO inhibitor, such as the antidepressants **Nardil** and **Parnate**.

If you are taking a tranquilizer such as **Valium** or **Xanax**, or a sleep aid such as **Halcion** or **Seconal**, do not take this medication without your doctor's approval; the combination could cause extreme drowsiness. For the same reason, avoid alcohol while taking this product.

Brand name:

TheraFlu Flu, Cold & Cough Medicine

Pronounced: THAIR-uh-flew
Generic ingredients: Acetaminophen, Chlorpheniramine maleate,
Dextromethorphan hydrobromide, Pseudoephedrine hydrochloride

What this drug is used for

TheraFlu Flu, Cold & Cough Medicine relieves the headache, body aches, minor sore throat pain, and fever that accompany colds and flu. It also unclogs stuffy nose and sinuses, combats runny nose and sneezing, and relieves coughs due to minor throat and bronchial irritation.

The product comes in regular-strength and maximum-strength-nighttime formulations. Both are available in powder form, packaged in foil packets. The maximum-strength variety is also available in caplets.

How should you take this medication?

For adults and children 12 years and over, the usual dosage is 1 packet or 2 caplets every 6 hours. Dissolve the powder in 6 ounces of hot water. Do not take more than 4 doses a day. For children under 12, consult your doctor.

Do not take this medication if...

Unless your doctor approves, do not take TheraFlu Flu, Cold & Cough Medicine if you have heart disease, high blood pressure, thyroid disease, diabetes, high pressure within the eye (glaucoma), an enlarged prostate gland, or a breathing problem such as emphysema or chronic bronchitis.

Also check with your doctor before using this product for the type of chronic cough that results from smoking or asthma, or for a cough that brings up lots of phlegm.

Special warnings about this medication

If you become dizzy or nervous, or have trouble sleeping, stop taking TheraFlu Flu, Cold & Cough Medicine and check with your doctor.

This medication may cause drowsiness. Be especially cautious when driving and when operating machinery. The product can also cause excitability, especially in children.

Do not take this product for more than 10 days for pain or 3 days for fever without your doctor's approval. If your pain or fever won't go away or gets worse, or if you develop new symptoms or notice any redness or swelling, check with your doctor; you might have a serious condition.

You should also check with your doctor immediately if you have a severe sore throat that lasts for more than 2 days, or if your sore throat is accompanied or followed by fever, headache, rash, nausea, or vomiting.

Likewise, call your doctor if you have a cough that lasts for more than 7 days or tends to come back, or a cough accompanied by rash, lasting headache, and fever. A lingering cough could signal a serious condition.

Possible food and drug interactions when taking this medication

Do not use TheraFlu Flu, Cold & Cough Medicine within 2 weeks of taking a drug classified as an MAO inhibitor, such as the antidepressants **Nardil** and **Parnate**.

If you are taking a tranquilizer such as **Valium** or **Xanax**, or a sleep aid such as **Halcion** or **Seconal**, do not take this medication without your doctor's approval; the combination could cause extreme drowsiness. For the same reason, avoid alcohol while taking this product.

Brand name:

TheraFlu Non-Drowsy Formulas

Pronounced: THAIR-uh-flew
Generic ingredients: Acetaminophen, Pseudoephedrine hydrochloride, Dextromethorphan (No-Drowsiness powder and Non-Drowsy caplets only)

What this drug is used for

The ingredients in the TheraFlu Non-Drowsy Formulas relieve the minor aches and pains of colds and flu, such as headache, body aches, minor sore throat pain, and sinus pain. They also reduce fever and unclog stuffy nose and sinuses.

In addition, the No-Drowsiness powder and the Non-Drowsy caplets contain dextromethorphan to relieve cough due to minor throat and bronchial irritation. The *Sinus* Non-Drowsy caplets do not.

Unlike other TheraFlu products, none of these formulas includes an antihistamine to relieve sneezing and runny nose, and therefore are unlikely to make you drowsy.

How should you take this medication?

For adults and children 12 years and over, the usual dosage is 1 packet or 2 caplets every 6 hours. Do not take more than 4 doses a day. The No-Drowsiness powder should be dissolved in 6 ounces of hot water and sipped while hot. For children under 12, consult your doctor.

■ STORAGE

Store at room temperature in a dry place.

Do not take this medication if...

Unless your doctor approves, do not take any of these products if you have heart disease, high blood pressure, thyroid disease, diabetes, or an enlarged prostate gland.

Also check with your doctor before using the No-Drowsiness powder and the Non-Drowsy caplets for the type of chronic cough that results from smoking or asthma, or for a cough that brings up lots of phlegm.

Special warnings about this medication

If you become dizzy or nervous, or have trouble sleeping, stop taking this medication and check with your doctor.

Do not take this product for more than 10 days for pain or 3 days for fever without your doctor's approval. If your pain or fever won't go away or gets worse, or if you develop new symptoms or notice any redness or swelling, check with your doctor; you might have a serious condition.

You should also check with your doctor immediately if you have a severe sore throat that lasts for more than 2 days, or if your sore throat is accompanied or followed by fever, headache, rash, nausea, or vomiting.

Likewise, call your doctor if you have a cough that lasts for more than 7 days or tends to come back, or a cough accompanied by rash, lasting headache, and fever.

Possible food and drug interactions
when taking this medication

Do not use TheraFlu Non-Drowsy Formulas within 2 weeks of taking a drug classified as an MAO inhibitor, such as the antidepressants **Nardil** and **Parnate**.

Brand name:

Titralac

See Tums

Brand name:

Titralac Plus

See Tums Antigas/Antacid Formula

Brand name:

Triaminic

Pronounced: TRY-uh-MIN-ik
Generic ingredients: Chlorpheniramine maleate,
*   Phenylpropanolamine hydrochloride*

What this drug is used for

Triaminic syrup unclogs stuffy nose and gives temporary relief from
the runny nose, itchy nose or throat, and itchy, watery eyes caused by
a cold or allergy.

How should you take this medication?

Doses may be repeated every 4 to 6 hours, up to a maximum of 6
doses each day. To assure accurate measurement, use the cup that
comes with each bottle. Check with your doctor before giving this
product to a child under 6 years of age.

■ ADULTS
For adults and children 12 years and over, the usual dosage is 4 teaspoonfuls.

■ CHILDREN
Age 6 to 12: 2 teaspoonfuls.
Age 2 to 6: 1 teaspoonful.
Age 1 to 2: ½ teaspoonful.
Infants 4 to 12 months: ¼ teaspoonful.

Do not take this medication if...

Unless your doctor approves, do not take Triaminic if you have heart
disease, high blood pressure, thyroid disease, diabetes, high pressure

within the eye (glaucoma), an enlarged prostate gland, or a breathing problem such as emphysema or chronic bronchitis.

Special warnings about this medication

If you become dizzy or nervous, or have trouble sleeping, stop taking Triaminic and check with your doctor.

If symptoms do not improve in 7 days, or include a fever, get in touch with your doctor.

This product may cause overexcitement, especially in children. On the other hand, Triaminic makes some people drowsy. Be especially careful when driving and when operating machinery.

Possible food and drug interactions when taking this medication

Do not use Triaminic within 2 weeks of taking a drug classified as an MAO inhibitor, such as the antidepressants **Nardil** and **Parnate**.

Check with your doctor before combining Triaminic with any other product containing phenylpropanolamine, including **Acutrim**, **Dimetane-DC**, **Dura-Vent**, **Ornade**, **Poly-Histine**, or **Sinuvent**.

Also avoid Triaminic if you are taking a tranquilizer such as **Valium** or **Xanax**, or a sleep aid such as **Halcion** or **Seconal**, unless your doctor approves. The combination could cause extreme drowsiness. For the same reason, avoid alcohol while taking this product.

Brand name:

Triaminic AM Cough and Decongestant Formula

Pronounced: TRY-uh-MIN-ik
Generic ingredients: Dextromethorphan hydrobromide, Pseudo-
  ephedrine hydrochloride

What this drug is used for

This member of the Triaminic line contains no antihistamines, and therefore won't cause drowsiness. It temporarily quiets coughs caused by minor irritation of the throat and bronchial tubes, and relieves stuffy nose.

How should you take this medication?

Doses may be repeated every 6 hours, up to a maximum of 4 doses each day. To assure accurate measurement, use the cup that comes with each bottle. Check with your doctor before giving the product to a child under 2 years of age.

■ ADULTS
For adults and children 12 years and over, the usual dose is 4 teaspoonfuls.

■ CHILDREN
Age 6 to 12: 2 teaspoonfuls
Age 2 to 6: 1 teaspoonful
Age 1 to 2: ½ teaspoonful
Infants 4 to 12 months: ¼ teaspoonful

Do not take this medication if...
Unless your doctor approves, do not take Triaminic AM if you have heart disease, high blood pressure, thyroid disease, diabetes, or an enlarged prostate gland.

Also check with your doctor before using Triaminic AM for the type of chronic cough that results from smoking, asthma, or emphysema, or for a cough that brings up lots of phlegm.

Special warnings about this medication
If you become dizzy or nervous, or have trouble sleeping, stop taking Triaminic AM and check with your doctor.

If cough and other symptoms don't improve within 7 days or tend to come back—or if you also have a fever, rash, or lasting headache— check with your doctor. A lingering cough could signal a serious condition.

Possible food and drug interactions
when taking this medication
Do not use Triaminic AM within 2 weeks of taking a drug classified as an MAO inhibitor, such as the antidepressants **Nardil** and **Parnate**.

Brand name:

Triaminic AM Decongestant Formula

See Sudafed

Brand name:

Triaminic DM

Pronounced: TRY-uh-MIN-ik
Generic ingredients: Dextromethorphan hydrobromide,
Phenylpropanolamine hydrochloride

What this drug is used for

Like all Triaminic products, Triaminic DM unclogs stuffy nose. This variety of Triaminic also temporarily quiets coughs caused by minor irritation of the throat and bronchial tubes.

How should you take this medication?

Doses may be repeated every 4 hours, up to a maximum of 6 doses a day. To assure accurate measurement, use the cup that comes with the bottle. Check with your doctor before giving the product to a child under 2 years of age.

■ ADULTS

For adults and children 12 years and over, the usual dose is 4 teaspoonfuls.

■ CHILDREN

Age 6 to 12: 2 teaspoonfuls
Age 2 to 6: 1 teaspoonful
Age 1 to 2: ½ teaspoonful
Infants 4 to 12 months: ¼ teaspoonful

Do not take this medication if...

Unless your doctor approves, do not take Triaminic DM if you have heart disease, high blood pressure, thyroid disease, diabetes, or an enlarged prostate gland.

Also check with your doctor before using Triaminic DM for the type of chronic cough that results from smoking, asthma, or emphysema, or for a cough that brings up lots of phlegm.

Special warnings about this medication

If you become dizzy or nervous, or have trouble sleeping, stop taking Triaminic DM and check with your doctor.

If cough and other symptoms don't improve within 7 days or tend to come back—or if you also have a fever, rash, or lasting headache—check with your doctor. A lingering cough could signal a serious condition.

Possible food and drug interactions when taking this medication

Do not use Triaminic DM within 2 weeks of taking a drug classified as an MAO inhibitor, such as the antidepressants **Nardil** and **Parnate**.

Check with your doctor before combining Triaminic DM with another product containing phenylpropanolamine, such as **Acutrim**, **Dimetane-DC**, **Dura-Vent**, **Ornade**, **Poly-Histine**, or **Sinuvent**.

Brand name:

Triaminic Expectorant

Pronounced: TRY-uh-MIN-ik
Generic ingredients: Guaifenesin, Phenylpropanolamine hydrochloride

What this drug is used for

Triaminic Expectorant relieves chest congestion by loosening mucus to help clear bronchial passageways. It also temporarily relieves a stuffy nose.

How should you take this medication?

Doses may be repeated every 4 hours, up to a maximum of 6 doses each day. To assure accuracy, use the dosage cup supplied with each bottle. Check with your doctor before giving the product to a child under 2 years of age.

■ ADULTS

For adults and children 12 years and over, the usual dose is 4 tea-spoonfuls.

■ CHILDREN

Age 6 to 12: 2 teaspoonfuls
Age 2 to 6: 1 teaspoonful
Age 1 to 2: ½ teaspoonful
Infants 4 to 12 months: ¼ teaspoonful

Do not take this medication if...

Unless your doctor approves, do not take Triaminic Expectorant if you have heart disease, high blood pressure, thyroid disease, diabetes, or an enlarged prostate gland.

Also check with your doctor before using Triaminic Expectorant for the type of lasting cough that results from smoking, asthma, chronic bronchitis, or emphysema, or for a cough that brings up lots of phlegm.

Special warnings about this medication

If you become dizzy or nervous, or have trouble sleeping, stop taking Triaminic Expectorant and check with your doctor.

If cough and other symptoms don't improve within 7 days or tend to come back—or if you also have a fever, rash, or lasting headache—check with your doctor. A lingering cough could signal a serious condition.

**Possible food and drug interactions
when taking this medication**

Do not use Triaminic Expectorant within 2 weeks of taking a drug classified as an MAO inhibitor, such as the antidepressants **Nardil** and **Parnate**.

Unless your doctor approves, do not use Triaminic Expectorant while taking another product containing phenylpropanolamine, such as **Acutrim, Dimetane-DC, Dura-Vent, Ornade, Poly-Histine,** or **Sinuvent**.

Brand name:

Triaminic Infant Oral Decongestant Drops

See Sudafed

Brand name:

Triaminic Night Time

Pronounced: TRY-uh-MIN-ik
*Generic ingredients: Chlorpheniramine maleate, Dextromethorphan
  hydrobromide, Pseudoephedrine hydrochloride*

What this drug is used for

Like its companion product, Triaminic AM, Triaminic Night Time unclogs stuffy nose and temporarily relieves coughs caused by minor irritation of the throat and bronchial tubes. However, Triaminic Night Time also contains an antihistamine to relieve runny nose and sneezing, itchy nose or throat, and itchy, watery eyes. This antihistamine can cause drowsiness; hence the "Night Time" in the name.

How should you take this medication?

Doses may be repeated every 6 hours, up to a maximum of 4 doses a day. To assure accurate measurement, use the cup that comes with the bottle. Check with your doctor before giving the product to a child under 6 years of age.

■ ADULTS

For adults and children 12 years and over, the usual dose is 4 tea-spoonfuls.

■ CHILDREN

Age 6 to 12: 2 teaspoonfuls
Age 2 to 6: 1 teaspoonful
Age 1 to 2: ½ teaspoonful
Infants 4 to 12 months: ¼ teaspoonful

Do not take this medication if...

Unless your doctor approves, do not take Triaminic Night Time if you have heart disease, high blood pressure, thyroid disease, diabetes, high pressure within the eye (glaucoma), an enlarged prostate gland, or breathing problems such as emphysema or chronic bronchitis.

Also check with your doctor before using Triaminic Night Time for the type of chronic cough that results from smoking or asthma, or for a cough that brings up lots of phlegm.

Special warnings about this medication

If you become dizzy or nervous, or have trouble sleeping, stop taking Triaminic Night Time and check with your doctor.

If cough and other symptoms don't improve within 7 days or tend to come back—or if you also have a fever, rash, or lasting headache—check with your doctor. A lingering cough could signal a serious condition.

The antihistamine in Triaminic Night Time may cause overexcitement, especially in children. It also has a tendency to make some people drowsy. Be especially cautious when driving and when operating machinery.

Possible food and drug interactions when taking this medication

Do not use Triaminic Night Time within 2 weeks of taking a drug classified as an MAO inhibitor, such as the antidepressants **Nardil** and **Parnate**.

If you are taking a tranquilizer such as **Valium** or **Xanax**, or a sleep aid such as **Halcion** or **Seconal**, do not take Triaminic Night Time without your doctor's approval; the combination could cause extreme drowsiness. For the same reason, avoid alcohol while taking this product.

Brand name:

Triaminic Sore Throat Formula

Pronounced: TRY-uh-MIN-ik
Generic ingredients: Acetaminophen, Dextromethorphan hydrobromide, Pseudoephedrine hydrochloride

What this drug is used for

Triaminic Sore Throat Formula temporarily relieves sore throat pain and other minor aches and pains. It also unclogs stuffy nose, reduces fever, and quiets coughs caused by minor irritation to the throat and bronchial tubes.

How should you take this medication?

Doses may be repeated every 6 hours, up to a maximum of 4 doses a day. To assure accurate measurement, use the cup that comes with the bottle. Check with your doctor before giving the product to a child under 2 years of age.

■ ADULTS

For adults and children 12 years and over, the usual dose is 4 teaspoonfuls.

■ CHILDREN

Age 6 to 12: 2 teaspoonfuls
Age 2 to 6: 1 teaspoonful
Age 1 to 2: ¹/₂ teaspoonful
Infants 4 to 12 months: ¹/₄ teaspoonful

Do not take this medication if...

Unless your doctor approves, avoid Triaminic Sore Throat Formula if you have heart disease, high blood pressure, thyroid disease, diabetes, or an enlarged prostate gland.

Also check with your doctor before using this product for the type of chronic cough that results from smoking, asthma, or emphysema, or for a cough that brings up lots of phlegm.

Special warnings about this medication

If you become dizzy or nervous, or have trouble sleeping, stop taking Triaminic Sore Throat Formula and check with your doctor.

You should check with your doctor immediately if you have a severe sore throat that lasts for more than 2 days, or if your sore throat is accompanied or followed by fever, headache, rash, nausea, or vomiting.

Likewise, call your doctor if you have a cough that lasts for more than 7 days or tends to come back, or your cough is accompanied by rash, lasting headache, and a 3-day fever.

Call, too, if your pain or fever won't go away or gets worse, or if you develop new symptoms or notice any redness or swelling. These could be signs of a serious condition.

In any event, do not take this product for more than 7 days, or give it to a child for more than 5 days.

Possible food and drug interactions when taking this medication

Do not use Triaminic Sore Throat Formula within 2 weeks of taking a drug classified as an MAO inhibitor, such as the antidepressants **Nardil** and **Parnate**.

Brand name:

Triaminicin

Pronounced: TRY-uh-MIN-ih-sin
Generic ingredients: Acetaminophen, Chlorpheniramine maleate,
Phenylpropanolamine hydrochloride

What this drug is used for

Like basic Triaminic syrup, Triaminicin tablets unclog stuffy nose and temporarily relieve allergy symptoms such as runny nose, sneezing, itchy nose or throat, and itchy, watery eyes. However, Triaminicin also contains acetaminophen for relief of the minor aches, pains, muscular aches, headache, and fever that often accompany a common cold.

How should you take this medication?

For adults and children 12 years and over, the usual dosage is 1 tablet every 4 to 6 hours. Do not take more than 6 tablets each 24 hours. For children under 12, consult your doctor.

Do not take this medication if...

Unless your doctor approves, do not take Triaminicin if you have heart disease, high blood pressure, thyroid disease, diabetes, high pressure within the eye (glaucoma), an enlarged prostate gland, or a breathing problem such as emphysema or chronic bronchitis.

Special warnings about this medication

If you become dizzy or nervous, or have trouble sleeping, stop taking Triaminicin and check with your doctor.

Do not take this product for more than 10 days for pain or 3 days for fever without your doctor's approval. If your pain or fever won't go away or gets worse, or if you develop new symptoms or notice any redness or swelling, check with your doctor; you might have a serious condition.

Triaminicin may cause overexcitement, especially in children. It also has a tendency to make some people drowsy. Be especially cautious when driving and when operating machinery.

Possible food and drug interactions when taking this medication

Do not use Triaminicin within 2 weeks of taking a drug classified as an MAO inhibitor, such as the antidepressants **Nardil** and **Parnate**.

Check with your doctor before combining Triaminicin with another product containing phenylpropanolamine, such as **Acutrim**, **Dimetane-DC**, **Dura-Vent**, **Ornade**, **Poly-Histine**, or **Sinuvent**.

If you are taking a tranquilizer such as **Valium** or **Xanax**, or a sleep aid such as **Halcion** or **Seconal**, do not take Triaminicin without your doctor's approval; the combination could cause extreme drowsiness. For the same reason, avoid alcohol while taking this product.

Brand name:

Triaminicol

Pronounced: TRY-uh-MIN-i-call
Generic ingredients: Chlorpheniramine maleate, Dextromethorphan
hydrobromide, Phenylpropanolamine hydrochloride

What this drug is used for

Like basic Triaminic syrup, Triaminicol unclogs stuffy nose and temporarily relieves allergy symptoms such as runny nose, sneezing, itchy nose or throat, and itchy, watery eyes. However, Triaminicol also contains dextromethorphan for relief of coughs due to minor throat and bronchial irritation.

How should you take this medication?

Doses may be repeated every 4 to 6 hours, up to a maximum of 6 doses a day. To assure accurate measurement, use the cup that comes with the bottle. Check with your doctor before giving the product to a child under 6 years of age.

■ ADULTS

For adults and children 12 years and over, the usual dose is 4 teaspoonfuls.

■ CHILDREN

Age 6 to 12: 2 teaspoonfuls
Age 2 to 6: 1 teaspoonful
Age 1 to 2: ½ teaspoonful
Infants 4 to 12 months: ¼ teaspoonful

Do not take this medication if...

Unless your doctor approves, do not take Triaminicol if you have heart disease, high blood pressure, thyroid disease, diabetes, high pressure within the eye (glaucoma), an enlarged prostate gland, or breathing problems such as emphysema or chronic bronchitis.

Also check with your doctor before using Triaminicol for the type of chronic cough that results from smoking or asthma, or for a cough that brings up lots of phlegm.

Special warnings about this medication

If you become dizzy or nervous, or have trouble sleeping, stop taking Triaminicol and check with your doctor.

If cough and other symptoms don't improve within 7 days or tend to come back—or if you also have a fever, rash, or lasting headache—check with your doctor. A lingering cough could signal a serious condition.

Triaminicol may cause overexcitement, especially in children. It also has a tendency to make some people drowsy. Be especially cautious when driving and when operating machinery.

**Possible food and drug interactions
when taking this medication**

Do not use Triaminicol within 2 weeks of taking a drug classified as
an MAO inhibitor, such as the antidepressants **Nardil** and **Parnate**.

Check with your doctor before combining Triaminicol with another
product containing phenylpropanolamine, such as **Acutrim**,
Dimetane-DC, **Dura-Vent**, **Ornade**, **Poly-Histine**, or **Sinuvent**.

If you are taking a tranquilizer such as **Valium** or **Xanax**, or a sleep
aid such as **Halcion** or **Seconal**, do not take Triaminicol without your
doctor's approval; the combination could cause extreme drowsiness.
For the same reason, avoid alcohol while taking this product.

Brand name:

Tums

Pronounced: TUMS
Generic name: Calcium carbonate
Other brand names: Alka-mints, Children's Mylanta, Mylanta
   Soothing Lozenges, Titralac

What this medication is used for

These products all consist of various amounts of the stomach-acid
neutralizer, calcium carbonate. They relieve acid indigestion, heartburn, sour stomach, and upset stomach. Tums is also sold for use as a
calcium supplement. Most brands are available in assorted flavors.

How should you take this medication?

Most tablets can be chewed. Titralac tablets can also be allowed to
melt in your mouth. Mylanta Soothing Lozenges should always be
dissolved in the mouth.

■ AS AN ANTACID

Tums and Tums E-X

1 to 4 tablets every hour as needed, but no more than 16 Tums tablets
or 10 Tums E-X tablets a day.

Tums Ultra

2 or 3 tablets every hour as needed, but no more than 8 tablets a day.

Alka-Mints
1 or 2 tablets every 2 hours, but no more than 9 tablets a day.

Mylanta Soothing Lozenges
1 lozenge followed by a second if needed, but no more than 12 lozenges a day.

Children's Mylanta
For children 6 to 11, the usual dosage is 2 tablets or teaspoonfuls up to 3 times a day (maximum: 6 a day); for children 2 to 5, the dosage is 1 tablet or teaspoonful up to 3 times a day (maximum: 3 a day); for children under 2, consult your doctor.

Titralac
2 tablets every 2 or 3 hours as needed, but no more than 19 tablets a day.

Titralac Extra Strength
1 or 2 tablets every 2 or 3 hours, but no more than 10 tablets a day.

■ AS A CALCIUM SUPPLEMENT
Tums, Tums E-X, and Tums Ultra
2 tablets twice a day. Do not take more than 12 Tums, 8 Tums E-X, or 6 Tums Ultra tablets a day.

Tums 500
1 tablet with meals, 2 or 3 times a day.

Special warnings when using this medication
Do not take the maximum daily dosage of any of these products continuously for more than 2 weeks without consulting a doctor.

Alka-Mints can cause constipation. If you must avoid phenylalanine, do not take Tums E-X Sugar Free tablets.

Possible food and drug interactions
when taking this medication
When taken at the same time, antacids interact with a variety of prescription drugs. However, an interaction is unlikely if you keep doses of the two at least 2 or 3 hours apart. Drugs that may interact include the following:

Alendronate (**Fosamax**)

Allopurinol (**Zyloprim**)

Antibiotics classified as quinolones, such as **Cipro**, **Floxin**, and **Noroxin**

Aspirin

Atenolol (**Tenormin**)

Captopril (**Capoten**)

Chlordiazepoxide (**Librium**)

Cimetidine (**Tagamet**)

Digoxin (**Lanoxin**)

Doxycycline (**Vibramycin**)

Fosfomycin (**Monurol**)

Gabapentin (**Neurontin**)

Glipizide (**Glucotrol**)

Glyburide (**Micronase**, **DiaBeta**)

Isoniazid (**Rifamate**)

Ketoconazole (**Nizoral**)

Levothyroxine (**Synthroid**)

Methenamine (**Urised**)

Metronidazole (**Flagyl**)

Misoprostol (**Cytotec**)

Mycophenolate mofetil (**CellCept**)

Nonsteroidal anti-inflammatory drugs such as **Dolobid**, **Motrin**, **Naprosyn**, and **Voltaren**

Penicillamine (**Cuprimine**)

Phenytoin (**Dilantin**)

Quinidine (**Quinidex**)

Sodium polystyrene sulfonate (**Kayexalate**)

Sucralfate (**Carafate**)

Tetracycline antibiotics such as **Achromycin V** and **Minocin**

Tilodronate (**Skelid**)

Ursodiol (**Actigall**)

Prolonged and heavy use of antacids such as Tums, combined with a high intake of calcium-rich foods such as milk, can lead to an overload of calcium in the system. Early symptoms are constipation, weakness, nausea, and vomiting; and a severe overload can cause kidney damage. If you need a high-calcium diet, check with your doctor about a substitute for Tums.

Brand name:

Tums Antigas/Antacid Formula

Generic ingredients: Calcium carbonate, Simethicone
Other brand name: Titralac Plus

What this drug is used for

These versions of Tums and Titralac add the antigas ingredient simethicone to their regular antacid formulations. They are used to relieve acid indigestion, heartburn, and sour stomach accompanied by gas.

How should you take this medication?

■ TUMS

Chew 1 or 2 tablets when you need them. No water is required. You can repeat the dosage every hour, but do not take more than 16 tablets each 24 hours.

■ TITRALAC PLUS TABLETS

Take 2 tablets every 2 or 3 hours. You can chew the tablets, swallow them whole, or let them melt in your mouth. Do not take more than 19 tablets each 24 hours.

■ TITRALAC PLUS LIQUID

Shake well before using. Take 2 teaspoonfuls between meals and at bedtime. Do not take more than 16 teaspoonfuls each 24 hours.

Special warnings about this medication

Do not take the maximum dosage of any of these products for more than 2 weeks without your doctor's approval.

Possible food and drug interactions
when taking this medication

Antacids interact with a variety of prescription drugs when taken at the same time. An interaction is unlikely, however, if you keep doses of the two at least 2 or 3 hours apart. Drugs that may interact include the following:

Alendronate (**Fosamax**)

Allopurinol (**Zyloprim**)

Antibiotics classified as quinolones, such as **Cipro**, **Floxin**, and **Noroxin**

Aspirin

Atenolol (**Tenormin**)

Captopril (**Capoten**)

Chlordiazepoxide (**Librium**)

Cimetidine (**Tagamet**)

Digoxin (**Lanoxin**)

Doxycycline (**Vibramycin**)

Fosfomycin (**Monurol**)

Gabapentin (**Neurontin**)

Glipizide (**Glucotrol**)

Glyburide (**Micronase**, **DiaBeta**)

Isoniazid (**Rifamate**)

Ketoconazole (**Nizoral**)

Levothyroxine (**Synthroid**)

Methenamine (**Urised**)

Metronidazole (**Flagyl**)

Misoprostol (**Cytotec**)

Mycophenolate mofetil (**CellCept**)

Nonsteroidal anti-inflammatory drugs such as **Dolobid**, **Motrin**, **Naprosyn**, and **Voltaren**

Penicillamine (**Cuprimine**)

Phenytoin (**Dilantin**)

Quinidine (**Quinidex**)

Sodium polystyrene sulfonate (**Kayexalate**)

Sucralfate (**Carafate**)

Tetracycline antibiotics such as **Achromycin V** and **Minocin**

Tilodronate (**Skelid**)

Ursodiol (**Actigall**)

Prolonged and heavy use of antacids such as Tums and Titralac, combined with a high intake of calcium-rich foods such as milk, can lead to an overload of calcium in the system. Early symptoms are constipation, weakness, nausea, and vomiting; and a severe overload can cause kidney damage. If you need a high-calcium diet, check with your doctor about a substitute for these products.

Brand name:

Tylenol

Pronounced: TYE-luh-naul
Generic name: Acetaminophen
Other brand name: Panadol

What this drug is used for

Tylenol and Panadol are brands of the widely used fever- and pain-relieving medication acetaminophen. They can be used for relief of simple headaches and muscle aches, the minor aches and pains of the common cold and flu, backache; toothache; minor pain of arthritis; and menstrual cramps.

Children's forms of these products are used to reduce fever and relieve pain due to colds, flu, teething, immunizations, tonsillectomy, and childhood illnesses. They also combat earache and headache.

Tylenol and Panadol are available in a variety of strengths and forms, including tablets, caplets, geltabs, gelcaps, and liquid.

How should you take this medication?

■ ADULTS AND CHILDREN 12 YEARS AND OVER

Regular Strength Tylenol
The usual dosage is 2 pills every 4 to 6 hours, up to a maximum of 12 pills each 24 hours.

Extra Strength Tylenol and Panadol
The usual dosage is 2 pills or tablespoonfuls every 4 to 6 hours, up to a maximum of 8 pills or tablespoonfuls each 24 hours.

Tylenol Extended Relief Caplets
The usual dosage is 2 caplets every 8 hours, up to a maximum of 6 caplets each 24 hours. Swallow each caplet whole. Do not crush, chew, or dissolve it.

■ CHILDREN
All doses may be given as frequently as every 4 hours, but give no more than 5 doses each 24 hours. Caplets should be taken with liquid; chewable tablets should be well chewed. Extra Strength and Extended Relief formulations are not for children under 12. Check with your doctor before giving liquid or drops to children under 2.

The usual doses are as follows:

Regular Strength Tylenol
Age 6 to 12: ¹/₂ to 1 pill

Junior Strength Tylenol
Age 12: 4 pills
Age 11: 3 pills
Age 9 to 10: 2¹/₂ pills
Age 6 to 8: 2 pills

Children's Tylenol and Children's Panadol Chewable Tablets
Age 11 to 12: 6 tablets
Age 9 to 10: 5 tablets
Age 6 to 8: 4 tablets
Age 4 to 5: 3 tablets
Age 2 to 3: 2 tablets

Children's Tylenol Elixir and Liquid and Children's Panadol Liquid
Age 11 to 12: 3 teaspoonfuls
Age 9 to 10: 2¹/₂ teaspoonfuls
Age 6 to 8: 2 teaspoonfuls
Age 4 to 5: 1¹/₂ teaspoonfuls
Age 2 to 3: 1 teaspoonful
Age 12 to 23 months: ³/₄ teaspoonful
Age 4 to 11 months: ¹/₂ teaspoonful

Infants' Tylenol and Infant's Panadol Drops
Age 4 to 5: 2.4 milliliters
Age 2 to 3: 1.6 milliliters
Age 12 to 23 months: 1.2 milliliters
Age 4 to 11 months: 0.8 milliliter
Under 3 months: 0.4 milliliter

Special warnings about this medication

Do not take these products for more than 10 days for pain (5-day limit for children) or 3 days for fever without your doctor's approval. If your pain or fever won't go away or gets worse, or if you develop new symptoms or notice any redness or swelling, check with your doctor; you might have a serious condition.

If you develop an allergic reaction, stop taking this medication. If your child must avoid phenyalanine, do not give the Tylenol grape or fruit burst chewable tablet.

Possible food and drug interactions when taking this medication

Do not take either of these products if you are using other medications containing acetaminophen, such as all other forms of **Tylenol, Excedrin Extra-Strength, Excedrin P.M., Percocet, Sinulin,** and **Sine-Aid.**

Check with your doctor before combining Tylenol or Panadol with the following:

The cholesterol-lowering drug cholestyramine (**Questran**)
The TB medication isoniazid (**Nydrazid**)
Nonsteroidal anti-inflammatory drugs (NSAIDs) such as **Dolobid** and **Motrin**
Oral contraceptives
The anti-seizure drug phenytoin (**Dilantin**)
The blood-thinning medication warfarin (**Coumadin**)
The HIV drug zidovudine (**Retrovir**)

Combined with heavy drinking, acetaminophen could conceivably cause liver damage. Check with your doctor before taking Tylenol or Panadol if you generally have more than 3 alcoholic beverages a day.

Overdosage

Particularly in heavy drinkers, a massive overdose of acetaminophen could cause liver damage. Early signs of an acetaminophen overdose include sweating, general discomfort, nausea, and vomiting. If you suspect an overdose, seek medical attention immediately.

Brand name:

Tylenol Allergy Sinus

Pronounced: TYE-luh-naul
Generic ingredients: Acetaminophen, Chlorpheniramine maleate, Pseudoephedrine hydrochloride

What this drug is used for

Tylenol Allergy Sinus temporarily relieves runny nose, sneezing, itchy nose or throat, and itchy, watery eyes caused by allergies such as hay fever. It also unclogs stuffy nose and sinuses, and relieves sinus pain and headaches.

The product is available in caplet, gelcap, and geltab form.

How should you take this medication?

The usual dosage is 2 pills every 6 hours. Do not take more than 8 pills each 24 hours.

Do not take this medication if...

Unless your doctor approves, do not take Tylenol Allergy Sinus if you have heart disease, high blood pressure, thyroid disease, diabetes, high pressure within the eye (glaucoma), an enlarged prostate gland, or a breathing problem such as emphysema or chronic bronchitis.

Not for children under 12.

Special warnings about this medication

If you become dizzy or nervous, or have trouble sleeping, stop taking Tylenol Allergy Sinus and check with your doctor. Do the same if you develop an allergic reaction to the product.

Do not take this product for more than 7 days for pain or 3 days for fever without your doctor's approval. If your pain or fever won't go away or gets worse, or if you develop new symptoms or notice any redness or swelling, check with your doctor; you might have a serious condition.

Tylenol Allergy Sinus may cause overexcitement, especially in children. It can also make some people drowsy. Be especially cautious when driving and when operating machinery.

Possible food and drug interactions when taking this medication

Do not use Tylenol Allergy Sinus while taking other medications containing acetaminophen, such as **Excedrin**, **Panadol**, **Percocet**, **Sine-Aid**, **Sinulin**, and all other forms of **Tylenol**.

Also avoid taking this product within 2 weeks of taking any drug classified as an MAO inhibitor, including the antidepressants **Nardil** and **Parnate**.

If you are taking a tranquilizer such as **Valium** or **Xanax**, or a sleep aid such as **Halcion** or **Seconal**, do not take Tylenol Allergy Sinus without your doctor's approval; the combination could cause extreme drowsiness. For the same reason, avoid alcohol while taking this product.

Overdosage

■ *Symptoms of Tylenol Allergy Sinus overdose may include:*
Feeling of general discomfort, mild anxiety, perspiration, rapid heartbeat, high blood pressure, nausea, vomiting

The mild anxiety, rapid heartbeat, and high blood pressure usually appear within 4 to 8 hours after the overdose and usually disappear without treatment.

Particularly in heavy drinkers, a massive overdose of acetaminophen could cause liver damage. If you suspect an overdose, seek medical attention immediately.

Brand name:

Tylenol Allergy Sinus NightTime

Pronounced: TYE-luh-naul
Generic ingredients: Acetaminophen, Diphenhydramine hydrochloride, Pseudoephedrine hydrochloride

What this drug is used for

Tylenol Allergy Sinus NightTime temporarily relieves runny nose, sneezing, itchy nose or throat, and itchy, watery eyes caused by allergies such as hay fever. It also unclogs stuffy nose and sinuses, and relieves sinus pain and headaches.

Because it contains a larger dose of antihistamine than regular Tylenol Allergy Sinus, it is more likely to cause drowsiness, and should be taken only at bedtime.

How should you take this medication?

Take 2 caplets at bedtime.

Do not take this medication if...

Unless your doctor approves, do not take Tylenol Allergy Sinus NightTime if you have heart disease, high blood pressure, thyroid disease, diabetes, high pressure within the eye (glaucoma), an enlarged prostate gland, or a breathing problem such as emphysema or chronic bronchitis.

Not for children under 12.

Special warnings about this medication

If you become dizzy or nervous, or have trouble sleeping, stop taking Tylenol Allergy Sinus NightTime and check with your doctor. Do the same if you develop an allergic reaction to the product.

Do not take this product for more than 7 days for pain or 3 days for fever without your doctor's approval. If your pain or fever won't go away or gets worse, or if you develop new symptoms or notice any redness or swelling, check with your doctor; you might have a serious condition.

Tylenol Allergy Sinus NightTime may cause overexcitement, especially in children. It can also make you drowsy. If you take this product during the day, be especially cautious when driving and when operating machinery.

Possible food and drug interactions when taking this medication

Do not use Tylenol Allergy Sinus NightTime while taking other medications containing acetaminophen, such as **Excedrin**, **Panadol**, **Percocet**, **Sine-Aid**, **Sinulin**, and all other forms of **Tylenol**.

Also avoid taking this product within 2 weeks of taking any drug classified as an MAO inhibitor, including the antidepressants **Nardil** and **Parnate**.

If you are taking a tranquilizer such as **Valium** or **Xanax**, or a sleep aid such as **Halcion** or **Seconal**, do not take Tylenol Allergy Sinus NightTime without your doctor's approval; the combination could cause extreme drowsiness. For the same reason, avoid alcohol while taking this product.

Overdosage

■ *Symptoms of Tylenol Allergy Sinus NightTime overdose may include:*
Feeling of general discomfort, mild anxiety, perspiration, rapid heartbeat, high blood pressure, nausea, vomiting

The mild anxiety, rapid heartbeat, and high blood pressure usually appear within 4 to 8 hours after the overdose and usually disappear without treatment.

Particularly in heavy drinkers, a massive overdose of acetaminophen could cause liver damage. If you suspect an overdose, seek medical attention immediately.

Brand name:

Tylenol Children's Cold Plus Cough

Pronounced: TYE-luh-naul
Generic ingredients: Acetaminophen, Chlorpheniramine maleate,
  Dextromethorphan hydrobromide, Pseudoephedrine hydrochloride

What this drug is used for

This medication temporarily relieves coughs, stuffy and runny nose, sore throat, sneezing, minor aches and pains, headaches, and fever caused by a common cold or an allergy such as hay fever. The product comes in chewable tablets and a liquid.

How should you take this medication?

Doses may be repeated every 4 to 6 hours, up to a maximum of 4 doses a day. A measuring cup is provided with the liquid form of the product.

■ CHILDREN 6 TO 12

The usual dosage is 4 tablets or 2 teaspoonfuls.

■ CHILDREN 2 TO 6

Check first with your doctor before giving this product to a child under 6. The usual dosage is 2 tablets or 1 teaspoonful.

Do not take this medication if...

Unless your doctor approves, do not use this medication if the child has heart disease, high blood pressure, thyroid disease, diabetes, high pressure within the eye (glaucoma), or a breathing problem such as chronic bronchitis.

Also check with your doctor before using this medication for the type of chronic cough that results from asthma, or for a cough that brings up lots of phlegm.

Special warnings about this medication

If the child develops an allergic reaction, becomes dizzy or nervous, or has trouble sleeping, stop using this medication and check with your doctor.

Do not give this product for more than 5 days for pain or 3 days for fever without your doctor's approval. If the pain or fever won't go away or gets worse, or if the child develops new symptoms or you notice any redness or swelling, check with your doctor; the child might have a serious condition.

You should also check with your doctor immediately if the child has a severe sore throat that lasts for more than 2 days, or if the sore throat is accompanied or followed by fever, headache, rash, nausea, or vomiting.

Likewise, call your doctor if the child has a cough that lasts for more than 7 days or tends to come back, or has a cough accompanied by rash, lasting headache, or a fever.

This medication can make children either overexcited or drowsy.

If the child must avoid phenylalanine, do not use the chewable tablets.

Possible food and drug interactions
when taking this medication

Do not use this medication if the child is taking other medications containing acetaminophen, such as **Excedrin**, **Panadol**, **Percocet**, **Sine-Aid**, **Sinulin**, and all other forms of **Tylenol**.

Do not use this medication within 2 weeks of giving the child a drug classified as an MAO inhibitor, such as the antidepressants **Nardil** and **Parnate**.

If the child is taking a tranquilizer such as **Valium** or **Xanax**, or a sleep aid such as **Halcion** or **Seconal**, do not use this medication without your doctor's approval; the combination could cause extreme drowsiness.

Overdosage

■ *Symptoms of Tylenol Children's Cold Plus Cough overdose may include:*
Feeling of general discomfort, mild anxiety, rapid heartbeat, high blood pressure, perspiration, nausea, vomiting

A massive overdose can also cause problems with the nervous system, trigger visual disturbances, and disrupt normal urination.

The anxiety, rapid heartbeat, and high blood pressure usually appear within 4 to 8 hours after the child has taken the overdose and usually go away without treatment. Nevertheless, if you suspect an overdose, seek medical attention immediately.

Brand name:

Tylenol Children's Cold Products

Pronounced: TYE-luh-naul
Generic ingredients: Acetaminophen, Chlorpheniramine maleate,
  Pseudoephedrine hydrochloride

What this drug is used for

Children's Tylenol Cold products relieve the stuffy nose, sore throat, minor aches and pains, headache, and fever of a cold, along with the sneezing and runny nose of a cold and allergies such as hay fever. They are available in chewable tablet and liquid form.

How should you take this medication?

Doses may be repeated every 4 to 6 hours, up to a maximum of 4 doses a day. A measuring cup is provided with the liquid form of this product.

■ CHILDREN 6 TO 12

The usual dose is 4 tablets or 2 teaspoonfuls.

■ CHILDREN 2 TO 6

Check with your doctor before giving these products to a child under 6. The usual dose is 2 tablets or 1 teaspoonful.

Do not take this medication if...

Unless your doctor approves, do not give either of these products if the child has a breathing problem such as chronic bronchitis, high pressure within the eye (glaucoma), heart disease, high blood pressure, thyroid disease, or diabetes.

Special warnings about this medication

If either of these products causes an allergic reaction, stop using it and call your doctor. These products may also cause either overexcitement or drowsiness.

Do not give either of these products for more than 5 days for pain or 3 days for fever without your doctor's approval. If the pain or fever won't go away or gets worse, or if you notice new symptoms or any redness or swelling, check with your doctor; the child might have a serious condition.

You should also check with your doctor immediately if the child has a severe sore throat that lasts for more than 2 days, or if the sore throat is accompanied or followed by fever, headache, rash, nausea, or vomiting.

If the child becomes nervous or dizzy, or has trouble sleeping, stop using this medication and call your doctor.

If the child must avoid phenylalanine, do not use the chewable tablets.

Possible food and drug interactions when taking this medication

Do not use these products while the child is taking other medications containing acetaminophen, such as **Excedrin**, **Panadol**, **Percocet**, **Sine-Aid**, **Sinulin**, and all other forms of **Tylenol**.

Children also should not be given these products within 2 weeks of taking a drug classified as an MAO inhibitor, such as the antidepressants **Nardil** and **Parnate**.

If the child is taking a tranquilizer such as **Valium** or **Xanax**, or a sleep aid such as **Halcion** or **Seconal**, do not use these products without your doctor's approval; the combination could cause extreme drowsiness.

Overdosage

■ *Symptoms of an overdose of Tylenol Children's Cold Products may include:*
Feeling of general discomfort, mild anxiety, perspiration, rapid heartbeat, high blood pressure, nausea, vomiting

The anxiety, rapid heartbeat, and high blood pressure usually appear within 4 to 8 hours after the overdose and usually disappear without treatment. Nevertheless, if you suspect an overdose, seek medical attention immediately.

Brand name:

Tylenol Children's Flu Liquid

Pronounced: TYE-luh-naul
Generic ingredients: Acetaminophen, Chlorpheniramine maleate, Dextromethorphan hydrobromide, Pseudoephedrine hydrochloride

What this drug is used for

Tylenol Children's Flu Liquid temporarily relieves fever, minor aches and pains, headaches, sore throat, stuffy and runny nose, and coughs caused by a cold or flu.

How should you take this medication?

For children 6 to 12 years of age, the usual dosage is 2 teaspoonfuls every 6 to 8 hours, up to a maximum of 4 doses a day. For children under 6, consult your doctor.

Do not take this medication if...

Unless your doctor approves, do not use Tylenol Children's Flu Liquid if the child has heart disease, high blood pressure, thyroid disease, diabetes, high pressure within the eye (glaucoma), or a breathing problem such as chronic bronchitis.

Also check with your doctor before using this medication for the type of chronic cough that results from asthma, or for a cough that brings up lots of phlegm.

Special warnings about this medication

If the child becomes dizzy or nervous, or has trouble sleeping, stop using this medication and check with your doctor.

Do not give Tylenol Children's Flu Liquid for more than 5 days for pain or 3 days for fever without your doctor's approval. If the pain or fever won't go away or gets worse, or if the child develops new symptoms or you notice any redness or swelling, check with your doctor; the child might have a serious condition.

You should also check with your doctor immediately if the child has a severe sore throat that lasts for more than 2 days, or if the sore throat is accompanied or followed by fever, headache, rash, nausea, or vomiting.

Likewise, call your doctor if the child has a cough that lasts for more than 7 days or tends to come back, or has a cough accompanied by rash, lasting headache, or a fever.

This medication can make children either overexcited or drowsy.

Possible food and drug interactions
when taking this medication

Do not use Tylenol Children's Flu Liquid if the child is taking other medications containing acetaminophen, such as **Excedrin**, **Panadol**, **Percocet**, **Sine-Aid**, **Sinulin**, and all other forms of **Tylenol**.

Do not use this medication within 2 weeks of giving the child a drug classified as an MAO inhibitor, such as the antidepressants **Nardil** and **Parnate**.

If the child is taking a tranquilizer such as **Valium** or **Xanax**, or a sleep aid such as **Halcion** or **Seconal**, do not use Tylenol Children's Flu Liquid without your doctor's approval; the combination could cause extreme drowsiness.

Overdosage

■ *Symptoms of an overdose of Tylenol Children's Flu Liquid may include:*

Feeling of general discomfort, mild anxiety, rapid heartbeat, high blood pressure, perspiration, nausea, vomiting

A massive overdose can also cause problems with the nervous system, trigger visual disturbances, and disrupt normal urination.

The anxiety, rapid heartbeat, and high blood pressure usually appear within 4 to 8 hours after the child has taken the overdose and usually go away without treatment. Nevertheless, if you suspect an overdose, seek medical attention immediately.

Brand name:

Tylenol Cold Medications

Pronounced: TYE-luh-naul
Generic ingredients: Acetaminophen, Dextromethorphan hydrobro-
  mide, Pseudoephedrine hydrochloride, Chlorpheniramine maleate
  (Multi-Symptom products only)

What this drug is used for

All three Tylenol Cold Medications—No Drowsiness Formula, Multi-Symptom Formula, and Multi-Symptom Hot Medication—temporarily relieve stuffy nose, cough, body aches and pains, headache, sore throat, and fever caused by a cold or flu. The Multi-Symptom products also relieve runny nose, sneezing, and watery, itchy eyes.

The No Drowsiness Formula and the Multi-Symptom Formula come in pill form. The Multi-Symptom Hot Medication is supplied in packets.

How should you take this medication?

Doses of all three medications can be repeated every 6 hours, up to a maximum of 4 doses a day.

■ ADULTS AND CHILDREN 12 YEARS AND OVER
No Drowsiness and Multi-Symptom Formulas
The usual dosage is 2 pills.

Hot Medication
Dissolve 1 packet in a 6-ounce cup of hot water. Sip while hot. Sweeten to taste, if you wish.

■ CHILDREN
No Drowsiness and Multi-Symptom Formulas
For children 6 to 12, the usual dosage is 1 pill. These formulas are not for children under 6.

Hot Medication
Not for children under 12.

Do not take this medication if...

Unless your doctor approves, do not take any of these products if you have heart disease, high blood pressure, thyroid disease, diabetes, or an enlarged prostate gland. In addition, avoid the Multi-Symptom products if you have high pressure within the eye (glaucoma) or a breathing problem such as emphysema or chronic bronchitis.

Also check with your doctor before using any of these products for the type of chronic cough that results from smoking or asthma, or for a cough that brings up lots of phlegm.

Special warnings about this medication

If any of these products give you an allergic reaction, stop taking the medicine and call your doctor.

Do not take any of these products for more than 7 days (3 days for fever) without your doctor's approval. If your pain or fever won't go away or gets worse, or if you develop new symptoms or notice any redness or swelling, check with your doctor; you might have a serious condition.

You should also check with your doctor immediately if you have a severe sore throat that lasts for more than 2 days, or if your sore throat is accompanied or followed by fever, headache, rash, nausea, or vomiting.

Likewise, call your doctor if you have a cough that lasts for more than 7 days or tends to come back, or a cough accompanied by rash, lasting headache, and fever.

The Multi-Symptom varieties contain an antihistamine that may cause overexcitement, especially in children. This ingredient also tends to make some people drowsy. Be especially cautious when driving, and when operating machinery. Remember, too, that if you take more than the recommended dosage of these varieties, they can make you nervous or dizzy, or interfere with your sleep.

If you must avoid phenylalanine, do not use the Hot Medication formula.

Possible food and drug interactions when taking this medication

Do not use any of these products while taking other medications containing acetaminophen, such as **Excedrin**, **Panadol**, **Percocet**, **Sine-Aid**, **Sinulin**, and all other forms of **Tylenol**.

Also avoid taking these products within 2 weeks of taking any drug classified as an MAO inhibitor, including the antidepressants **Nardil** and **Parnate**.

If you are taking a tranquilizer such as **Valium** or **Xanax**, or a sleep aid such as **Halcion** or **Seconal**, do not take the Multi-Symptom varieties without your doctor's approval; the combination could cause extreme drowsiness. For the same reason, avoid alcohol while taking these varieties.

Overdosage

■ *Symptoms of an overdose of Tylenol Cold Medications may include:*

Feeling of general discomfort, mild anxiety, nervous system problems, perspiration, rapid heartbeat, high blood pressure, visual problems, nausea, vomiting

The anxiety, rapid heartbeat, and high blood pressure usually appear within 4 to 8 hours after the overdose and usually disappear without treatment.

Particularly in heavy drinkers, a massive overdose of the acetaminophen in these products could cause liver damage. If you suspect an overdose, seek medical attention immediately.

Brand name:

Tylenol Cold Severe Congestion

Pronounced: TYE-luh-naul
Generic ingredients: Acetaminophen, Dextromethorphan hydrobro-
mide, Guaifenesin, Pseudoephedrine hydrochloride

What this drug is used for

Tylenol Cold Severe Congestion temporarily relieves a stuffy nose, congestion in the chest, coughing, sore throat, headaches, body aches, and fever. Because it does not contain an antihistamine for sneezing and runny nose, it won't cause drowsiness.

How should you take this medication?

■ ADULTS

For adults and children 12 years and over, the usual dosage is 2 caplets every 6 to 8 hours. Do not take more than 8 caplets each 24 hours.

■ CHILDREN

For children 6 to 12, the usual dosage is 1 caplet every 6 to 8 hours. Do not give more than 4 caplets each 24 hours.

Do not take this medication if...

Unless your doctor approves, do not take this product if you have heart disease, high blood pressure, thyroid disease, diabetes, or an enlarged prostate gland.

Also check with your doctor before using this product for the type of chronic cough that results from smoking, emphysema, or asthma, or for a cough that brings up lots of phlegm.

Not for children under 6.

Special warnings about this medication

If you develop an allergic reaction, become dizzy or nervous, or have trouble sleeping, stop taking this product and check with your doctor.

Do not take this product for more than 7 days for pain or 3 days for fever without your doctor's approval. If your pain or fever won't go away or gets worse, or if you develop new symptoms or notice any redness or swelling, check with your doctor; you might have a serious condition.

You should also check with your doctor immediately if you have a severe sore throat that lasts for more than 2 days, or if your sore throat is accompanied or followed by fever, headache, rash, nausea, or vomiting.

Likewise, call your doctor if you have a cough that lasts for more than 7 days or tends to come back, or your cough is accompanied by rash, lasting headache, or fever.

Possible food and drug interactions when taking this medication

Do not use Tylenol Cold Severe Congestion while taking other products that contain acetaminophen, such as Excedrin, Panadol, Percocet, Sine-Aid, Sinulin, and all other forms of Tylenol.

Do not use this medication within 2 weeks of taking a drug classified as an MAO inhibitor, such as the antidepressants **Nardil** and **Parnate**.

Combined with heavy drinking, the acetaminophen in Tylenol Cold Severe Congestion could conceivably cause liver damage. Check with your doctor before taking this product if you generally have more than 3 alcoholic beverages a day.

Overdosage

■ *Symptoms of an overdose of Tylenol Cold Severe Congestion may include:*
Feeling of general discomfort, mild anxiety, perspiration, rapid heartbeat, high blood pressure, nausea and vomiting

A massive overdose can also cause problems with the nervous system, trigger visual disturbances, and disrupt normal urination.

The anxiety, rapid heartbeat, and high blood pressure usually appear within 4 to 8 hours after the overdose and disappear without treatment. Nevertheless, if you suspect an overdose, seek medical attention immediately.

Brand name:

Tylenol Cough Medications

Pronounced: TYE-luh-naul
Generic ingredients: Acetaminophen, Dextromethorphan hydrobromide, Pseudoephedrine hydrochloride (Tylenol Cough Medication with Decongestant only)

What this drug is used for

Both forms of Tylenol Cough Medication temporarily relieve coughing and the aches, pains, and sore throat that may accompany a cough caused by a cold. Tylenol Cough Medication with Decongestant contains an extra ingredient that helps to unclog stuffy nose.

Both products come in liquid form.

How should you take this medication?

Doses may be repeated every 6 to 8 hours, up to a maximum of 4 doses a day.

■ ADULTS

For adults and children 12 years and over, the usual dose is 1 tablespoonful.

■ CHILDREN

For children 6 to 12, the usual dose is 1½ teaspoonfuls.

Do not take this medication if...

Unless your doctor approves, do not use either of these medications for the type of chronic cough that results from smoking, asthma, or emphysema, or for a cough that brings up lots of phlegm.

In addition, you need to avoid the Cough Medication with Decongestant formulation if you have heart disease, high blood pressure, thyroid disease, diabetes, or an enlarged prostate gland.

Neither formulation is for children under 6.

Special warnings about this medication

If either product gives you an allergic reaction, stop taking it and call your doctor.

Limit use of the Cough Medication formulation to 10 days, and the Cough Medication with Decongestant formula to 7 days. Take neither product for more than 3 days if you have a fever. If your symptoms do not improve, or include severe pain or lasting fever, call your doctor.

You should also check with your doctor immediately if you have a severe sore throat that lasts for more than 2 days, or if your sore throat is accompanied or followed by fever, headache, rash, nausea, or vomiting.

Likewise, call your doctor if you have a cough that lasts for more than 7 days or tends to come back, or a cough accompanied by rash, lasting headache, and fever.

Taking more than the maximum dosage of the Cough Medication with Decongestant formula can make you nervous or dizzy, or interfere with your sleep.

Possible food and drug interactions when taking this medication

Do not use either of these products while taking other medications containing acetaminophen, such as **Excedrin, Panadol, Percocet, Sine-Aid, Sinulin**, and all other forms of **Tylenol**.

Also avoid taking these products within 2 weeks of taking any drug classified as an MAO inhibitor, including the antidepressants **Nardil** and **Parnate**.

In addition, do not take the Cough Medication with Decongestant formula if you are taking a medication for high blood pressure.

Combined with heavy drinking, the acetaminophen in these products could conceivably cause liver damage. Check with your doctor before taking either of these products if you generally have more than 3 alcoholic beverages a day.

Overdosage

■ *Symptoms of an overdose of either product may include:*
Feeling of general discomfort, inability to urinate, perspiration, visual problems, nervous system problems, nausea, vomiting

■ *An overdose of Tylenol Cough Medication with Decongestant may also produce:*
Mild anxiety, rapid heartbeat, and high blood pressure that usually appear within 4 to 8 hours after the overdose and disappear without treatment.

Particularly in heavy drinkers, a massive overdose of acetaminophen could cause liver damage. If you suspect an overdose, seek medical attention immediately.

Brand name:

Tylenol Flu Medications

Pronounced: TYE-luh-naul
Generic ingredients: Acetaminophen, Pseudoephedrine hydrochloride,
Dextromethorphan hydrobromide (No Drowsiness Formula only),
Diphenhydramine hydrochloride (NightTime Medications only)

What this drug is used for

All three Tylenol Flu Medications—No Drowsiness Formula, NightTime Medication, and NightTime Hot Medication—temporarily relieve body aches, headaches, fever, sore throat, and stuffy nose. The No Drowsiness Formula also relieves coughing, while the two NightTime Medications contain an antihistamine to relieve runny nose and sneezing.

How should you take this medication?

You can take any of the Tylenol Flu Medications every 6 hours, up to a maximum of 4 doses a day. The usual dosage for adults and children 12 years and over is 2 gelcaps or 1 packet.

Dissolve the NightTime Hot Medication in a 6-ounce cup of hot water. Sip while hot. Sweeten to taste, if you wish.

Do not take this medication if...

Unless your doctor approves, do not take any of the Tylenol Flu Medications if you have heart disease, high blood pressure, thyroid disease, diabetes, or an enlarged prostate gland, Avoid the NightTime Medications if you have high pressure within the eye (glaucoma) or a breathing problem such as emphysema or chronic bronchitis.

Check with your doctor before using the No Drowsiness Formula for the type of chronic cough that results from smoking, emphysema, or asthma, or for a cough that brings up lots of phlegm.

None of these medications is for children under 12.

Special warnings about this medication

If any of these products gives you an allergic reaction, stop using it and call your doctor. Taking more than the recommended dosage can make you nervous or dizzy, or interfere with your sleep.

Do not take these products for more than 7 days (3 days for fever) without your doctor's approval. Get in touch with your doctor if your symptoms do not improve or you have a fever.

You should also check with your doctor immediately if you have a severe sore throat that lasts for more than 2 days, or if your sore throat is accompanied or followed by fever, headache, rash, nausea, or vomiting.

Likewise, call your doctor if you have a cough that lasts for more than 7 days or tends to come back, or your cough is accompanied by rash, lasting headache, or fever.

The antihistamine in the two NightTime Medications may cause overexcitement, especially in children. It can also cause drowsiness, so be cautious when driving and when operating machinery.

If you must avoid phenylalanine, do not use the NightTime Hot Medication.

Possible food and drug interactions when taking this medication

Do not use any of the Tylenol Flu Medications while taking other products that contain acetaminophen, such as **Excedrin**, **Panadol**, **Percocet**, **Sine-Aid**, **Sinulin**, and all other forms of **Tylenol**.

Do not use any of these medications within 2 weeks of taking a drug classified as an MAO inhibitor, such as the antidepressants **Nardil** and **Parnate**.

Combined with heavy drinking, the acetaminophen in these Tylenol Flu Medications could conceivably cause liver damage. Check with your doctor before taking any of them if you generally have more than 3 alcoholic beverages a day.

If you are taking a tranquilizer such as **Valium** or **Xanax**, or a sleep aid such as **Halcion** or **Seconal**, do not take either of the NightTime Medications without your doctor's approval; the combination could cause extreme drowsiness. For the same reason, avoid alcohol while taking the NightTime Medications.

Overdosage

■ *Symptoms of an overdose of Tylenol Flu Medications may include:* Feeling of general discomfort, mild anxiety, perspiration, rapid heartbeat, high blood pressure, nausea, vomiting. A massive overdose of the No Drowsiness Formula can also cause problems with the nervous system, trigger visual disturbances, and disrupt normal urination.

The anxiety, rapid heartbeat, and high blood pressure usually appear within 4 to 8 hours after the overdose and disappear without treatment. Nevertheless, if you suspect an overdose, seek medical attention immediately.

Brand name:

Tylenol Infants' Cold Drops

Pronounced: TYE-luh-naul
Generic ingredients: Acetaminophen, Pseudoephedrine hydrochloride

What this drug is used for

Tylenol Infants' Cold Drops temporarily relieve stuffy nose, minor aches and pains, headaches, and fever caused by the common cold or allergies such as hay fever.

How should you take this medication?

Doses may be repeated every 4 to 6 hours, up to a maximum of 4 times a day. Check with your doctor before giving the drops to children under 2. The usual doses are:

Children 4 to 5 years: 2.4 milligrams
Children 2 to 3 years: 1.6 milligrams
Children 12 to 23 months: 1.2 milligrams
Infants 4 to 11 months: 0.8 milligram
Birth to 3 months: 0.4 milligram

Do not take this medication if...

Unless your doctor approves, do not use this product if the child has heart disease, high blood pressure, thyroid disease, or diabetes.

Special warnings about this medication

If the child becomes nervous or dizzy, or has trouble sleeping, stop giving the drops and call your doctor. Do the same if the drops cause an allergic reaction.

Do not give this product for more than 5 days for pain or 3 days for fever without your doctor's approval. If the pain or fever won't go away or gets worse, or if you notice any new symptoms, redness, or swelling, check with your doctor; the child might have a serious condition.

Possible food and drug interactions
when taking this medication

Do not use these drops while giving other medications containing acetaminophen, such as **Excedrin**, **Panadol**, **Percocet**, **Sine-Aid**, **Sinulin**, and all other forms of **Tylenol**.

Also avoid using the drops within 2 weeks of giving the child a drug classified as an MAO inhibitor, such as the antidepressants **Nardil** and **Parnate**.

Overdosage

■ *Symptoms of an overdose of Tylenol Infants' Cold Drops may include:*

Feeling of general discomfort, mild anxiety, perspiration, rapid heartbeat, high blood pressure, nausea, vomiting

The anxiety, rapid heartbeat, and high blood pressure usually appear within 4 to 8 hours after the overdose and disappear without treatment.

If you suspect an overdose, seek medical attention immediately.

Brand name:

Tylenol PM

Pronounced: TYE-luh-naul
Generic ingredients: Acetaminophen, Diphenhydramine hydrochloride
Other brand names: Legatrin PM, Unisom with Pain Relief

What this drug is used for

The acetaminophen in these products provides temporary relief of minor aches and pains such as headache, muscle aches, and leg cramps. They also contain an antihistamine to help fight sleeplessness. Of the three, Unisom contains the highest amount of both ingredients.

How should you take this medication?

■ TYLENOL PM

The usual dosage is 2 pills at bedtime.

■ UNISOM WITH PAIN RELIEF AND LEGATRIN PM

The usual dosage is 1 pill at bedtime.

Do not take this medication if...

Unless your doctor approves, do not take these products if you have high pressure within the eye (glaucoma), an enlarged prostate gland, or a breathing problem such as emphysema or chronic bronchitis.

Do not take Unisom if you are pregnant or nursing a baby; check with your doctor before taking the others. Also, do not use Unisom for arthritis unless your doctor approves.

None of these products is for children under 12.

Special warnings about this medication

Do not take this product for more than 10 days for pain or 3 days for fever without your doctor's approval. If your pain or fever won't go away or gets worse, or if you develop new symptoms or notice any redness or swelling, check with your doctor; you might have a serious condition.

Also check with your doctor if you are troubled by sleeplessness for more than 2 weeks.

These products are designed to make you sleepy and should be used only at bedtime. Do not drive or operate machinery after taking them.

Possible food and drug interactions
when taking this medication

Do not use these products while taking other medications containing acetaminophen, such as **Excedrin**, **Panadol**, **Percocet**, **Sine-Aid**, **Sinulin**, and all other forms of **Tylenol**. Check with your doctor before combining the products with a drug classified as an MAO inhibitor, such as the antidepressants **Nardil** and **Parnate**.

If you are taking a tranquilizer such as **Valium** or **Xanax**, or a sleep aid such as **Halcion** or **Seconal**, do not take any of these products without your doctor's approval; the combination could cause extreme drowsiness. For the same reason, avoid alcohol while taking one of these products.

Overdosage

Particularly in heavy drinkers, a massive overdose of acetaminophen could cause liver damage.

■ *Early signs of acetaminophen overdose include:*
Feeling of general discomfort, perspiration, nausea, vomiting

If you suspect an overdose, seek medical attention immediately.

Brand name:

Tylenol Severe Allergy

Pronounced: TYE-luh-naul
Generic ingredients: Acetaminophen, Diphenhydramine hydrochloride

What this drug is used for

Tylenol Severe Allergy temporarily relieves runny nose, sneezing, itchy nose or throat, and itchy, watery eyes caused by allergies such as hay fever, and can also be used for sore or scratchy throat.

Unlike Tylenol Allergy *Sinus* products, this medication does not include a decongestant to unclog stuffy nose and sinuses.

How should you take this medication?

The usual dosage is 2 caplets every 4 to 6 hours. Do not take more than 8 caplets each 24 hours.

Do not take this medication if...

Unless your doctor approves, avoid Tylenol Severe Allergy if you have high pressure within the eye (glaucoma), an enlarged prostate gland, or a breathing problem such as emphysema or chronic bronchitis.

Not for children under 12.

Special warnings about this medication

If you have an allergic reaction to this product, stop taking it and call your doctor.

Do not take this product for more than 10 days for pain or 3 days for fever without your doctor's approval. If your pain or fever won't go away or gets worse, or if you develop new symptoms or notice any redness or swelling, check with your doctor; you might have a serious condition.

You should also check with your doctor immediately if you have a severe sore throat that lasts for more than 2 days, or if your sore throat is accompanied or followed by fever, headache, rash, nausea, or vomiting.

Tylenol Severe Allergy may cause overexcitement, especially in children. It can also make some people drowsy. Be especially cautious when driving, and when operating machinery.

Possible food and drug interactions
when taking this medication

Do not use Tylenol Severe Allergy while taking other medications containing acetaminophen, such as **Excedrin**, **Panadol**, **Percocet**, **Sine-Aid**, **Sinulin**, and all other forms of **Tylenol**.

If you are taking a tranquilizer such as **Valium** or **Xanax**, or a sleep aid such as **Halcion** or **Seconal**, do not take Tylenol Severe Allergy without your doctor's approval; the combination could cause extreme drowsiness. For the same reason, avoid alcohol while taking this product.

Overdosage
■ *Symptoms of Tylenol Severe Allergy overdose may include:*
Feeling of general discomfort, perspiration, nausea, vomiting

Particularly in heavy drinkers, a massive overdose of acetaminophen could cause liver damage. If you suspect an overdose, seek medical attention immediately.

Brand name:
Tylenol Sinus

See Sine-Aid

Brand name:
Unifiber

See Citrucel

Brand name:
Unisom

Pronounced: YOU-ni-sahm
Generic name: Doxylamine succinate

What this drug is used for
Unisom is a sleep aid. Another variety of Unisom, labeled "Maximum Strength Unisom," contains a different active ingredient, but shares similar concerns and precautions.

How should you take this medication?
Take 1 tablet 30 minutes before going to bed.

Do not take this medication if...
Do not take Unisom while pregnant or nursing a baby; and do not give it to children under 12 years of age.

Unless your doctor approves, do not take Unisom if you have high pressure within the eye (glaucoma), an enlarged prostate gland, or a breathing problem such as asthma, emphysema, or chronic bronchitis.

Special warnings about this medication

Unisom is for occasional use. If you have problems sleeping for more than 2 weeks, talk to your doctor. There may be a serious underlying problem.

Possible food and drug interactions
when taking this medication

If you are taking a tranquilizer such as **Valium** or **Xanax**, or a sleep aid such as **Halcion** or **Seconal**, do not take Unisom without your doctor's approval; the combination could cause extreme drowsiness. For the same reason, avoid alcohol while using this product.

Overdosage

An overdose of antihistamines can cause severe problems. If you suspect an overdose, seek medical help immediately.

■ *Symptoms of overdose may include:*

Coma, convulsion, delirium, difficulty breathing, dilated pupils, dry mouth, flushed skin, loss of appetite, low blood pressure, nausea, tremor, vomiting

In a child, initial sleepiness may be followed by overexcitement.

Brand name:

Unisom with Pain Relief

See Tylenol PM

Brand name:

Vagistat-1

Pronounced: VAJ-i-stat
Generic name: Tioconazole

What this drug is used for

A single dose of Vagistat-1 cures common vaginal yeast infections. The ointment comes in a prefilled applicator.

How should you take this medication?

Insert 1 applicatorful of Vagistat-1 into the vagina, preferably just prior to bedtime. Apply it as soon as you open the applicator. For vaginal use only.

■ STORAGE

Store at room temperature.

Do not take this medication if...

If you are pregnant or have diabetes, check with your doctor before using Vagistat-1. Do not use Vagistat-1 while breast-feeding. Avoid the product if you have had an allergic reaction to other medications classified as imadozoles.

Special warnings about this medication

Vagistat-1 may weaken the latex in condoms and vaginal diaphragms. After a dose of Vagistat-1, it's best to wait 3 days before using one of these products.

Vagistat-1 causes burning and itching in a few women. Very rarely, it causes vaginal pain or dryness, swelling, irritation, discharge, peeling, painful urination, nighttime urination, or pain during sex.

Possible food and drug interactions when taking this medication

No interactions have been reported.

Brand name:

Vanquish

Pronounced: VAN-kwish
Generic ingredients: Acetaminophen, Aluminum hydroxide, Aspirin, Caffeine, Magnesium hydroxide

What this drug is used for

Vanquish provides temporary relief of headaches, backaches, muscle aches, menstrual pain, minor arthritis pain, and aches and pains associated with colds and flu.

How should you take this medication?

The usual dose for adults and children 12 years and over is 2 caplets with water every 4 hours as needed, up to a maximum of 12 caplets each 24 hours. For children under 12, consult a doctor.

Do not take this medication if...

Unless your doctor approves, do not use Vanquish if you are allergic to aspirin, or if you have asthma, ulcers or bleeding problems, or stomach problems—heartburn, upset stomach, or stomach pain—that do not get better or that go away and come back again.

Special warnings about this medication

The aspirin in Vanquish has been known to trigger a serious illness called Reye's syndrome in children and teenagers who catch a virus. If your child gets chickenpox or flu, do not treat the symptoms with Vanquish.

Do not take Vanquish for more than 10 days for pain or 3 days for fever, unless your doctor recommends. Call your doctor immediately if you develop new symptoms, your pain or fever continues or gets worse, or you notice redness or swelling.

Do not take this product during the last 3 months of pregnancy. It could harm the baby or cause complications during delivery. Earlier during pregnancy, and while nursing a baby, check with your doctor before taking Vanquish.

If you notice ringing in your ears or you begin to lose your hearing, check with your doctor before taking any more of this product.

Possible food and drug interactions when taking this medication

Aspirin-containing products such as Vanquish can interact with a number of prescription drugs. Check with your doctor before combining Vanquish with any of the following:

Acetazolamide (**Diamox**)
ACE-inhibitor-type blood pressure medications such as **Capoten**
Anti-gout drugs such as **Anturane**, **Benemid**, and **Zyloprim**
Arthritis preparations such as **Aleve**, **Anaprox**, **Ecotrin**, **Indocin**, **Motrin**, **Naprosyn**, and **Orudis**
Blood-thinning drugs such as **Coumadin**
Certain diuretics (water pills), including **Lasix**
Diabetes medications, including **DiaBeta**, **Diabinese**, **Micronase**, and **Glucotrol**
Diltiazem (**Cardizem**)
Dipyridamole (**Persantine**)
Seizure medications such as **Depakene**
Steroids such as prednisone (**Deltasone**, **Orasone**)

Brand name:

Vasocon-A

Pronounced: VAZ-oh-kon
Generic ingredients: Antazoline phosphate, Naphazoline hydro-
chloride

What this drug is used for

Vasocon-A temporarily relieves minor allergic symptoms of the eye, including itching and redness due to pollen and animal hair.

How should you take this medication?

Put 1 or 2 drops in the affected eye up to 4 times daily. Remove contact lenses before using. For children under 6, consult your doctor.

■ STORAGE

Store at room temperature. Keep away from light.

Do not use this medication if...

Unless your doctor approves, do not use Vasocon-A if you have heart disease, high blood pressure, or high pressure within the eye (glaucoma). Avoid this product if you've had a reaction to any of its ingredients.

Special warnings about this medication

The drops may sting briefly when first applied. However, if you experience eye pain, changes in vision, or continued redness or irritation—or if the condition gets worse or lasts more than 3 days—stop using the drops and call your doctor.

To avoid contaminating the eyedrops, do not touch the tip of the container to any surface. Replace the cap after using. If the solution becomes cloudy or changes color, do not use it.

Overdosage

Overuse of Vasocon-A can make the redness worse. If an infant or child drinks the solution, it could lead to coma and a marked loss of body temperature.

Brand name:

Vicks 44 Cough Relief

See Benylin Adult Formula Cough Suppressant

Brand name:

Vicks 44D

Pronounced: VIX 44-D
Generic ingredients: Dextromethorphan hydrobromide, Pseudo-
    ephedrine hydrochloride

What this drug is used for

Vicks 44D liquid temporarily relieves coughs and stuffy nose from the common cold. It shares two of the ingredients in Vicks Dayquil, but omits the acetaminophen that Dayquil provides for relief of fever and pain.

How should you take this medication?

Doses may be repeated every 6 hours as needed. Do not take more than 4 doses a day.

■ ADULTS

For adults and children 12 years and over, the usual dose is 3 teaspoonfuls.

■ CHILDREN

For children 6 to 12, the usual dose is 1½ teaspoonfuls. For children under 6, consult your doctor.

Do not take this medication if...

Unless your doctor approves, do not take Vicks 44D if you have heart disease, high blood pressure, thyroid disease, diabetes, an enlarged prostate gland, or a breathing problem such as emphysema or chronic bronchitis.

Also check with your doctor before using Vicks 44D for the type of chronic cough that results from smoking or asthma, or for a cough that brings up lots of phlegm.

Special warnings about this medication

If you become dizzy or nervous, or have trouble sleeping, stop taking Vicks 44D and check with your doctor.

If cough and other symptoms don't improve within 7 days or tend to come back—or if you also have a fever, rash, or lasting headache—check with your doctor. A lingering cough could signal a serious condition.

**Possible food and drug interactions
when taking this medication**

Do not use Vicks 44D within 2 weeks of taking a drug classified as an
MAO inhibitor, such as the antidepressants **Nardil** and **Parnate**.

Brand name:

Vicks 44E

See Robitussin-DM

Brand name:

Vicks 44M

Pronounced: VIX 44-M
Generic ingredients: Acetaminophen, Chlorpheniramine maleate,
Dextromethorphan hydrobromide, Pseudoephedrine hydrochloride

What this drug is used for

Vicks 44M liquid temporarily relieves the fever and minor aches and
pains of a cold or flu, including muscular aches, headache, and sore throat
pain. It also combats stuffy nose, cough, and runny nose and sneezing.

The product is similar to Vicks Nyquil, but contains a different antihistamine for relief of sneezing and runny nose.

How should you take this medication?

The usual dose for adults and children 12 years and older is 4 teaspoonfuls. Repeat doses every 6 hours as needed, but do not take more
than 4 doses per day. For children under 12, consult your doctor.

Do not take this medication if...

Unless your doctor approves, do not take Vicks 44M if you have heart
disease, high blood pressure, thyroid disease, diabetes, high pressure
within the eye (glaucoma), an enlarged prostate gland, or a breathing
problem such as emphysema or chronic bronchitis.

Also check with your doctor before using Vicks 44M for the type of
chronic cough that results from smoking or asthma, or for a cough that
brings up lots of phlegm.

If you are on a sodium-restricted diet, do not use this product without
your doctor's approval.

Special warnings about this medication

If you become dizzy or nervous, or have trouble sleeping, stop taking Vicks 44M and check with your doctor.

Because Vicks 44M may cause drowsiness, be especially cautious when driving, and when operating machinery. The product could also cause excitability, especially in children.

Do not take Vicks 44M for more than 7 days. If your symptoms do not improve or include a fever that lasts more than 3 days—or if new symptoms appear—call your doctor.

You should also check with your doctor immediately if you have a severe sore throat that lasts for more than 2 days, or if your sore throat is accompanied or followed by fever, headache, rash, nausea, or vomiting.

Likewise, call your doctor if you have a cough that lasts for more than 7 days or tends to come back, or a cough accompanied by rash, lasting headache, and fever.

Possible food and drug interactions when taking this medication

Do not use Vicks 44M within 2 weeks of taking a drug classified as an MAO inhibitor, such as the antidepressants **Nardil** and **Parnate**.

If you are taking a tranquilizer such as **Valium** or **Xanax**, or a sleep aid such as **Halcion** or **Seconal**, do not take Vicks 44M without your doctor's approval; the combination could cause extreme drowsiness. For the same reason, avoid alcohol while taking this product.

Brand name:

Vicks Chloraseptic Cough & Throat Drops

See Halls Cough Suppressant

Brand name:

Vicks Chloraseptic Sore Throat Lozenges

Pronounced: KLOR-uh-SEP-tick
Generic ingredients: Benzocaine, Menthol

What this drug is used for

These lozenges provide temporary relief from sore mouth or throat.

They also ease occasional minor mouth irritation and pain, and the pain of canker sores.

How should you take this medication?
Allow 1 lozenge to dissolve slowly in your mouth every 2 hours as needed or as directed by a doctor or dentist.

Do not take this medication if...
Avoid this product if you have a history of allergy to local anesthetics with "caine" in their names (for example, procaine, butacaine, or benzocaine).

Special warnings about this medication
Check with a doctor or dentist before giving this product to a child under the age of 5.

If your sore mouth does not improve in 7 days, or if irritation, pain, or redness continues or gets worse, contact your doctor.

Call your doctor if a sore throat is severe or lasts for more than 2 days, or if you have difficulty breathing. Also contact a doctor if your sore throat is accompanied or followed by fever, headache, rash, swelling, nausea, or vomiting.

Brand name:
Vicks Chloraseptic Sore Throat Spray

See Cepastat

Brand name:
Vicks Cough Drops

See Halls Cough Suppressant

Brand name:
Vicks DayQuil

Pronounced: VIX DAY-kwill
Generic ingredients: Acetaminophen, Dextromethorphan hydrobro-
mide, Pseudoephedrine hydrochloride

What this drug is used for
Vicks DayQuil temporarily relieves the fever and minor aches and pains of a cold or flu, including headache, muscular aches, and sore

throat pain. It also combats cough and unclogs stuffy nose. However, it does not contain an antihistamine to fight sneezing and runny nose, because antihistamines can make you drowsy. For this added ingredient, you can turn to the companion product, Vicks NyQuil.

DayQuil comes in liquid and softgel forms.

How should you take this medication?
Doses may be repeated every 4 hours, but limit doses of DayQuil—or DayQuil and NyQuil together—to 4 per day.

■ ADULTS

For adults and children 12 years and over, the usual dose is 2 pills or tablespoonfuls.

■ CHILDREN

For children 6 to 12, the usual dose is 1 pill or tablespoonful. For children under 6, consult your doctor.

Do not take this medication if...
Unless your doctor approves, do not take DayQuil if you have heart disease, high blood pressure, thyroid disease, diabetes, an enlarged prostate gland, or a breathing problem such as emphysema or chronic bronchitis.

Also check with your doctor before using DayQuil for the type of chronic cough that results from smoking or asthma, or for a cough that brings up lots of phlegm.

Special warnings about this medication
If you become dizzy or nervous, or have trouble sleeping, stop taking DayQuil and check with your doctor.

Do not take DayQuil for more than 7 days (5-day limit for children). If your symptoms do not improve or include a fever that lasts more than 3 days—or if new symptoms appear—call your doctor.

You should also check with your doctor immediately if you have a severe sore throat that lasts for more than 2 days, or if your sore throat is accompanied or followed by fever, headache, rash, nausea, or vomiting.

Likewise, call your doctor if you have a cough that lasts for more than 7 days (5 for children) or tends to come back, or a cough accompanied by rash, lasting headache, and fever.

Possible food and drug interactions when taking this medication

Do not use DayQuil within 2 weeks of taking a drug classified as an MAO inhibitor, such as the antidepressants **Nardil** and **Parnate**.

Brand name:

Vicks DayQuil Allergy

Pronounced: VIX DAY-kwill
Generic ingredients: Brompheniramine maleate, Phenylpropanolamine hydrochloride

What this drug is used for

Vicks DayQuil Allergy tablets temporarily relieve the runny nose, sneezing, and itchy, watery eyes that result from allergies such as hay fever. They also unclog the stuffy nose associated with colds, hay fever, and inflamed sinuses.

Although it shares the DayQuil name, this product has none of the same ingredients. Unlike DayQuil, it includes an allergy-fighting antihistamine that may cause drowsiness.

How should you take this medication?

For adults and children 12 years and over, the usual dose is 1 tablet every 12 hours. Allow at least 12 hours between doses. Do not take more than 2 tablets each 24 hours. For children under 12, consult your doctor.

Do not take this medication if...

Unless your doctor approves, do not take Vicks DayQuil Allergy if you have heart disease, high blood pressure, thyroid disease, diabetes, high pressure within the eye (glaucoma), an enlarged prostate gland, or a breathing problem such as emphysema or chronic bronchitis.

Also avoid this product if you've ever had an allergic reaction to any of its ingredients.

Special warnings about this medication

Exceeding the recommended dosage can make you nervous or dizzy, and could interfere with your sleep. Excitability can be problem, especially in children.

This medicine can also cause drowsiness. Avoid driving a car or operating machinery while using it.

If your symptoms do not improve within 7 days or include a fever, call your doctor.

Possible food and drug interactions when taking this medication

Do not use Vicks DayQuil Allergy within 2 weeks of taking a drug classified as an MAO inhibitor, such as the antidepressants **Nardil** and **Parnate**.

Also avoid combining Vicks DayQuil Allergy with prescription blood pressure medications such as **Calan**, **Lotensin**, and **Zestril**, and do not drink alcoholic beverages while using the product.

Brand name:

Vicks DayQuil Sinus Pressure & Pain Relief

See Advil Cold and Sinus

Brand name:

Vicks DayQuil, Children's Allergy

Pronounced: VIX DAY-kwill
Generic ingredients: Chlorpheniramine maleate, Pseudoephedrine hydrochloride

What this drug is used for

Children's Vicks DayQuil Allergy temporarily relieves the runny nose, sneezing, and itchy, watery eyes that result from allergies such as hay fever. It also unclogs stuffy nose and sinuses.

Children's DayQuil Allergy is similar to the adult version, though it employs a different set of ingredients. Both products contain an allergy-fighting antihistamine that may cause drowsiness.

How should you take this medication?

Doses may be given every 6 hours as needed, up to a maximum of 4 doses a day. Check with your doctor before giving this medication to children under 6. The usual doses are as follows:

12 years and over: 2 tablespoonfuls
6 to 12 years: 1 tablespoonful

2 to 6 years: half a tablespoonful
1 to 2 years: 1¼ teaspoonfuls
6 months to 1 year: 1 teaspoonful

Do not take this medication if...

Unless your doctor approves, do not use Children's DayQuil Allergy if the child has heart disease, high blood pressure, thyroid disease, diabetes, high pressure within the eye (glaucoma), or a breathing problem such as chronic bronchitis.

Special warnings about this medication

If the child becomes dizzy or nervous, or has trouble sleeping, stop giving Children's DayQuil Allergy and check with your doctor.

This medicine can cause excitability, especially in children. It can also cause drowsiness.

Do not use this product for more than 7 days. If the child's symptoms do not improve or include a fever, call your doctor.

Possible food and drug interactions when taking this medication

Do not use Children's DayQuil Allergy within 2 weeks of giving the child a drug classified as an MAO inhibitor, such as the antidepressants **Nardil** and **Parnate**.

If the child is taking a tranquilizer such as **Valium** or **Xanax**, or a sleep aid such as **Halcion** or **Seconal**, do not use Children's DayQuil Allergy without your doctor's approval; the combination could cause extreme drowsiness.

Brand name:

Vicks NyQuil

Pronounced: VIX NYE-kwill
Generic ingredients: Acetaminophen, Dextromethorphan hydrobromide, Doxylamine succinate, Pseudoephedrine hydrochloride

What this drug is used for

Vicks NyQuil temporarily relieves the fever and minor aches and pains of a cold or flu, including muscular aches, headache, and sore throat pain. It also combats stuffy nose, cough, and runny nose and sneezing.

NyQuil is a companion product to Vicks DayQuil, which has a similar formula except for the antihistamine doxylamine succinate. This ingredient in NyQuil fights runny nose and sneezing, but tends to make you drowsy.

NyQuil is available in liquid and Liquicap form, and as a powder called Vicks NyQuil Hot Therapy Adult Nighttime Cold/Flu Hot Liquid Medicine.

How should you take this medication?

NyQuil is for adults and children 12 years and over. Consult your doctor for younger children. Limit doses of NyQuil—or DayQuil and NyQuil together—to 4 per day.

■ LIQUID

The usual dose is 2 tablespoonfuls every 6 hours.

■ LIQUICAPS

The usual dose is 2 pills, swallowed with water, every 4 hours.

■ HOT THERAPY

The usual dose is 1 packet dissolved in 6 ounces of hot water at bedtime. If you are confined to bed because of cold or flu symptoms, doses may be repeated every 6 hours. You can sweeten the mixture, if desired. Sip the medicine while it is hot.

Do not take this medication if...

Unless your doctor approves, do not take NyQuil if you have heart disease, high blood pressure, thyroid disease, diabetes, high pressure within the eye (glaucoma), an enlarged prostate gland, or a breathing problem such as emphysema or chronic bronchitis.

Also check with your doctor before using NyQuil for the type of chronic cough that results from smoking or asthma, or for a cough that brings up lots of phlegm.

Special warnings about this medication

If you become dizzy or nervous, or have trouble sleeping, stop taking NyQuil and check with your doctor.

Because NyQuil may cause drowsiness, be especially cautious when driving, and when operating machinery. The product could also cause excitability, especially in children.

Do not take NyQuil for more than 7 days. If your symptoms do not improve or include a fever that lasts more than 3 days—or if new symptoms appear—call your doctor.

You should also check with your doctor immediately if you have a severe sore throat that lasts for more than 2 days, or if your sore throat is accompanied or followed by fever, headache, rash, nausea, or vomiting.

Likewise, call your doctor if you have a cough that lasts for more than 7 days or tends to come back, or a cough accompanied by rash, lasting headache, and fever.

Possible food and drug interactions when taking this medication

Do not use NyQuil within 2 weeks of taking a drug classified as an MAO inhibitor, such as the antidepressants **Nardil** and **Parnate**.

If you are taking a tranquilizer such as **Valium** or **Xanax**, or a sleep aid such as **Halcion** or **Seconal**, do not take NyQuil without your doctor's approval; the combination could cause extreme drowsiness. For the same reason, avoid alcohol while taking this product.

Brand name:

Vicks NyQuil, Children's

Pronounced: VIX NYE-qwill
Generic ingredients: Chlorpheniramine maleate, Dextromethorphan hydrobromide, Pseudoephedrine hydrochloride
Other brand name: Pediatric Vicks 44M

What this drug is used for

Children's NyQuil and Pediatric 44M share the same set of ingredients. They provide temporary relief of stuffy nose, cough, sneezing, and runny nose. Both products lack the acetaminophen contained in their adult counterparts, and therefore cannot be used for relief of pain and fever.

How should you take this medication?

Doses may be given every 6 hours as needed, but do not give more than 4 doses a day. Check with your doctor before giving either medication to children under 6. The usual dosages are as follows:

12 years and over: 2 tablespoonfuls
6 to 12 years: 1 tablespoonful
2 to 5 years: half a tablespoonful
1 to 2 years: 1¼ teaspoonfuls
6 months to 1 year: 1 teaspoonful

Do not take this medication if...

Unless your doctor approves, do not use these products if the child has heart disease, high blood pressure, thyroid disease, diabetes, high pressure within the eye (glaucoma), or a breathing problem such as chronic bronchitis.

Also check with your doctor before using these products for the type of chronic cough that results from asthma, or for a cough that brings up lots of phlegm.

Special warnings about this medication

If the child becomes dizzy or nervous, or has trouble sleeping, stop giving the medicine and check with your doctor.

These products can cause excitability, especially in children. They may also cause drowsiness.

Do not use these products for more than 7 days. If the child's symptoms do not improve or include a fever, call your doctor.

You should also check with your doctor immediately if the child has a cough that lasts for more than 7 days or tends to come back, or a cough accompanied by rash, lasting headache, and fever.

Possible food and drug interactions when taking this medication

Do not use either product within 2 weeks of giving the child a drug classified as an MAO inhibitor, such as the antidepressants **Nardil** and **Parnate**.

If the child is taking a tranquilizer such as **Valium** or **Xanax**, or a sleep aid such as **Halcion** or **Seconal**, do not use these products without your doctor's approval; the combination could cause extreme drowsiness.

Brand name:

Vicks Sinex

See Neo-Synephrine

Brand name:

Vicks Sinex 12-Hour

See Afrin 12 Hour

Brand name:

Zantac 75

Pronounced: ZAN-tack
Generic name: Ranitidine hydrochloride

What this drug is used for

Zantac 75 relieves heartburn, acid indigestion, and sour stomach. It is part of a family of acid-blocking prescription drugs recently released in over-the-counter formulations. Other members of the family are Axid AR, Mylanta AR, Pepcid AC, and Tagamet HB.

How should you take this medication?

Swallow 1 tablet with water. Do not chew. Take no more than 2 tablets a day.

■ STORAGE

Store at room temperature. Protect from high heat or humidity.

Do not take this medication if...

Not for children under 12, unless your doctor approves.

Special warnings about this medication

Do not take 2 tablets of Zantac 75 every day for more than 2 weeks without your doctor's approval.

If you have trouble swallowing, or if you have stomach pain that does not go away, see your doctor right away. You may have a serious condition that needs different treatment.

Possible food and drug interactions
when taking this medication

Check with your doctor before combining Zantac 75 with the following:

Alcohol
Blood-thinning drugs such as **Coumadin**
Diabetes medications such as **Glucotrol**, **DiaBeta**, and **Micronase**
Itraconazole (**Sporanox**)
Ketoconazole (**Nizoral**)
Metoprolol (**Lopressor**)
Nifedipine (**Procardia**)
Phenytoin (**Dilantin**)
Procainamide (**Procan SR**)
Sucralfate (**Carafate**)
Theophylline (**Theo-Dur**)

3. Interaction Tables

When you're taking several medicines at the same time, there is very real possibility that their actions may clash. In some cases, one drug may reduce the effects of another. In other cases, the two drugs may act in concert to increase the severity of a side effect.

There are thousands of drugs on the market, and millions of possible combinations. Although most are completely harmless, that still leaves a substantial number you should do your best to avoid. The tables in this section are designed to make that as easy as possible. For each over-the-counter remedy, they list the specific medications that tend to interact, and tell what to do about it or what to expect.

In most cases, the best policy is to simply avoid combining the drugs. In a few instances, you can eliminate the conflict just by allowing an hour or two to pass between your dose of each. However, if you have any doubt over what to do, a call to your doctor should resolve the matter.

The drug listings in these tables are drawn primarily from the manufacturer's package labeling as published in *PDR for Nonprescription Drugs*, the professional over-the-counter guide for physicians. Where appropriate, the listings have be augmented with information from other sources the publisher has found reliable. Because in some cases a number of brands share the same active ingredient, drugs have been listed by their generic names to conserve space. If you're not sure of a prescription's generic name, check the handout that came with it, or ask your pharmacist.

Actifed Allergy Daytime/Nighttime Caplets

And:	Action:
Alcohol	May cause extra drowsiness. Do not combine.
Alprazolam	May cause extra drowsiness. Check with your doctor.
Buspirone	May cause extra drowsiness. Check with your doctor.
Chlordiazepoxide	May cause extra drowsiness. Check with your doctor.
Chlorpromazine	May cause extra drowsiness. Check with your doctor.
Chlorprothixene	May cause extra drowsiness. Check with your doctor.
Clorazepate	May cause extra drowsiness. Check with your doctor.
Diazepam	May cause extra drowsiness. Check with your doctor.
Droperidol	May cause extra drowsiness. Check with your doctor.
Estazolam	May cause extra drowsiness. Check with your doctor.
Ethchlorvynol	May cause extra drowsiness. Check with your doctor.
Ethinamate	May cause extra drowsiness. Check with your doctor.
Fluphenazine	May cause extra drowsiness. Check with your doctor.
Flurazepam	May cause extra drowsiness. Check with your doctor.
Furazolidone	Do not combine. Wait 2 weeks after using Furazolidone.
Glutethimide	May cause extra drowsiness. Check with your doctor.
Haloperidol	May cause extra drowsiness. Check with your doctor.
Hydroxyzine	May cause extra drowsiness. Check with your doctor.
Isocarboxazid	Do not combine. Wait 2 weeks after using Isocarboxazid.
Lorazepam	May cause extra drowsiness. Check with your doctor.
Loxapine	May cause extra drowsiness. Check with your doctor.
Meprobamate	May cause extra drowsiness. Check with your doctor.
Mesoridazine	May cause extra drowsiness. Check with your doctor.
Midazolam	May cause extra drowsiness. Check with your doctor.
Molindone	May cause extra drowsiness. Check with your doctor.
Oxazepam	May cause extra drowsiness. Check with your doctor.
Perphenazine	May cause extra drowsiness. Check with your doctor.
Phenelzine	Do not combine. Wait 2 weeks after using Phenelzine.
Prazepam	May cause extra drowsiness. Check with your doctor.
Prochlorperazine	May cause extra drowsiness. Check with your doctor.
Promethazine	May cause extra drowsiness. Check with your doctor.
Propofol	May cause extra drowsiness. Check with your doctor.
Quazepam	May cause extra drowsiness. Check with your doctor.
Secobarbital	May cause extra drowsiness. Check with your doctor.

Selegiline	Do not combine. Wait 2 weeks after using Selegiline.
Temazepam	May cause extra drowsiness. Check with your doctor.
Thioridazine	May cause extra drowsiness. Check with your doctor.
Thiothixene	May cause extra drowsiness. Check with your doctor.
Tranylcypromine	Do not combine. Wait 2 weeks after using Tranylcypromine.
Triazolam	May cause extra drowsiness. Check with your doctor.
Trifluoperazine	May cause extra drowsiness. Check with your doctor.
Zolpidem	May cause extra drowsiness. Check with your doctor.

Actifed Cold & Allergy

See Actifed Allergy Daytime/Nighttime Caplets

Actifed Cold & Sinus

See Actifed Allergy Daytime/Nighttime Caplets

Actifed Sinus Daytime/Nighttime

See Actifed Allergy Daytime/Nighttime Caplets

Actron

And:	Action:
Dicumarol	Do not combine without your doctor's approval.
Diuretics	Do not combine without your doctor's approval.
Lithium	Do not combine without your doctor's approval.
Methotrexate	Do not combine without your doctor's approval.
Other Pain and Fever Reducers	Do not combine with Actron.
Other Ketoprofen-Containing Products	Do not combine with Actron.
Probenecid	Do not combine without your doctor's approval.
Warfarin	Do not combine without your doctor's approval.

Acutrim

And:	Action:
Ephedrine-Containing Products	Do not combine.
Furazolidone	Do not combine. Wait 2 weeks after using Furazolidone.
Isocarboxazid	Do not combine. Wait 2 weeks after using Isocarboxazid.
Phenelzine	Do not combine. Wait 2 weeks after using Phenelzine.
Phenylephrine-Containing Products	Do not combine.
Phenylpropanolamine-Containing Products	Do not combine.

Pseudoephedrine-Containing Products	Do not combine.
Selegiline	Do not combine. Wait 2 weeks after using Selegiline.
Tranylcypromine	Do not combine. Wait 2 weeks after using Tranylcypromine.

Advil

And:	Action:
Acetaminophen	Do not combine without your doctor's approval.
Aspirin	Do not combine without your doctor's approval.

Advil Cold and Sinus

And:	Action:
Furazolidone	Do not combine. Wait 2 weeks after using Furazolidone.
Isocarboxazid	Do not combine. Wait 2 weeks after using Isocarboxazid.
Phenelzine	Do not combine. Wait 2 weeks after using Phenelzine.
Selegiline	Do not combine. Wait 2 weeks after using Selegiline.
Tranylcypromine	Do not combine. Wait 2 weeks after using Tranylcypromine.

Afrin 4 Hour

No interactions reported.

Afrin 12 Hour

No interactions reported.

Aleve

And:	Action:
Acetaminophen	Do not combine without your doctor's approval.
Alcohol	Do not combine without your doctor's approval.
Aspirin	Do not combine without your doctor's approval.
Ibuprofen	Do not combine without your doctor's approval.
Naproxen	Do not combine without your doctor's approval.

Alka-Mints

See Tums

Alka-Seltzer

And:	Action:
Acarbose	Do not combine without your doctor's approval.
Alendronate	Allow 2 to 3 hours between doses of the antacid and the drug.
Allopurinol	Allow 2 to 3 hours between doses of the antacid and the drug.
Arthritis Medications	Do not combine without your doctor's approval.
Aspirin	Allow 2 to 3 hours between doses of the antacid and the drug.
Atenolol	Allow 2 to 3 hours between doses of the antacid and the drug.

Captopril	Allow 2 to 3 hours between doses of the antacid and the drug.
Chlordiazepoxide	Allow 2 to 3 hours between doses of the antacid and the drug.
Chlorpropamide	Do not combine without your doctor's approval.
Cimetidine	Allow 2 to 3 hours between doses of the antacid and the drug.
Ciprofloxacin	Allow 2 to 3 hours between doses of the antacid and the drug.
Demeclocycline	Allow 2 to 3 hours between doses of the antacid and the drug.
Dicumarol	Do not combine without your doctor's approval.
Digoxin	Allow 2 to 3 hours between doses of the antacid and the drug.
Doxycycline	Allow 2 to 3 hours between doses of the antacid and the drug.
Enoxacin	Allow 2 to 3 hours between doses of the antacid and the drug.
Fosfomycin	Allow 2 to 3 hours between doses of the antacid and the drug.
Gabapentin	Allow 2 to 3 hours between doses of the antacid and the drug.
Glimepiride	Do not combine without your doctor's approval.
Glipizide	Do not combine without your doctor's approval.
Glyburide	Do not combine without your doctor's approval.
Isoniazid	Allow 2 to 3 hours between doses of the antacid and the drug.
Ketoconazole	Allow 2 to 3 hours between doses of the antacid and the drug.
Levothyroxine	Allow 2 to 3 hours between doses of the antacid and the drug.
Lomefloxacin	Allow 2 to 3 hours between doses of the antacid and the drug.
Metformin	Do not combine without your doctor's approval.
Methacycline	Allow 2 to 3 hours between doses of the antacid and the drug.
Methenamine	Allow 2 to 3 hours between doses of the antacid and the drug.
Metronidazole	Allow 2 to 3 hours between doses of the antacid and the drug.
Miglitol	Do not combine without your doctor's approval.
Minocycline	Allow 2 to 3 hours between doses of the antacid and the drug.
Misoprostol	Allow 2 to 3 hours between doses of the antacid and the drug.
Mycophenolate	Allow 2 to 3 hours between doses of the antacid and the drug.
Norfloxacin	Allow 2 to 3 hours between doses of the antacid and the drug.
Ofloxacin	Allow 2 to 3 hours between doses of the antacid and the drug.
Oxytetracycline	Allow 2 to 3 hours between doses of the antacid and the drug.
Penicillamine	Allow 2 to 3 hours between doses of the antacid and the drug.
Phenytoin	Allow 2 to 3 hours between doses of the antacid and the drug.
Probenecid	Do not combine without your doctor's approval.
Quinidine	Allow 2 to 3 hours between doses of the antacid and the drug.
Sodium Polystyrene Sulfonate	Allow 2 to 3 hours between doses of the antacid and the drug.
Sucralfate	Allow 2 to 3 hours between doses of the antacid and the drug.

Sulfinpyrazone	Do not combine without your doctor's approval.
Tetracycline	Allow 2 to 3 hours between doses of the antacid and the drug.
Tilodronate	Allow 2 to 3 hours between doses of the antacid and the drug.
Tolazamide	Do not combine without your doctor's approval.
Tolbutamide	Do not combine without your doctor's approval.
Troglitazone	Do not combine without your doctor's approval.
Ursodiol	Allow 2 to 3 hours between doses of the antacid and the drug.
Warfarin	Do not combine without your doctor's approval.

Alka-Seltzer Gold

See Alka-Seltzer

Alka-Seltzer Plus Cold & Cough Medicine Liqui-Gels

See Alka-Seltzer Plus Night-Time Cold Medicine Liqui-Gels

Alka-Seltzer Plus Cold & Cough Medicine Tablets

And:	Action:
Acarbose	Do not combine.
Alcohol	May cause extra drowsiness. Do not combine.
Allopurinol	Do not combine.
Alprazolam	May cause extra drowsiness. Check with your doctor.
Arthritis Medications	Do not combine.
Buspirone	May cause extra drowsiness. Check with your doctor.
Chlordiazepoxide	May cause extra drowsiness. Check with your doctor.
Chlorpromazine	May cause extra drowsiness. Check with your doctor.
Chlorpropamide	Do not combine.
Chlorprothixene	May cause extra drowsiness. Check with your doctor.
Clorazepate	May cause extra drowsiness. Check with your doctor.
Diazepam	May cause extra drowsiness. Check with your doctor.
Dicumarol	Do not combine.
Droperidol	May cause extra drowsiness. Check with your doctor.
Estazolam	May cause extra drowsiness. Check with your doctor.
Ethchlorvynol	May cause extra drowsiness. Check with your doctor.
Ethinamate	May cause extra drowsiness. Check with your doctor.
Fluphenazine	May cause extra drowsiness. Check with your doctor.
Flurazepam	May cause extra drowsiness. Check with your doctor.
Furazolidone	Do not combine. Wait 2 weeks after using Furazolidone.
Glimepiride	Do not combine.
Glipizide	Do not combine.

Glutethimide	May cause extra drowsiness. Check with your doctor.
Glyburide	Do not combine.
Haloperidol	May cause extra drowsiness. Check with your doctor.
Hydroxyzine	May cause extra drowsiness. Check with your doctor.
Insulin	Do not combine.
Isocarboxazid	Do not combine. Wait 2 weeks after using Isocarboxazid.
Lorazepam	May cause extra drowsiness. Check with your doctor.
Loxapine	May cause extra drowsiness. Check with your doctor.
Meprobamate	May cause extra drowsiness. Check with your doctor.
Mesoridazine	May cause extra drowsiness. Check with your doctor.
Metformin	Do not combine.
Midazolam	May cause extra drowsiness. Check with your doctor.
Molindone	May cause extra drowsiness. Check with your doctor.
Oxazepam	May cause extra drowsiness. Check with your doctor.
Perphenazine	May cause extra drowsiness. Check with your doctor.
Phenelzine	Do not combine. Wait 2 weeks after using Phenelzine.
Prazepam	May cause extra drowsiness. Check with your doctor.
Probenecid	Do not combine.
Prochlorperazine	May cause extra drowsiness. Check with your doctor.
Promethazine	May cause extra drowsiness. Check with your doctor.
Propofol	May cause extra drowsiness. Check with your doctor.
Quazepam	May cause extra drowsiness. Check with your doctor.
Secobarbital	May cause extra drowsiness. Check with your doctor.
Selegiline	Do not combine. Wait 2 weeks after using Selegiline.
Sulfinpyrazone	Do not combine.
Temazepam	May cause extra drowsiness. Check with your doctor.
Thioridazine	May cause extra drowsiness. Check with your doctor.
Thiothixene	May cause extra drowsiness. Check with your doctor.
Tolazamide	Do not combine.
Tolbutamide	Do not combine.
Tranylcypromine	Do not combine. Wait 2 weeks after using Tranylcypromine.
Triazolam	May cause extra drowsiness. Check with your doctor.
Trifluoperazine	May cause extra drowsiness. Check with your doctor.
Troglitazone	Do not combine.
Warfarin	Do not combine.
Zolpidem	May cause extra drowsiness. Check with your doctor.

Alka-Seltzer Plus Cold Medicine Liqui-Gels

See Alka-Seltzer Plus Night-Time Cold Medicine Liqui-Gels

Alka-Seltzer Plus Cold Medicine Tablets

See Alka-Seltzer Plus Cold & Cough Medicine Tablets

Alka-Seltzer Plus Flu & Body Aches Liqui-Gels

And:	Action:
Furazolidone	Do not combine. Wait 2 weeks after using Furazolidone.
Isocarboxazid	Do not combine. Wait 2 weeks after using Isocarboxazid.
Phenelzine	Do not combine. Wait 2 weeks after using Phenelzine.
Selegiline	Do not combine. Wait 2 weeks after using Selegiline.
Tranylcypromine	Do not combine. Wait 2 weeks after using Tranylcypromine.

Alka-Seltzer Plus Flu & Body Aches Tablets

And:	Action:
Alcohol	May cause extra drowsiness. Do not combine.
Alprazolam	May cause extra drowsiness. Check with your doctor.
Buspirone	May cause extra drowsiness. Check with your doctor.
Chlordiazepoxide	May cause extra drowsiness. Check with your doctor.
Chlorpromazine	May cause extra drowsiness. Check with your doctor.
Chlorprothixene	May cause extra drowsiness. Check with your doctor.
Clorazepate	May cause extra drowsiness. Check with your doctor.
Diazepam	May cause extra drowsiness. Check with your doctor.
Droperidol	May cause extra drowsiness. Check with your doctor.
Estazolam	May cause extra drowsiness. Check with your doctor.
Ethchlorvynol	May cause extra drowsiness. Check with your doctor.
Ethinamate	May cause extra drowsiness. Check with your doctor.
Fluphenazine	May cause extra drowsiness. Check with your doctor.
Flurazepam	May cause extra drowsiness. Check with your doctor.
Furazolidone	Do not combine. Wait 2 weeks after using Furazolidone.
Glutethimide	May cause extra drowsiness. Check with your doctor.
Haloperidol	May cause extra drowsiness. Check with your doctor.
Hydroxyzine	May cause extra drowsiness. Check with your doctor.
Isocarboxazid	Do not combine. Wait 2 weeks after using Isocarboxazid.
Lorazepam	May cause extra drowsiness. Check with your doctor.
Loxapine	May cause extra drowsiness. Check with your doctor.
Meprobamate	May cause extra drowsiness. Check with your doctor.

Mesoridazine	May cause extra drowsiness. Check with your doctor.
Midazolam	May cause extra drowsiness. Check with your doctor.
Molindone	May cause extra drowsiness. Check with your doctor.
Oxazepam	May cause extra drowsiness. Check with your doctor.
Perphenazine	May cause extra drowsiness. Check with your doctor.
Phenelzine	Do not combine. Wait 2 weeks after using Phenelzine.
Prazepam	May cause extra drowsiness. Check with your doctor.
Prochlorperazine	May cause extra drowsiness. Check with your doctor.
Promethazine	May cause extra drowsiness. Check with your doctor.
Propofol	May cause extra drowsiness. Check with your doctor.
Quazepam	May cause extra drowsiness. Check with your doctor.
Secobarbital	May cause extra drowsiness. Check with your doctor.
Selegiline	Do not combine. Wait 2 weeks after using Selegiline.
Temazepam	May cause extra drowsiness. Check with your doctor.
Thioridazine	May cause extra drowsiness. Check with your doctor.
Thiothixene	May cause extra drowsiness. Check with your doctor.
Tranylcypromine	Do not combine. Wait 2 weeks after using Tranylcypromine.
Triazolam	May cause extra drowsiness. Check with your doctor.
Trifluoperazine	May cause extra drowsiness. Check with your doctor.
Zolpidem	May cause extra drowsiness. Check with your doctor.

Alka-Seltzer Plus Night-Time Cold Medicine Liqui-Gels

And:	Action:
Alcohol	May cause extra drowsiness. Do not combine.
Alprazolam	May cause extra drowsiness. Check with your doctor.
Buspirone	May cause extra drowsiness. Check with your doctor.
Chlordiazepoxide	May cause extra drowsiness. Check with your doctor.
Chlorpromazine	May cause extra drowsiness. Check with your doctor.
Chlorprothixene	May cause extra drowsiness. Check with your doctor.
Clorazepate	May cause extra drowsiness. Check with your doctor.
Diazepam	May cause extra drowsiness. Check with your doctor.
Droperidol	May cause extra drowsiness. Check with your doctor.
Estazolam	May cause extra drowsiness. Check with your doctor.
Ethchlorvynol	May cause extra drowsiness. Check with your doctor.
Ethinamate	May cause extra drowsiness. Check with your doctor.
Fluphenazine	May cause extra drowsiness. Check with your doctor.

Flurazepam	May cause extra drowsiness. Check with your doctor.
Furazolidone	Do not combine. Wait 2 weeks after using Furazolidone.
Glutethimide	May cause extra drowsiness. Check with your doctor.
Haloperidol	May cause extra drowsiness. Check with your doctor.
Hydroxyzine	May cause extra drowsiness. Check with your doctor.
Isocarboxazid	Do not combine. Wait 2 weeks after using Isocarboxazid.
Lorazepam	May cause extra drowsiness. Check with your doctor.
Loxapine	May cause extra drowsiness. Check with your doctor.
Meprobamate	May cause extra drowsiness. Check with your doctor.
Mesoridazine	May cause extra drowsiness. Check with your doctor.
Midazolam	May cause extra drowsiness. Check with your doctor.
Molindone	May cause extra drowsiness. Check with your doctor.
Oxazepam	May cause extra drowsiness. Check with your doctor.
Perphenazine	May cause extra drowsiness. Check with your doctor.
Phenelzine	Do not combine. Wait 2 weeks after using Phenelzine.
Prazepam	May cause extra drowsiness. Check with your doctor.
Prochlorperazine	May cause extra drowsiness. Check with your doctor.
Promethazine	May cause extra drowsiness. Check with your doctor.
Propofol	May cause extra drowsiness. Check with your doctor.
Quazepam	May cause extra drowsiness. Check with your doctor.
Secobarbital	May cause extra drowsiness. Check with your doctor.
Selegiline	Do not combine. Wait 2 weeks after using Selegiline.
Temazepam	May cause extra drowsiness. Check with your doctor.
Thioridazine	May cause extra drowsiness. Check with your doctor.
Thiothixene	May cause extra drowsiness. Check with your doctor.
Tranylcypromine	Do not combine. Wait 2 weeks after using Tranylcypromine.
Triazolam	May cause extra drowsiness. Check with your doctor.
Trifluoperazine	May cause extra drowsiness. Check with your doctor.
Zolpidem	May cause extra drowsiness. Check with your doctor.

Alka-Seltzer Plus Night-Time Cold Medicine Tablets

See Alka-Seltzer Plus Cold & Cough Medicine Tablets

Alka-Seltzer Plus Sinus Medicine Tablets

See Alka-Seltzer Plus Cold & Cough Medicine Tablets

Allerest

And:	Action:
Furazolidone	Do not combine. Wait 2 weeks after using Furazolidone.
Isocarboxazid	Do not combine. Wait 2 weeks after using Isocarboxazid.
Phenelzine	Do not combine. Wait 2 weeks after using Phenelzine.
Selegiline	Do not combine. Wait 2 weeks after using Selegiline.
Tranylcypromine	Do not combine. Wait 2 weeks after using Tranylcypromine.

ALternaGEL

And:	Action:
Alendronate	Allow 2 to 3 hours between doses of the antacid and the drug.
Allopurinol	Allow 2 to 3 hours between doses of the antacid and the drug.
Arthritis Drugs	Allow 2 to 3 hours between doses of the antacid and the drug.
Aspirin	Allow 2 to 3 hours between doses of the antacid and the drug.
Atenolol	Allow 2 to 3 hours between doses of the antacid and the drug.
Captopril	Allow 2 to 3 hours between doses of the antacid and the drug.
Chlordiazepoxide	Allow 2 to 3 hours between doses of the antacid and the drug.
Cimetidine	Allow 2 to 3 hours between doses of the antacid and the drug.
Ciprofloxacin	Allow 2 to 3 hours between doses of the antacid and the drug.
Demeclocycline	Allow 2 to 3 hours between doses of the antacid and the drug.
Digoxin	Allow 2 to 3 hours between doses of the antacid and the drug.
Doxycycline	Allow 2 to 3 hours between doses of the antacid and the drug.
Enoxacin	Allow 2 to 3 hours between doses of the antacid and the drug.
Fosfomycin	Allow 2 to 3 hours between doses of the antacid and the drug.
Gabapentin	Allow 2 to 3 hours between doses of the antacid and the drug.
Glipizide	Allow 2 to 3 hours between doses of the antacid and the drug.
Glyburide	Allow 2 to 3 hours between doses of the antacid and the drug.
Isoniazid	Allow 2 to 3 hours between doses of the antacid and the drug.
Ketoconazole	Allow 2 to 3 hours between doses of the antacid and the drug.
Levothyroxine	Allow 2 to 3 hours between doses of the antacid and the drug.
Lomefloxacin	Allow 2 to 3 hours between doses of the antacid and the drug.
Meat	Antacid action reduced by high-protein foods.
Methacycline	Allow 2 to 3 hours between doses of the antacid and the drug.
Methenamine	Allow 2 to 3 hours between doses of the antacid and the drug.
Metronidazole	Allow 2 to 3 hours between doses of the antacid and the drug.
Minocycline	Allow 2 to 3 hours between doses of the antacid and the drug.
Misoprostol	Allow 2 to 3 hours between doses of the antacid and the drug.

Mycophenolate	Allow 2 to 3 hours between doses of the antacid and the drug.
Norfloxacin	Allow 2 to 3 hours between doses of the antacid and the drug.
Ofloxacin	Allow 2 to 3 hours between doses of the antacid and the drug.
Oxytetracycline	Allow 2 to 3 hours between doses of the antacid and the drug.
Penicillamine	Allow 2 to 3 hours between doses of the antacid and the drug.
Phenytoin	Allow 2 to 3 hours between doses of the antacid and the drug.
Quinidine	Allow 2 to 3 hours between doses of the antacid and the drug.
Sodium Polystyrene Sulfonate	Allow 2 to 3 hours between doses of the antacid and the drug.
Sucralfate	Allow 2 to 3 hours between doses of the antacid and the drug.
Tetracycline	Allow 2 to 3 hours between doses of the antacid and the drug.
Tilodronate	Allow 2 to 3 hours between doses of the antacid and the drug.
Ursodiol	Allow 2 to 3 hours between doses of the antacid and the drug.

Amphojel

And:	Action:
Alendronate	Allow 2 to 3 hours between doses of the antacid and the drug.
Allopurinol	Allow 2 to 3 hours between doses of the antacid and the drug.
Arthritis Drugs	Allow 2 to 3 hours between doses of the antacid and the drug.
Aspirin	Allow 2 to 3 hours between doses of the antacid and the drug.
Atenolol	Allow 2 to 3 hours between doses of the antacid and the drug.
Captopril	Allow 2 to 3 hours between doses of the antacid and the drug.
Chlordiazepoxide	Allow 2 to 3 hours between doses of the antacid and the drug.
Cimetidine	Allow 2 to 3 hours between doses of the antacid and the drug.
Ciprofloxacin	Allow 2 to 3 hours between doses of the antacid and the drug.
Demeclocycline	Do not combine.
Digoxin	Allow 2 to 3 hours between doses of the antacid and the drug.
Doxycycline	Do not combine.
Enoxacin	Allow 2 to 3 hours between doses of the antacid and the drug.
Fosfomycin	Allow 2 to 3 hours between doses of the antacid and the drug.
Gabapentin	Allow 2 to 3 hours between doses of the antacid and the drug.
Glipizide	Allow 2 to 3 hours between doses of the antacid and the drug.
Glyburide	Allow 2 to 3 hours between doses of the antacid and the drug.
Isoniazid	Allow 2 to 3 hours between doses of the antacid and the drug.
Ketoconazole	Allow 2 to 3 hours between doses of the antacid and the drug.
Levothyroxine	Allow 2 to 3 hours between doses of the antacid and the drug.
Lomefloxacin	Allow 2 to 3 hours between doses of the antacid and the drug.

Meat	Antacid action reduced by high-protein foods.
Methacycline	Do not combine.
Methenamine	Allow 2 to 3 hours between doses of the antacid and the drug.
Metronidazole	Allow 2 to 3 hours between doses of the antacid and the drug.
Minocycline	Do not combine.
Misoprostol	Allow 2 to 3 hours between doses of the antacid and the drug.
Mycophenolate	Allow 2 to 3 hours between doses of the antacid and the drug.
Norfloxacin	Allow 2 to 3 hours between doses of the antacid and the drug.
Ofloxacin	Allow 2 to 3 hours between doses of the antacid and the drug.
Oxytetracycline	Do not combine.
Penicillamine	Allow 2 to 3 hours between doses of the antacid and the drug.
Phenytoin	Allow 2 to 3 hours between doses of the antacid and the drug.
Quinidine	Allow 2 to 3 hours between doses of the antacid and the drug.
Sodium Polystyrene Sulfonate	Allow 2 to 3 hours between doses of the antacid and the drug.
Sucralfate	Allow 2 to 3 hours between doses of the antacid and the drug.
Tetracycline	Do not combine.
Tilodronate	Allow 2 to 3 hours between doses of the antacid and the drug.
Ursodiol	Allow 2 to 3 hours between doses of the antacid and the drug.

Arco-Lase

No interactions reported.

Arthritis Strength Bufferin

See Bufferin

Ascriptin

And:	Action:
Acarbose	Do not combine without your doctor's approval.
Arthritis Medications	Do not combine without your doctor's approval.
Chlorpropamide	Do not combine without your doctor's approval.
Dicumarol	Do not combine without your doctor's approval.
Glimepiride	Do not combine without your doctor's approval.
Glipizide	Do not combine without your doctor's approval.
Glyburide	Do not combine without your doctor's approval.
Metformin	Do not combine without your doctor's approval.
Miglitol	Do not combine without your doctor's approval.
Probenecid	Do not combine without your doctor's approval.

Sulfinpyrazone	Do not combine without your doctor's approval.
Tolazamide	Do not combine without your doctor's approval.
Tolbutamide	Do not combine without your doctor's approval.
Troglitazone	Do not combine without your doctor's approval.
Warfarin	Do not combine without your doctor's approval.

Aspirin Regimen Bayer

See Bayer Aspirin

Axid AR

No interactions reported.

Backache Caplets

And:	Action:
Acarbose	Do not combine without your doctor's approval.
Arthritis Medications	Do not combine without your doctor's approval.
Chlorpropamide	Do not combine without your doctor's approval.
Dicumarol	Do not combine without your doctor's approval.
Glimepiride	Do not combine without your doctor's approval.
Glipizide	Do not combine without your doctor's approval.
Glyburide	Do not combine without your doctor's approval.
Metformin	Do not combine without your doctor's approval.
Miglitol	Do not combine without your doctor's approval.
Probenecid	Do not combine without your doctor's approval.
Sulfinpyrazone	Do not combine without your doctor's approval.
Tolazamide	Do not combine without your doctor's approval.
Tolbutamide	Do not combine without your doctor's approval.
Troglitazone	Do not combine without your doctor's approval.
Warfarin	Do not combine without your doctor's approval.

Basaljel

And:	Action:
Alendronate	Allow 2 to 3 hours between doses of the antacid and the drug.
Allopurinol	Allow 2 to 3 hours between doses of the antacid and the drug.
Arthritis Drugs	Allow 2 to 3 hours between doses of the antacid and the drug.
Aspirin	Allow 2 to 3 hours between doses of the antacid and the drug.
Atenolol	Allow 2 to 3 hours between doses of the antacid and the drug.
Captopril	Allow 2 to 3 hours between doses of the antacid and the drug.
Chlordiazepoxide	Allow 2 to 3 hours between doses of the antacid and the drug.

Cimetidine	Allow 2 to 3 hours between doses of the antacid and the drug.
Ciprofloxacin	Allow 2 to 3 hours between doses of the antacid and the drug.
Demeclocycline	Do not combine.
Digoxin	Allow 2 to 3 hours between doses of the antacid and the drug.
Doxycycline	Do not combine.
Enoxacin	Allow 2 to 3 hours between doses of the antacid and the drug.
Fosfomycin	Allow 2 to 3 hours between doses of the antacid and the drug.
Gabapentin	Allow 2 to 3 hours between doses of the antacid and the drug.
Glipizide	Allow 2 to 3 hours between doses of the antacid and the drug.
Glyburide	Allow 2 to 3 hours between doses of the antacid and the drug.
Isoniazid	Allow 2 to 3 hours between doses of the antacid and the drug.
Ketoconazole	Allow 2 to 3 hours between doses of the antacid and the drug.
Levothyroxine	Allow 2 to 3 hours between doses of the antacid and the drug.
Lomefloxacin	Allow 2 to 3 hours between doses of the antacid and the drug.
Methacycline	Do not combine.
Methenamine	Allow 2 to 3 hours between doses of the antacid and the drug.
Metronidazole	Allow 2 to 3 hours between doses of the antacid and the drug.
Minocycline	Do not combine.
Misoprostol	Allow 2 to 3 hours between doses of the antacid and the drug.
Mycophenolate	Allow 2 to 3 hours between doses of the antacid and the drug.
Norfloxacin	Allow 2 to 3 hours between doses of the antacid and the drug.
Ofloxacin	Allow 2 to 3 hours between doses of the antacid and the drug.
Oxytetracycline	Do not combine.
Penicillamine	Allow 2 to 3 hours between doses of the antacid and the drug.
Phenytoin	Allow 2 to 3 hours between doses of the antacid and the drug.
Quinidine	Allow 2 to 3 hours between doses of the antacid and the drug.
Sodium Polystyrene Sulfonate	Allow 2 to 3 hours between doses of the antacid and the drug.
Sucralfate	Allow 2 to 3 hours between doses of the antacid and the drug.
Tetracycline	Do not combine.
Tilodronate	Allow 2 to 3 hours between doses of the antacid and the drug.
Ursodiol	Allow 2 to 3 hours between doses of the antacid and the drug.

Bayer Arthritis Pain Regimen Formula

See Bayer Aspirin

Bayer Aspirin

And:	Action:
Acarbose	Do not combine without your doctor's approval.
Arthritis Medications	Do not combine without your doctor's approval.
Chlorpropamide	Do not combine without your doctor's approval.
Dicumarol	Do not combine without your doctor's approval.
Glimepiride	Do not combine without your doctor's approval.
Glipizide	Do not combine without your doctor's approval.
Glyburide	Do not combine without your doctor's approval.
Metformin	Do not combine without your doctor's approval.
Miglitol	Do not combine without your doctor's approval.
Probenecid	Do not combine without your doctor's approval.
Sulfinpyrazone	Do not combine without your doctor's approval.
Tolazamide	Do not combine without your doctor's approval.
Tolbutamide	Do not combine without your doctor's approval.
Troglitazone	Do not combine without your doctor's approval.
Warfarin	Do not combine without your doctor's approval.

Bayer Plus

See Bayer Aspirin

Bayer PM

And:	Action:
Acarbose	Do not combine without your doctor's approval.
Alcohol	Do not combine.
Alprazolam	Do not combine.
Arthritis Medications	Do not combine without your doctor's approval.
Buspirone	Do not combine.
Chlordiazepoxide	Do not combine.
Chlorpromazine	Do not combine.
Chlorpropamide	Do not combine without your doctor's approval.
Chlorprothixene	Do not combine.
Clorazepate	Do not combine.
Diazepam	Do not combine.
Dicumarol	Do not combine without your doctor's approval.
Droperidol	Do not combine.
Estazolam	Do not combine.

Ethchlorvynol	Do not combine.
Ethinamate	Do not combine.
Fluphenazine	Do not combine.
Flurazepam	Do not combine.
Glimepiride	Do not combine without your doctor's approval.
Glipizide	Do not combine without your doctor's approval.
Glutethimide	Do not combine.
Glyburide	Do not combine without your doctor's approval.
Haloperidol	Do not combine.
Hydroxyzine	Do not combine.
Lorazepam	Do not combine.
Loxapine	Do not combine.
Meprobamate	Do not combine.
Mesoridazine	Do not combine.
Metformin	Do not combine without your doctor's approval.
Midazolam	Do not combine.
Miglitol	Do not combine without your doctor's approval.
Molindone	Do not combine.
Oxazepam	Do not combine.
Perphenazine	Do not combine.
Prazepam	Do not combine.
Probenecid	Do not combine.
Prochlorperazine	Do not combine.
Promethazine	Do not combine.
Propofol	Do not combine.
Quazepam	Do not combine.
Secobarbital	Do not combine.
Sulfinpyrazone	Do not combine.
Temazepam	Do not combine.
Thioridazine	Do not combine.
Thiothixene	Do not combine.
Tolazamide	Do not combine without your doctor's approval.
Tolbutamide	Do not combine without your doctor's approval.
Triazolam	Do not combine.
Trifluoperazine	Do not combine.
Troglitazone	Do not combine without your doctor's approval.

Warfarin	Do not combine without your doctor's approval.
Zolpidem	Do not combine.

BC Allergy Sinus Cold Powder

And:	Action:
Furazolidone	Do not combine. Wait 2 weeks after using Furazolidone.
Isocarboxazid	Do not combine. Wait 2 weeks after using Isocarboxazid.
Phenelzine	Do not combine. Wait 2 weeks after using Phenelzine.
Selegiline	Do not combine. Wait 2 weeks after using Selegiline.
Tranylcypromine	Do not combine. Wait 2 weeks after using Tranylcypromine.

BC Powder

See BC Allergy Sinus Cold Powder

BC Powder, Arthritis Strength

See BC Allergy Sinus Cold Powder

BC Sinus Cold Powder

See BC Allergy Sinus Cold Powder

Beano

And:	Action:
Furazolidone	Do not combine.
Isocarboxazid	Do not combine.
Phenelzine	Do not combine.
Selegiline	Do not combine.
Tranylcypromine	Do not combine.

Benadryl Allergy

And:	Action:
Alcohol	May cause extra drowsiness. Do not combine.
Alprazolam	May cause extra drowsiness. Check with your doctor.
Buspirone	May cause extra drowsiness. Check with your doctor.
Chlordiazepoxide	May cause extra drowsiness. Check with your doctor.
Chlorpromazine	May cause extra drowsiness. Check with your doctor.
Chlorprothixene	May cause extra drowsiness. Check with your doctor.
Clorazepate	May cause extra drowsiness. Check with your doctor.
Diazepam	May cause extra drowsiness. Check with your doctor.
Droperidol	May cause extra drowsiness. Check with your doctor.
Estazolam	May cause extra drowsiness. Check with your doctor.
Ethchlorvynol	May cause extra drowsiness. Check with your doctor.

Ethinamate	May cause extra drowsiness. Check with your doctor.
Fluphenazine	May cause extra drowsiness. Check with your doctor.
Flurazepam	May cause extra drowsiness. Check with your doctor.
Furazolidone	Do not combine. Wait 2 weeks after using Furazolidone.
Glutethimide	May cause extra drowsiness. Check with your doctor.
Haloperidol	May cause extra drowsiness. Check with your doctor.
Hydroxyzine	May cause extra drowsiness. Check with your doctor.
Isocarboxazid	Do not combine. Wait 2 weeks after using Isocarboxazid.
Lorazepam	May cause extra drowsiness. Check with your doctor.
Loxapine	May cause extra drowsiness. Check with your doctor.
Meprobamate	May cause extra drowsiness. Check with your doctor.
Mesoridazine	May cause extra drowsiness. Check with your doctor.
Midazolam	May cause extra drowsiness. Check with your doctor.
Molindone	May cause extra drowsiness. Check with your doctor.
Oxazepam	May cause extra drowsiness. Check with your doctor.
Perphenazine	May cause extra drowsiness. Check with your doctor.
Phenelzine	Do not combine. Wait 2 weeks after using Phenelzine.
Prazepam	May cause extra drowsiness. Check with your doctor.
Prochlorperazine	May cause extra drowsiness. Check with your doctor.
Promethazine	May cause extra drowsiness. Check with your doctor.
Propofol	May cause extra drowsiness. Check with your doctor.
Quazepam	May cause extra drowsiness. Check with your doctor.
Secobarbital	May cause extra drowsiness. Check with your doctor.
Selegiline	Do not combine. Wait 2 weeks after using Selegiline.
Temazepam	May cause extra drowsiness. Check with your doctor.
Thioridazine	May cause extra drowsiness. Check with your doctor.
Thiothixene	May cause extra drowsiness. Check with your doctor.
Tranylcypromine	Do not combine. Wait 2 weeks after using Tranylcypromine.
Triazolam	May cause extra drowsiness. Check with your doctor.
Trifluoperazine	May cause extra drowsiness. Check with your doctor.
Zolpidem	May cause extra drowsiness. Check with your doctor.

Benadryl Allergy/Cold Tablets

See Benadryl Allergy

Benadryl Allergy Decongestant

See Benadryl Allergy

Benadryl Allergy Sinus Headache Caplets

See Benadryl Allergy

Benadryl Dye-Free Allergy

See Benadryl Allergy

Benylin Adult Formula Cough Suppressant

And:	Action:
Furazolidone	Do not combine. Wait 2 weeks after using Furazolidone.
Isocarboxazid	Do not combine. Wait 2 weeks after using Isocarboxazid.
Phenelzine	Do not combine. Wait 2 weeks after using Phenelzine.
Selegiline	Do not combine. Wait 2 weeks after using Selegiline.
Tranylcypromine	Do not combine. Wait 2 weeks after using Tranylcypromine.

Benylin Cough Suppressant Expectorant

See Benylin Adult Formula Cough Suppressant

Benylin Multisymptom

See Benylin Adult Formula Cough Suppressant

Benylin Pediatric Cough Suppressant

See Benylin Adult Formula Cough Suppressant

Benzedrex

No interactions reported.

Bonine

And:	Action:
Alcohol	May cause extra drowsiness. Do not combine.
Alprazolam	May cause extra drowsiness. Check with your doctor.
Buspirone	May cause extra drowsiness. Check with your doctor.
Chlordiazepoxide	May cause extra drowsiness. Check with your doctor.
Chlorpromazine	May cause extra drowsiness. Check with your doctor.
Chlorprothixene	May cause extra drowsiness. Check with your doctor.
Clorazepate	May cause extra drowsiness. Check with your doctor.
Diazepam	May cause extra drowsiness. Check with your doctor.
Droperidol	May cause extra drowsiness. Check with your doctor.
Estazolam	May cause extra drowsiness. Check with your doctor.
Ethchlorvynol	May cause extra drowsiness. Check with your doctor.
Ethinamate	May cause extra drowsiness. Check with your doctor.
Fluphenazine	May cause extra drowsiness. Check with your doctor.
Flurazepam	May cause extra drowsiness. Check with your doctor.

Glutethimide	May cause extra drowsiness. Check with your doctor.
Haloperidol	May cause extra drowsiness. Check with your doctor.
Hydroxyzine	May cause extra drowsiness. Check with your doctor.
Lorazepam	May cause extra drowsiness. Check with your doctor.
Loxapine	May cause extra drowsiness. Check with your doctor.
Meprobamate	May cause extra drowsiness. Check with your doctor.
Mesoridazine	May cause extra drowsiness. Check with your doctor.
Midazolam	May cause extra drowsiness. Check with your doctor.
Molindone	May cause extra drowsiness. Check with your doctor.
Oxazepam	May cause extra drowsiness. Check with your doctor.
Perphenazine	May cause extra drowsiness. Check with your doctor.
Prazepam	May cause extra drowsiness. Check with your doctor.
Prochlorperazine	May cause extra drowsiness. Check with your doctor.
Promethazine	May cause extra drowsiness. Check with your doctor.
Propofol	May cause extra drowsiness. Check with your doctor.
Quazepam	May cause extra drowsiness. Check with your doctor.
Secobarbital	May cause extra drowsiness. Check with your doctor.
Temazepam	May cause extra drowsiness. Check with your doctor.
Thioridazine	May cause extra drowsiness. Check with your doctor.
Thiothixene	May cause extra drowsiness. Check with your doctor.
Triazolam	May cause extra drowsiness. Check with your doctor.
Trifluoperazine	May cause extra drowsiness. Check with your doctor.
Zolpidem	May cause extra drowsiness. Check with your doctor.

Bufferin

And:	Action:
Acarbose	Do not combine without your doctor's approval.
Aluminum Carbonate	This antacid may change the rate of aspirin absorption.
Aluminum Hydroxide	This antacid may change the rate of aspirin absorption.
Aluminum Hydroxide Gel	This antacid may change the rate of aspirin absorption.
Arthritis Medications	Do not combine without your doctor's approval.
Chlorpropamide	Do not combine without your doctor's approval.
Dicumarol	Do not combine without your doctor's approval.
Glimepiride	Do not combine without your doctor's approval.
Glipizide	Do not combine without your doctor's approval.
Glyburide	Do not combine without your doctor's approval.

Magnesium Hydroxide	This antacid may change the rate of aspirin absorption.
Magnesium Oxide	This antacid may change the rate of aspirin absorption.
Metformin	Do not combine without your doctor's approval.
Miglitol	Do not combine without your doctor's approval.
Probenecid	Do not combine.
Sodium Bicarbonate	This antacid may lower aspirin levels.
Sulfinpyrazone	Do not combine.
Tolazamide	Do not combine without your doctor's approval.
Tolbutamide	Do not combine without your doctor's approval.
Troglitazone	Do not combine without your doctor's approval.
Warfarin	Do not combine without your doctor's approval.

Cepacol Sore Throat Lozenges

No interactions reported.

Cepacol Sore Throat Spray

No interactions reported.

Cepastat

No interactions reported.

Cerose DM

And:	Action:
Alcohol	May cause extra drowsiness. Do not combine.
Alprazolam	May cause extra drowsiness. Check with your doctor.
Buspirone	May cause extra drowsiness. Check with your doctor.
Chlordiazepoxide	May cause extra drowsiness. Check with your doctor.
Chlorpromazine	May cause extra drowsiness. Check with your doctor.
Chlorprothixene	May cause extra drowsiness. Check with your doctor.
Clorazepate	May cause extra drowsiness. Check with your doctor.
Diazepam	May cause extra drowsiness. Check with your doctor.
Droperidol	May cause extra drowsiness. Check with your doctor.
Estazolam	May cause extra drowsiness. Check with your doctor.
Ethchlorvynol	May cause extra drowsiness. Check with your doctor.
Ethinamate	May cause extra drowsiness. Check with your doctor.
Fluphenazine	May cause extra drowsiness. Check with your doctor.
Flurazepam	May cause extra drowsiness. Check with your doctor.
Furazolidone	Do not combine. Wait 2 weeks after using Furazolidone.
Glutethimide	May cause extra drowsiness. Check with your doctor.

Haloperidol	May cause extra drowsiness. Check with your doctor.
Hydroxyzine	May cause extra drowsiness. Check with your doctor.
Isocarboxazid	Do not combine. Wait 2 weeks after using Isocarboxazid.
Lorazepam	May cause extra drowsiness. Check with your doctor.
Loxapine	May cause extra drowsiness. Check with your doctor.
Meprobamate	May cause extra drowsiness. Check with your doctor.
Mesoridazine	May cause extra drowsiness. Check with your doctor.
Midazolam	May cause extra drowsiness. Check with your doctor.
Molindone	May cause extra drowsiness. Check with your doctor.
Oxazepam	May cause extra drowsiness. Check with your doctor.
Perphenazine	May cause extra drowsiness. Check with your doctor.
Phenelzine	Do not combine. Wait 2 weeks after using Phenelzine.
Prazepam	May cause extra drowsiness. Check with your doctor.
Prochlorperazine	May cause extra drowsiness. Check with your doctor.
Promethazine	May cause extra drowsiness. Check with your doctor.
Propofol	May cause extra drowsiness. Check with your doctor.
Quazepam	May cause extra drowsiness. Check with your doctor.
Secobarbital	May cause extra drowsiness. Check with your doctor.
Selegiline	Do not combine. Wait 2 weeks after using Selegiline.
Temazepam	May cause extra drowsiness. Check with your doctor.
Thioridazine	May cause extra drowsiness. Check with your doctor.
Thiothixene	May cause extra drowsiness. Check with your doctor.
Tranylcypromine	Do not combine. Wait 2 weeks after using Tranylcypromine.
Triazolam	May cause extra drowsiness. Check with your doctor.
Trifluoperazine	May cause extra drowsiness. Check with your doctor.
Zolpidem	May cause extra drowsiness. Check with your doctor.

Cheracol D

And:	Action:
Furazolidone	Do not combine. Wait 2 weeks after using Furazolidone.
Isocarboxazid	Do not combine. Wait 2 weeks after using Isocarboxazid.
Phenelzine	Do not combine. Wait 2 weeks after using Phenelzine.
Selegiline	Do not combine. Wait 2 weeks after using Selegiline.
Tranylcypromine	Do not combine. Wait 2 weeks after using Tranylcypromine.

Cheracol Plus

See Cheracol D

Children's Mylanta

See Tums

Chlor-Trimeton Allergy

And:	Action:
Alcohol	May cause extra drowsiness. Do not combine.
Alprazolam	May cause extra drowsiness. Check with your doctor.
Buspirone	May cause extra drowsiness. Check with your doctor.
Chlordiazepoxide	May cause extra drowsiness. Check with your doctor.
Chlorpromazine	May cause extra drowsiness. Check with your doctor.
Chlorprothixene	May cause extra drowsiness. Check with your doctor.
Clorazepate	May cause extra drowsiness. Check with your doctor.
Diazepam	May cause extra drowsiness. Check with your doctor.
Droperidol	May cause extra drowsiness. Check with your doctor.
Estazolam	May cause extra drowsiness. Check with your doctor.
Ethchlorvynol	May cause extra drowsiness. Check with your doctor.
Ethinamate	May cause extra drowsiness. Check with your doctor.
Fluphenazine	May cause extra drowsiness. Check with your doctor.
Flurazepam	May cause extra drowsiness. Check with your doctor.
Glutethimide	May cause extra drowsiness. Check with your doctor.
Haloperidol	May cause extra drowsiness. Check with your doctor.
Hydroxyzine	May cause extra drowsiness. Check with your doctor.
Lorazepam	May cause extra drowsiness. Check with your doctor.
Loxapine	May cause extra drowsiness. Check with your doctor.
Meprobamate	May cause extra drowsiness. Check with your doctor.
Mesoridazine	May cause extra drowsiness. Check with your doctor.
Midazolam	May cause extra drowsiness. Check with your doctor.
Molindone	May cause extra drowsiness. Check with your doctor.
Oxazepam	May cause extra drowsiness. Check with your doctor.
Perphenazine	May cause extra drowsiness. Check with your doctor.
Prazepam	May cause extra drowsiness. Check with your doctor.
Prochlorperazine	May cause extra drowsiness. Check with your doctor.
Promethazine	May cause extra drowsiness. Check with your doctor.
Propofol	May cause extra drowsiness. Check with your doctor.
Quazepam	May cause extra drowsiness. Check with your doctor.
Secobarbital	May cause extra drowsiness. Check with your doctor.
Temazepam	May cause extra drowsiness. Check with your doctor.

Thioridazine	May cause extra drowsiness. Check with your doctor.
Thiothixene	May cause extra drowsiness. Check with your doctor.
Triazolam	May cause extra drowsiness. Check with your doctor.
Trifluoperazine	May cause extra drowsiness. Check with your doctor.
Zolpidem	May cause extra drowsiness. Check with your doctor.

Chlor-Trimeton Allergy/Decongestant

And:	Action:
Alcohol	May cause extra drowsiness. Do not combine.
Alprazolam	May cause extra drowsiness. Check with your doctor.
Buspirone	May cause extra drowsiness. Check with your doctor.
Chlordiazepoxide	May cause extra drowsiness. Check with your doctor.
Chlorpromazine	May cause extra drowsiness. Check with your doctor.
Chlorprothixene	May cause extra drowsiness. Check with your doctor.
Clorazepate	May cause extra drowsiness. Check with your doctor.
Diazepam	May cause extra drowsiness. Check with your doctor.
Droperidol	May cause extra drowsiness. Check with your doctor.
Estazolam	May cause extra drowsiness. Check with your doctor.
Ethchlorvynol	May cause extra drowsiness. Check with your doctor.
Ethinamate	May cause extra drowsiness. Check with your doctor.
Fluphenazine	May cause extra drowsiness. Check with your doctor.
Flurazepam	May cause extra drowsiness. Check with your doctor.
Furazolidone	Do not combine. Wait 2 weeks after using Furazolidone.
Glutethimide	May cause extra drowsiness. Check with your doctor.
Haloperidol	May cause extra drowsiness. Check with your doctor.
Hydroxyzine	May cause extra drowsiness. Check with your doctor.
Isocarboxazid	Do not combine. Wait 2 weeks after using Isocarboxazid.
Lorazepam	May cause extra drowsiness. Check with your doctor.
Loxapine	May cause extra drowsiness. Check with your doctor.
Meprobamate	May cause extra drowsiness. Check with your doctor.
Mesoridazine	May cause extra drowsiness. Check with your doctor.
Midazolam	May cause extra drowsiness. Check with your doctor.
Molindone	May cause extra drowsiness. Check with your doctor.
Oxazepam	May cause extra drowsiness. Check with your doctor.
Perphenazine	May cause extra drowsiness. Check with your doctor.
Phenelzine	Do not combine. Wait 2 weeks after using Phenelzine.
Prazepam	May cause extra drowsiness. Check with your doctor.

Prochlorperazine	May cause extra drowsiness. Check with your doctor.
Promethazine	May cause extra drowsiness. Check with your doctor.
Propofol	May cause extra drowsiness. Check with your doctor.
Quazepam	May cause extra drowsiness. Check with your doctor.
Secobarbital	May cause extra drowsiness. Check with your doctor.
Selegiline	Do not combine. Wait 2 weeks after using Selegiline.
Temazepam	May cause extra drowsiness. Check with your doctor.
Thioridazine	May cause extra drowsiness. Check with your doctor.
Thiothixene	May cause extra drowsiness. Check with your doctor.
Tranylcypromine	Do not combine. Wait 2 weeks after using Tranylcypromine.
Triazolam	May cause extra drowsiness. Check with your doctor.
Trifluoperazine	May cause extra drowsiness. Check with your doctor.
Zolpidem	May cause extra drowsiness. Check with your doctor.

Citrucel

No interactions reported.

Colace

No interactions reported.

Comtrex Allergy-Sinus

And:	Action:
Alcohol	May cause extra drowsiness. The acetaminophen in this medication may cause liver damage in heavy drinkers.
Alprazolam	May cause extra drowsiness. Check with your doctor.
Buspirone	May cause extra drowsiness. Check with your doctor.
Chlordiazepoxide	May cause extra drowsiness. Check with your doctor.
Chlorpromazine	May cause extra drowsiness. Check with your doctor.
Chlorprothixene	May cause extra drowsiness. Check with your doctor.
Clorazepate	May cause extra drowsiness. Check with your doctor.
Diazepam	May cause extra drowsiness. Check with your doctor.
Droperidol	May cause extra drowsiness. Check with your doctor.
Estazolam	May cause extra drowsiness. Check with your doctor.
Ethchlorvynol	May cause extra drowsiness. Check with your doctor.
Ethinamate	May cause extra drowsiness. Check with your doctor.
Fluphenazine	May cause extra drowsiness. Check with your doctor.
Flurazepam	May cause extra drowsiness. Check with your doctor.
Furazolidone	Do not combine. Wait 2 weeks after using Furazolidone.
Glutethimide	May cause extra drowsiness. Check with your doctor.

Haloperidol	May cause extra drowsiness. Check with your doctor.
Hydroxyzine	May cause extra drowsiness. Check with your doctor.
Isocarboxazid	Do not combine. Wait 2 weeks after using Isocarboxazid.
Lorazepam	May cause extra drowsiness. Check with your doctor.
Loxapine	May cause extra drowsiness. Check with your doctor.
Meprobamate	May cause extra drowsiness. Check with your doctor.
Mesoridazine	May cause extra drowsiness. Check with your doctor.
Midazolam	May cause extra drowsiness. Check with your doctor.
Molindone	May cause extra drowsiness. Check with your doctor.
Oxazepam	May cause extra drowsiness. Check with your doctor.
Perphenazine	May cause extra drowsiness. Check with your doctor.
Phenelzine	Do not combine. Wait 2 weeks after using Phenelzine.
Prazepam	May cause extra drowsiness. Check with your doctor.
Prochlorperazine	May cause extra drowsiness. Check with your doctor.
Promethazine	May cause extra drowsiness. Check with your doctor.
Propofol	May cause extra drowsiness. Check with your doctor.
Quazepam	May cause extra drowsiness. Check with your doctor.
Secobarbital	May cause extra drowsiness. Check with your doctor.
Selegiline	Do not combine. Wait 2 weeks after using Selegiline.
Temazepam	May cause extra drowsiness. Check with your doctor.
Thioridazine	May cause extra drowsiness. Check with your doctor.
Thiothixene	May cause extra drowsiness. Check with your doctor.
Tranylcypromine	Do not combine. Wait 2 weeks after using Tranylcypromine.
Triazolam	May cause extra drowsiness. Check with your doctor.
Trifluoperazine	May cause extra drowsiness. Check with your doctor.
Zolpidem	May cause extra drowsiness. Check with your doctor.

Comtrex Cold & Flu Reliever

And:	Action:
Alcohol	May cause extra drowsiness. Do not combine.
Alprazolam	May cause extra drowsiness. Check with your doctor.
Buspirone	May cause extra drowsiness. Check with your doctor.
Chlordiazepoxide	May cause extra drowsiness. Check with your doctor.
Chlorpromazine	May cause extra drowsiness. Check with your doctor.
Chlorprothixene	May cause extra drowsiness. Check with your doctor.
Clorazepate	May cause extra drowsiness. Check with your doctor.
Diazepam	May cause extra drowsiness. Check with your doctor.

Droperidol	May cause extra drowsiness. Check with your doctor.
Estazolam	May cause extra drowsiness. Check with your doctor.
Ethchlorvynol	May cause extra drowsiness. Check with your doctor.
Ethinamate	May cause extra drowsiness. Check with your doctor.
Fluphenazine	May cause extra drowsiness. Check with your doctor.
Flurazepam	May cause extra drowsiness. Check with your doctor.
Furazolidone	Do not combine. Wait 2 weeks after using Furazolidone.
Glutethimide	May cause extra drowsiness. Check with your doctor.
Haloperidol	May cause extra drowsiness. Check with your doctor.
Hydroxyzine	May cause extra drowsiness. Check with your doctor.
Isocarboxazid	Do not combine. Wait 2 weeks after using Isocarboxazid.
Lorazepam	May cause extra drowsiness. Check with your doctor.
Loxapine	May cause extra drowsiness. Check with your doctor.
Meprobamate	May cause extra drowsiness. Check with your doctor.
Mesoridazine	May cause extra drowsiness. Check with your doctor.
Midazolam	May cause extra drowsiness. Check with your doctor.
Molindone	May cause extra drowsiness. Check with your doctor.
Oxazepam	May cause extra drowsiness. Check with your doctor.
Perphenazine	May cause extra drowsiness. Check with your doctor.
Phenelzine	Do not combine. Wait 2 weeks after using Phenelzine.
Prazepam	May cause extra drowsiness. Check with your doctor.
Prochlorperazine	May cause extra drowsiness. Check with your doctor.
Promethazine	May cause extra drowsiness. Check with your doctor.
Propofol	May cause extra drowsiness. Check with your doctor.
Quazepam	May cause extra drowsiness. Check with your doctor.
Secobarbital	May cause extra drowsiness. Check with your doctor.
Selegiline	Do not combine. Wait 2 weeks after using Selegiline.
Temazepam	May cause extra drowsiness. Check with your doctor.
Thioridazine	May cause extra drowsiness. Check with your doctor.
Thiothixene	May cause extra drowsiness. Check with your doctor.
Tranylcypromine	Do not combine. Wait 2 weeks after using Tranylcypromine.
Triazolam	May cause extra drowsiness. Check with your doctor.
Trifluoperazine	May cause extra drowsiness. Check with your doctor.
Zolpidem	May cause extra drowsiness. Check with your doctor.

Comtrex Deep Chest Cold

And:	Action:
Alcohol	The acetaminophen in the medication may cause liver damage in heavy drinkers.
Furazolidone	Do not combine. Wait 2 weeks after using Furazolidone.
Isocarboxazid	Do not combine. Wait 2 weeks after using Isocarboxazid.
Phenelzine	Do not combine. Wait 2 weeks after using Phenelzine.
Selegiline	Do not combine. Wait 2 weeks after using Selegiline.
Tranylcypromine	Do not combine. Wait 2 weeks after using Tranylcypromine.

Comtrex Non-Drowsy

See Comtrex Deep Chest Cold

Contac

And:	Action:
Alcohol	May cause extra drowsiness. Do not combine.
Alprazolam	May cause extra drowsiness. Check with your doctor.
Buspirone	May cause extra drowsiness. Check with your doctor.
Chlordiazepoxide	May cause extra drowsiness. Check with your doctor.
Chlorpromazine	May cause extra drowsiness. Check with your doctor.
Chlorprothixene	May cause extra drowsiness. Check with your doctor.
Clorazepate	May cause extra drowsiness. Check with your doctor.
Diazepam	May cause extra drowsiness. Check with your doctor.
Droperidol	May cause extra drowsiness. Check with your doctor.
Estazolam	May cause extra drowsiness. Check with your doctor.
Ethchlorvynol	May cause extra drowsiness. Check with your doctor.
Ethinamate	May cause extra drowsiness. Check with your doctor.
Fluphenazine	May cause extra drowsiness. Check with your doctor.
Flurazepam	May cause extra drowsiness. Check with your doctor.
Furazolidone	Do not combine. Wait 2 weeks after using Furazolidone.
Glutethimide	May cause extra drowsiness. Check with your doctor.
Haloperidol	May cause extra drowsiness. Check with your doctor.
Hydroxyzine	May cause extra drowsiness. Check with your doctor.
Isocarboxazid	Do not combine. Wait 2 weeks after using Isocarboxazid.
Lorazepam	May cause extra drowsiness. Check with your doctor.
Loxapine	May cause extra drowsiness. Check with your doctor.
Meprobamate	May cause extra drowsiness. Check with your doctor.
Mesoridazine	May cause extra drowsiness. Check with your doctor.

Midazolam	May cause extra drowsiness. Check with your doctor.
Molindone	May cause extra drowsiness. Check with your doctor.
Oxazepam	May cause extra drowsiness. Check with your doctor.
Perphenazine	May cause extra drowsiness. Check with your doctor.
Phenelzine	Do not combine. Wait 2 weeks after using Phenelzine.
Prazepam	May cause extra drowsiness. Check with your doctor.
Prochlorperazine	May cause extra drowsiness. Check with your doctor.
Promethazine	May cause extra drowsiness. Check with your doctor.
Propofol	May cause extra drowsiness. Check with your doctor.
Quazepam	May cause extra drowsiness. Check with your doctor.
Secobarbital	May cause extra drowsiness. Check with your doctor.
Selegiline	Do not combine. Wait 2 weeks after using Selegiline.
Temazepam	May cause extra drowsiness. Check with your doctor.
Thioridazine	May cause extra drowsiness. Check with your doctor.
Thiothixene	May cause extra drowsiness. Check with your doctor.
Tranylcypromine	Do not combine. Wait 2 weeks after using Tranylcypromine.
Triazolam	May cause extra drowsiness. Check with your doctor.
Trifluoperazine	May cause extra drowsiness. Check with your doctor.
Zolpidem	May cause extra drowsiness. Check with your doctor.

Contac Day & Night Cold/Flu

See Contac

Contac Severe Cold and Flu

See Contac

Contac Severe Cold and Flu Non-Drowsy

And:	Action:
Furazolidone	Do not combine. Wait 2 weeks after using Furazolidone.
Isocarboxazid	Do not combine. Wait 2 weeks after using Isocarboxazid.
Phenelzine	Do not combine. Wait 2 weeks after using Phenelzine.
Selegiline	Do not combine. Wait 2 weeks after using Selegiline.
Tranylcypromine	Do not combine. Wait 2 weeks after using Tranylcypromine.

Coricidin 'D'

And:	Action:
Alcohol	May cause extra drowsiness. Do not combine.
Alprazolam	May cause extra drowsiness. Check with your doctor.
Buspirone	May cause extra drowsiness. Check with your doctor.

Chlordiazepoxide	May cause extra drowsiness. Check with your doctor.
Chlorpromazine	May cause extra drowsiness. Check with your doctor.
Chlorprothixene	May cause extra drowsiness. Check with your doctor.
Clorazepate	May cause extra drowsiness. Check with your doctor.
Diazepam	May cause extra drowsiness. Check with your doctor.
Droperidol	May cause extra drowsiness. Check with your doctor.
Estazolam	May cause extra drowsiness. Check with your doctor.
Ethchlorvynol	May cause extra drowsiness. Check with your doctor.
Ethinamate	May cause extra drowsiness. Check with your doctor.
Fluphenazine	May cause extra drowsiness. Check with your doctor.
Flurazepam	May cause extra drowsiness. Check with your doctor.
Furazolidone	Do not combine. Wait 2 weeks after using Furazolidone.
Glutethimide	May cause extra drowsiness. Check with your doctor.
Haloperidol	May cause extra drowsiness. Check with your doctor.
Hydroxyzine	May cause extra drowsiness. Check with your doctor.
Isocarboxazid	Do not combine. Wait 2 weeks after using Isocarboxazid.
Lorazepam	May cause extra drowsiness. Check with your doctor.
Loxapine	May cause extra drowsiness. Check with your doctor.
Meprobamate	May cause extra drowsiness. Check with your doctor.
Mesoridazine	May cause extra drowsiness. Check with your doctor.
Midazolam	May cause extra drowsiness. Check with your doctor.
Molindone	May cause extra drowsiness. Check with your doctor.
Oxazepam	May cause extra drowsiness. Check with your doctor.
Perphenazine	May cause extra drowsiness. Check with your doctor.
Phenelzine	Do not combine. Wait 2 weeks after using Phenelzine.
Phenylpropanolamine	Do not combine with diet pills containing Phenylpropanolamine.
Prazepam	May cause extra drowsiness. Check with your doctor.
Prochlorperazine	May cause extra drowsiness. Check with your doctor.
Promethazine	May cause extra drowsiness. Check with your doctor.
Propofol	May cause extra drowsiness. Check with your doctor.
Quazepam	May cause extra drowsiness. Check with your doctor.
Secobarbital	May cause extra drowsiness. Check with your doctor.
Selegiline	Do not combine. Wait 2 weeks after using Selegiline.
Temazepam	May cause extra drowsiness. Check with your doctor.
Thioridazine	May cause extra drowsiness. Check with your doctor.
Thiothixene	May cause extra drowsiness. Check with your doctor.

Tranylcypromine	Do not combine. Wait 2 weeks after using Tranylcypromine.
Triazolam	May cause extra drowsiness. Check with your doctor.
Trifluoperazine	May cause extra drowsiness. Check with your doctor.
Zolpidem	May cause extra drowsiness. Check with your doctor.

Coricidin Cold & Flu Tablets

And:	Action:
Alcohol	May cause extra drowsiness. Do not combine.
Alprazolam	May cause extra drowsiness. Check with your doctor.
Buspirone	May cause extra drowsiness. Check with your doctor.
Chlordiazepoxide	May cause extra drowsiness. Check with your doctor.
Chlorpromazine	May cause extra drowsiness. Check with your doctor.
Chlorprothixene	May cause extra drowsiness. Check with your doctor.
Clorazepate	May cause extra drowsiness. Check with your doctor.
Diazepam	May cause extra drowsiness. Check with your doctor.
Droperidol	May cause extra drowsiness. Check with your doctor.
Estazolam	May cause extra drowsiness. Check with your doctor.
Ethchlorvynol	May cause extra drowsiness. Check with your doctor.
Ethinamate	May cause extra drowsiness. Check with your doctor.
Fluphenazine	May cause extra drowsiness. Check with your doctor.
Flurazepam	May cause extra drowsiness. Check with your doctor.
Glutethimide	May cause extra drowsiness. Check with your doctor.
Haloperidol	May cause extra drowsiness. Check with your doctor.
Hydroxyzine	May cause extra drowsiness. Check with your doctor.
Lorazepam	May cause extra drowsiness. Check with your doctor.
Loxapine	May cause extra drowsiness. Check with your doctor.
Meprobamate	May cause extra drowsiness. Check with your doctor.
Mesoridazine	May cause extra drowsiness. Check with your doctor.
Midazolam	May cause extra drowsiness. Check with your doctor.
Molindone	May cause extra drowsiness. Check with your doctor.
Oxazepam	May cause extra drowsiness. Check with your doctor.
Perphenazine	May cause extra drowsiness. Check with your doctor.
Prazepam	May cause extra drowsiness. Check with your doctor.
Prochlorperazine	May cause extra drowsiness. Check with your doctor.
Promethazine	May cause extra drowsiness. Check with your doctor.
Propofol	May cause extra drowsiness. Check with your doctor.

Quazepam	May cause extra drowsiness. Check with your doctor.
Secobarbital	May cause extra drowsiness. Check with your doctor.
Temazepam	May cause extra drowsiness. Check with your doctor.
Thioridazine	May cause extra drowsiness. Check with your doctor.
Thiothixene	May cause extra drowsiness. Check with your doctor.
Triazolam	May cause extra drowsiness. Check with your doctor.
Trifluoperazine	May cause extra drowsiness. Check with your doctor.
Zolpidem	May cause extra drowsiness. Check with your doctor.

Coricidin Cough & Cold Tablets

See Coricidin 'D'

Coricidin Nighttime Cold & Cough Liquid

See Coricidin Cold & Flu Tablets

Correctol

And:	Action:
Aluminum Carbonate	Do not combine. Wait 1 hour before taking Correctol.
Aluminum Hydroxide	Do not combine. Wait 1 hour before taking Correctol.
Aluminum Hydroxide Gel	Do not combine. Wait 1 hour before taking Correctol.
Dairy products	Do not combine. Wait 1 hour before taking Correctol.
Magaldrate	Do not combine. Wait 1 hour before taking Correctol.
Magnesium Hydroxide	Do not combine. Wait 1 hour before taking Correctol.
Magnesium Oxide	Do not combine. Wait 1 hour before taking Correctol.
Sodium Bicarbonate	Do not combine. Wait 1 hour before taking Correctol.

Correctol Herbal Tea

And:	Action:
Other Laxatives	Do not combine

Correctol Stool Softener

And:	Action:
Mineral Oil	Do not combine without your doctor's approval.

Delsym Cough Formula

And:	Action:
Furazolidone	Do not combine. Wait 2 weeks after using Furazolidone.
Isocarboxazid	Do not combine. Wait 2 weeks after using Isocarboxazid.
Phenelzine	Do not combine. Wait 2 weeks after using Phenelzine.
Selegiline	Do not combine. Wait 2 weeks after using Selegiline.

| Tranylcypromine | Do not combine. Wait 2 weeks after using Tranylcypromine. |

Dexatrim

And:	Action:
Furazolidone	Do not combine. Wait 2 weeks after using Furazolidone.
Isocarboxazid	Do not combine. Wait 2 weeks after using Isocarboxazid.
Phenelzine	Do not combine. Wait 2 weeks after using Phenelzine.
Phenylpropanolamine-Containing Diet Pills	Do not combine.
Selegiline	Do not combine. Wait 2 weeks after using Selegiline.
Tranylcypromine	Do not combine. Wait 2 weeks after using Tranylcypromine.

Dexatrim Plus Vitamin C

See Dexatrim

Dexatrim Plus Vitamins

See Dexatrim

Di-Gel

And:	Action:
Alendronate	Allow 2 to 3 hours between doses of the antacid and the drug.
Allopurinol	Allow 2 to 3 hours between doses of the antacid and the drug.
Arthritis Drugs	Allow 2 to 3 hours between doses of the antacid and the drug.
Aspirin	Allow 2 to 3 hours between doses of the antacid and the drug.
Atenolol	Allow 2 to 3 hours between doses of the antacid and the drug.
Captopril	Allow 2 to 3 hours between doses of the antacid and the drug.
Chlordiazepoxide	Allow 2 to 3 hours between doses of the antacid and the drug.
Cimetidine	Allow 2 to 3 hours between doses of the antacid and the drug.
Ciprofloxacin	Allow 2 to 3 hours between doses of the antacid and the drug.
Demeclocycline	Allow 2 to 3 hours between doses of the antacid and the drug.
Digoxin	Allow 2 to 3 hours between doses of the antacid and the drug.
Doxycycline	Allow 2 to 3 hours between doses of the antacid and the drug.
Enoxacin	Allow 2 to 3 hours between doses of the antacid and the drug.
Fosfomycin	Allow 2 to 3 hours between doses of the antacid and the drug.
Gabapentin	Allow 2 to 3 hours between doses of the antacid and the drug.
Glipizide	Allow 2 to 3 hours between doses of the antacid and the drug.
Glyburide	Allow 2 to 3 hours between doses of the antacid and the drug.
Isoniazid	Allow 2 to 3 hours between doses of the antacid and the drug.
Ketoconazole	Allow 2 to 3 hours between doses of the antacid and the drug.
Levothyroxine	Allow 2 to 3 hours between doses of the antacid and the drug.

Lomefloxacin	Allow 2 to 3 hours between doses of the antacid and the drug.
Meat	Antacid action reduced by high-protein foods.
Methacycline	Allow 2 to 3 hours between doses of the antacid and the drug.
Methenamine	Allow 2 to 3 hours between doses of the antacid and the drug.
Metronidazole	Allow 2 to 3 hours between doses of the antacid and the drug.
Minocycline	Allow 2 to 3 hours between doses of the antacid and the drug.
Misoprostol	Allow 2 to 3 hours between doses of the antacid and the drug.
Mycophenolate	Allow 2 to 3 hours between doses of the antacid and the drug.
Norfloxacin	Allow 2 to 3 hours between doses of the antacid and the drug.
Ofloxacin	Allow 2 to 3 hours between doses of the antacid and the drug.
Oxytetracycline	Allow 2 to 3 hours between doses of the antacid and the drug.
Penicillamine	Allow 2 to 3 hours between doses of the antacid and the drug.
Phenytoin	Allow 2 to 3 hours between doses of the antacid and the drug.
Quinidine	Allow 2 to 3 hours between doses of the antacid and the drug.
Sodium Polystyrene Sulfonate	Allow 2 to 3 hours between doses of the antacid and the drug.
Sucralfate	Allow 2 to 3 hours between doses of the antacid and the drug.
Tetracycline	Allow 2 to 3 hours between doses of the antacid and the drug.
Tilodronate	Allow 2 to 3 hours between doses of the antacid and the drug.
Ursodiol	Allow 2 to 3 hours between doses of the antacid and the drug.

Diabe-Tuss DM

And:	Action:
Furazolidone	Do not combine. Wait 2 weeks after using Furazolidone.
Isocarboxazid	Do not combine. Wait 2 weeks after using Isocarboxazid.
Phenelzine	Do not combine. Wait 2 weeks after using Phenelzine.
Phenylpropanolamine-Containing Diet Pills	Do not combine.
Selegiline	Do not combine. Wait 2 weeks after using Selegiline.
Tranylcypromine	Do not combine. Wait 2 weeks after using Tranylcypromine.

Dialose

And:	Action:
Mineral Oil	Do not combine.
Prescription Drugs	Do not combine.

Dialose Plus

And:	Action:
Mineral Oil	Do not combine.

Prescription Drugs	Do not combine.

Diarrid

And:	Action:
Antibiotics	Do not combine without your doctor's approval.

Dimetapp

And:	Action:
Alcohol	May cause extra drowsiness. Do not combine.
Alprazolam	May cause extra drowsiness. Check with your doctor.
Buspirone	May cause extra drowsiness. Check with your doctor.
Chlordiazepoxide	May cause extra drowsiness. Check with your doctor.
Chlorpromazine	May cause extra drowsiness. Check with your doctor.
Chlorprothixene	May cause extra drowsiness. Check with your doctor.
Clorazepate	May cause extra drowsiness. Check with your doctor.
Diazepam	May cause extra drowsiness. Check with your doctor.
Droperidol	May cause extra drowsiness. Check with your doctor.
Estazolam	May cause extra drowsiness. Check with your doctor.
Ethchlorvynol	May cause extra drowsiness. Check with your doctor.
Ethinamate	May cause extra drowsiness. Check with your doctor.
Fluphenazine	May cause extra drowsiness. Check with your doctor.
Flurazepam	May cause extra drowsiness. Check with your doctor.
Furazolidone	Do not combine. Wait 2 weeks after using Furazolidone.
Glutethimide	May cause extra drowsiness. Check with your doctor.
Haloperidol	May cause extra drowsiness. Check with your doctor.
Hydroxyzine	May cause extra drowsiness. Check with your doctor.
Isocarboxazid	Do not combine. Wait 2 weeks after using Isocarboxazid.
Lorazepam	May cause extra drowsiness. Check with your doctor.
Loxapine	May cause extra drowsiness. Check with your doctor.
Meprobamate	May cause extra drowsiness. Check with your doctor.
Mesoridazine	May cause extra drowsiness. Check with your doctor.
Midazolam	May cause extra drowsiness. Check with your doctor.
Molindone	May cause extra drowsiness. Check with your doctor.
Oxazepam	May cause extra drowsiness. Check with your doctor.
Perphenazine	May cause extra drowsiness. Check with your doctor.
Phenelzine	Do not combine. Wait 2 weeks after using Phenelzine.
Prazepam	May cause extra drowsiness. Check with your doctor.

Prochlorperazine	May cause extra drowsiness. Check with your doctor.
Promethazine	May cause extra drowsiness. Check with your doctor.
Propofol	May cause extra drowsiness. Check with your doctor.
Quazepam	May cause extra drowsiness. Check with your doctor.
Secobarbital	May cause extra drowsiness. Check with your doctor.
Selegiline	Do not combine. Wait 2 weeks after using Selegiline.
Temazepam	May cause extra drowsiness. Check with your doctor.
Thioridazine	May cause extra drowsiness. Check with your doctor.
Thiothixene	May cause extra drowsiness. Check with your doctor.
Tranylcypromine	Do not combine. Wait 2 weeks after using Tranylcypromine.
Triazolam	May cause extra drowsiness. Check with your doctor.
Trifluoperazine	May cause extra drowsiness. Check with your doctor.
Zolpidem	May cause extra drowsiness. Check with your doctor.

Dimetapp Allergy

And:	Action:
Alcohol	May cause extra drowsiness. Do not combine.
Alprazolam	May cause extra drowsiness. Check with your doctor.
Buspirone	May cause extra drowsiness. Check with your doctor.
Chlordiazepoxide	May cause extra drowsiness. Check with your doctor.
Chlorpromazine	May cause extra drowsiness. Check with your doctor.
Chlorprothixene	May cause extra drowsiness. Check with your doctor.
Clorazepate	May cause extra drowsiness. Check with your doctor.
Diazepam	May cause extra drowsiness. Check with your doctor.
Droperidol	May cause extra drowsiness. Check with your doctor.
Estazolam	May cause extra drowsiness. Check with your doctor.
Ethchlorvynol	May cause extra drowsiness. Check with your doctor.
Ethinamate	May cause extra drowsiness. Check with your doctor.
Fluphenazine	May cause extra drowsiness. Check with your doctor.
Flurazepam	May cause extra drowsiness. Check with your doctor.
Glutethimide	May cause extra drowsiness. Check with your doctor.
Haloperidol	May cause extra drowsiness. Check with your doctor.
Hydroxyzine	May cause extra drowsiness. Check with your doctor.
Lorazepam	May cause extra drowsiness. Check with your doctor.
Loxapine	May cause extra drowsiness. Check with your doctor.
Meprobamate	May cause extra drowsiness. Check with your doctor.

Mesoridazine	May cause extra drowsiness. Check with your doctor.
Midazolam	May cause extra drowsiness. Check with your doctor.
Molindone	May cause extra drowsiness. Check with your doctor.
Oxazepam	May cause extra drowsiness. Check with your doctor.
Perphenazine	May cause extra drowsiness. Check with your doctor.
Prazepam	May cause extra drowsiness. Check with your doctor.
Prochlorperazine	May cause extra drowsiness. Check with your doctor.
Promethazine	May cause extra drowsiness. Check with your doctor.
Propofol	May cause extra drowsiness. Check with your doctor.
Quazepam	May cause extra drowsiness. Check with your doctor.
Secobarbital	May cause extra drowsiness. Check with your doctor.
Temazepam	May cause extra drowsiness. Check with your doctor.
Thioridazine	May cause extra drowsiness. Check with your doctor.
Thiothixene	May cause extra drowsiness. Check with your doctor.
Triazolam	May cause extra drowsiness. Check with your doctor.
Trifluoperazine	May cause extra drowsiness. Check with your doctor.
Zolpidem	May cause extra drowsiness. Check with your doctor.

Dimetapp Allergy Sinus

See Dimetapp

Dimetapp Cold & Allergy

And:	*Action:*
Alprazolam	May cause extra drowsiness. Check with your doctor.
Buspirone	May cause extra drowsiness. Check with your doctor.
Chlordiazepoxide	May cause extra drowsiness. Check with your doctor.
Chlorpromazine	May cause extra drowsiness. Check with your doctor.
Chlorprothixene	May cause extra drowsiness. Check with your doctor.
Clorazepate	May cause extra drowsiness. Check with your doctor.
Diazepam	May cause extra drowsiness. Check with your doctor.
Droperidol	May cause extra drowsiness. Check with your doctor.
Estazolam	May cause extra drowsiness. Check with your doctor.
Ethchlorvynol	May cause extra drowsiness. Check with your doctor.
Ethinamate	May cause extra drowsiness. Check with your doctor.
Fluphenazine	May cause extra drowsiness. Check with your doctor.
Flurazepam	May cause extra drowsiness. Check with your doctor.
Furazolidone	Do not combine. Wait 2 weeks after using Furazolidone.

Glutethimide	May cause extra drowsiness. Check with your doctor.
Haloperidol	May cause extra drowsiness. Check with your doctor.
Hydroxyzine	May cause extra drowsiness. Check with your doctor.
Isocarboxazid	Do not combine. Wait 2 weeks after using Isocarboxazid.
Lorazepam	May cause extra drowsiness. Check with your doctor.
Loxapine	May cause extra drowsiness. Check with your doctor.
Meprobamate	May cause extra drowsiness. Check with your doctor.
Mesoridazine	May cause extra drowsiness. Check with your doctor.
Midazolam	May cause extra drowsiness. Check with your doctor.
Molindone	May cause extra drowsiness. Check with your doctor.
Oxazepam	May cause extra drowsiness. Check with your doctor.
Perphenazine	May cause extra drowsiness. Check with your doctor.
Phenelzine	Do not combine. Wait 2 weeks after using Phenelzine.
Prazepam	May cause extra drowsiness. Check with your doctor.
Prochlorperazine	May cause extra drowsiness. Check with your doctor.
Promethazine	May cause extra drowsiness. Check with your doctor.
Propofol	May cause extra drowsiness. Check with your doctor.
Quazepam	May cause extra drowsiness. Check with your doctor.
Secobarbital	May cause extra drowsiness. Check with your doctor.
Selegiline	Do not combine. Wait 2 weeks after using Selegiline.
Temazepam	May cause extra drowsiness. Check with your doctor.
Thioridazine	May cause extra drowsiness. Check with your doctor.
Thiothixene	May cause extra drowsiness. Check with your doctor.
Tranylcypromine	Do not combine. Wait 2 weeks after using Tranylcypromine.
Triazolam	May cause extra drowsiness. Check with your doctor.
Trifluoperazine	May cause extra drowsiness. Check with your doctor.
Zolpidem	May cause extra drowsiness. Check with your doctor.

Dimetapp Cold & Cough Liqui-Gels

See Dimetapp

Dimetapp Cold and Fever

See Dimetapp

Dimetapp Decongestant Pediatric Drops

And:	Action:
Furazolidone	Do not combine. Wait 2 weeks after using Furazolidone.
Isocarboxazid	Do not combine. Wait 2 weeks after using Isocarboxazid.

Phenelzine	Do not combine. Wait 2 weeks after using Phenelzine.
Selegiline	Do not combine. Wait 2 weeks after using Selegiline.
Tranylcypromine	Do not combine. Wait 2 weeks after using Tranylcypromine.

Dimetapp DM Elixir

See Dimetapp

Doan's

And:	Action:
Acarbose	Do not combine without your doctor's approval.
Arthritis Medications	Do not combine without your doctor's approval.
Chlorpropamide	Do not combine without your doctor's approval.
Dicumarol	Do not combine without your doctor's approval.
Glimepiride	Do not combine without your doctor's approval.
Glipizide	Do not combine without your doctor's approval.
Glyburide	Do not combine without your doctor's approval.
Metformin	Do not combine without your doctor's approval.
Miglitol	Do not combine without your doctor's approval.
Probenecid	Do not combine without your doctor's approval.
Sulfinpyrazone	Do not combine without your doctor's approval.
Tolazamide	Do not combine without your doctor's approval.
Tolbutamide	Do not combine without your doctor's approval.
Troglitazone	Do not combine without your doctor's approval.
Warfarin	Do not combine without your doctor's approval.

Doan's P.M.

And:	Action:
Acarbose	Do not combine without your doctor's approval.
Alcohol	May cause extra drowsiness. Do not combine.
Alprazolam	May cause extra drowsiness. Check with your doctor.
Arthritis Medications	Do not combine without your doctor's approval.
Buspirone	May cause extra drowsiness. Check with your doctor.
Chlordiazepoxide	May cause extra drowsiness. Check with your doctor.
Chlorpromazine	May cause extra drowsiness. Check with your doctor.
Chlorpropamide	Do not combine without your doctor's approval.
Chlorprothixene	May cause extra drowsiness. Check with your doctor.
Clorazepate	May cause extra drowsiness. Check with your doctor.
Diazepam	May cause extra drowsiness. Check with your doctor.

Dicumarol	Do not combine without your doctor's approval.
Droperidol	May cause extra drowsiness. Check with your doctor.
Estazolam	May cause extra drowsiness. Check with your doctor.
Ethchlorvynol	May cause extra drowsiness. Check with your doctor.
Ethinamate	May cause extra drowsiness. Check with your doctor.
Fluphenazine	May cause extra drowsiness. Check with your doctor.
Flurazepam	May cause extra drowsiness. Check with your doctor.
Glimepiride	Do not combine without your doctor's approval.
Glipizide	Do not combine without your doctor's approval.
Glutethimide	May cause extra drowsiness. Check with your doctor.
Glyburide	Do not combine without your doctor's approval.
Haloperidol	May cause extra drowsiness. Check with your doctor.
Hydroxyzine	May cause extra drowsiness. Check with your doctor.
Lorazepam	May cause extra drowsiness. Check with your doctor.
Loxapine	May cause extra drowsiness. Check with your doctor.
Meprobamate	May cause extra drowsiness. Check with your doctor.
Mesoridazine	May cause extra drowsiness. Check with your doctor.
Metformin	Do not combine without your doctor's approval.
Midazolam	May cause extra drowsiness. Check with your doctor.
Miglitol	Do not combine without your doctor's approval.
Molindone	May cause extra drowsiness. Check with your doctor.
Oxazepam	May cause extra drowsiness. Check with your doctor.
Perphenazine	May cause extra drowsiness. Check with your doctor.
Prazepam	May cause extra drowsiness. Check with your doctor.
Probenecid	Do not combine without your doctor's approval.
Prochlorperazine	May cause extra drowsiness. Check with your doctor.
Promethazine	May cause extra drowsiness. Check with your doctor.
Propofol	May cause extra drowsiness. Check with your doctor.
Quazepam	May cause extra drowsiness. Check with your doctor.
Secobarbital	May cause extra drowsiness. Check with your doctor.
Sulfinpyrazone	Do not combine without your doctor's approval.
Temazepam	May cause extra drowsiness. Check with your doctor.
Thioridazine	May cause extra drowsiness. Check with your doctor.
Thiothixene	May cause extra drowsiness. Check with your doctor.
Tolazamide	Do not combine without your doctor's approval.
Tolbutamide	Do not combine without your doctor's approval.

Triazolam	May cause extra drowsiness. Check with your doctor.
Trifluoperazine	May cause extra drowsiness. Check with your doctor.
Troglitazone	Do not combine without your doctor's approval.
Warfarin	Do not combine without your doctor's approval.
Zolpidem	May cause extra drowsiness. Check with your doctor.

Donnagel

No interactions reported.

Doxidan

| And: | Action: |
| Mineral Oil | Do not combine without your doctor's approval. |

Dramamine

And:	Action:
Alcohol	May cause extra drowsiness. Do not combine.
Alprazolam	May cause extra drowsiness. Check with your doctor.
Buspirone	May cause extra drowsiness. Check with your doctor.
Chlordiazepoxide	May cause extra drowsiness. Check with your doctor.
Chlorpromazine	May cause extra drowsiness. Check with your doctor.
Chlorprothixene	May cause extra drowsiness. Check with your doctor.
Clorazepate	May cause extra drowsiness. Check with your doctor.
Diazepam	May cause extra drowsiness. Check with your doctor.
Droperidol	May cause extra drowsiness. Check with your doctor.
Estazolam	May cause extra drowsiness. Check with your doctor.
Ethchlorvynol	May cause extra drowsiness. Check with your doctor.
Ethinamate	May cause extra drowsiness. Check with your doctor.
Fluphenazine	May cause extra drowsiness. Check with your doctor.
Flurazepam	May cause extra drowsiness. Check with your doctor.
Glutethimide	May cause extra drowsiness. Check with your doctor.
Haloperidol	May cause extra drowsiness. Check with your doctor.
Hydroxyzine	May cause extra drowsiness. Check with your doctor.
Lorazepam	May cause extra drowsiness. Check with your doctor.
Loxapine	May cause extra drowsiness. Check with your doctor.
Meprobamate	May cause extra drowsiness. Check with your doctor.
Mesoridazine	May cause extra drowsiness. Check with your doctor.
Midazolam	May cause extra drowsiness. Check with your doctor.
Molindone	May cause extra drowsiness. Check with your doctor.

Oxazepam	May cause extra drowsiness. Check with your doctor.
Perphenazine	May cause extra drowsiness. Check with your doctor.
Prazepam	May cause extra drowsiness. Check with your doctor.
Prochlorperazine	May cause extra drowsiness. Check with your doctor.
Promethazine	May cause extra drowsiness. Check with your doctor.
Propofol	May cause extra drowsiness. Check with your doctor.
Quazepam	May cause extra drowsiness. Check with your doctor.
Secobarbital	May cause extra drowsiness. Check with your doctor.
Temazepam	May cause extra drowsiness. Check with your doctor.
Thioridazine	May cause extra drowsiness. Check with your doctor.
Thiothixene	May cause extra drowsiness. Check with your doctor.
Triazolam	May cause extra drowsiness. Check with your doctor.
Trifluoperazine	May cause extra drowsiness. Check with your doctor.
Zolpidem	May cause extra drowsiness. Check with your doctor.

Dramamine II

See Dramamine

Drixoral Allergy/Sinus

And:	Action:
Alcohol	May cause extra drowsiness. Do not combine.
Alprazolam	May cause extra drowsiness. Check with your doctor.
Buspirone	May cause extra drowsiness. Check with your doctor.
Chlordiazepoxide	May cause extra drowsiness. Check with your doctor.
Chlorpromazine	May cause extra drowsiness. Check with your doctor.
Chlorprothixene	May cause extra drowsiness. Check with your doctor.
Clorazepate	May cause extra drowsiness. Check with your doctor.
Diazepam	May cause extra drowsiness. Check with your doctor.
Droperidol	May cause extra drowsiness. Check with your doctor.
Estazolam	May cause extra drowsiness. Check with your doctor.
Ethchlorvynol	May cause extra drowsiness. Check with your doctor.
Ethinamate	May cause extra drowsiness. Check with your doctor.
Fluphenazine	May cause extra drowsiness. Check with your doctor.
Flurazepam	May cause extra drowsiness. Check with your doctor.
Furazolidone	Do not combine. Wait 2 weeks after using Furazolidone.
Glutethimide	May cause extra drowsiness. Check with your doctor.
Haloperidol	May cause extra drowsiness. Check with your doctor.

Hydroxyzine	May cause extra drowsiness. Check with your doctor.
Isocarboxazid	Do not combine. Wait 2 weeks after using Isocarboxazid.
Lorazepam	May cause extra drowsiness. Check with your doctor.
Loxapine	May cause extra drowsiness. Check with your doctor.
Meprobamate	May cause extra drowsiness. Check with your doctor.
Mesoridazine	May cause extra drowsiness. Check with your doctor.
Midazolam	May cause extra drowsiness. Check with your doctor.
Molindone	May cause extra drowsiness. Check with your doctor.
Oxazepam	May cause extra drowsiness. Check with your doctor.
Perphenazine	May cause extra drowsiness. Check with your doctor.
Phenelzine	Do not combine. Wait 2 weeks after using Phenelzine.
Prazepam	May cause extra drowsiness. Check with your doctor.
Prochlorperazine	May cause extra drowsiness. Check with your doctor.
Promethazine	May cause extra drowsiness. Check with your doctor.
Propofol	May cause extra drowsiness. Check with your doctor.
Quazepam	May cause extra drowsiness. Check with your doctor.
Secobarbital	May cause extra drowsiness. Check with your doctor.
Selegiline	Do not combine. Wait 2 weeks after using Selegiline.
Temazepam	May cause extra drowsiness. Check with your doctor.
Thioridazine	May cause extra drowsiness. Check with your doctor.
Thiothixene	May cause extra drowsiness. Check with your doctor.
Tranylcypromine	Do not combine. Wait 2 weeks after using Tranylcypromine.
Triazolam	May cause extra drowsiness. Check with your doctor.
Trifluoperazine	May cause extra drowsiness. Check with your doctor.
Zolpidem	May cause extra drowsiness. Check with your doctor.

Drixoral Cold & Allergy

See Drixoral Allergy/Sinus

Drixoral Cold & Flu

See Drixoral Allergy/Sinus

Drixoral Nasal Decongestant

And:	Action:
Furazolidone	Do not combine. Wait 2 weeks after using Furazolidone.
Isocarboxazid	Do not combine. Wait 2 weeks after using Isocarboxazid.
Phenelzine	Do not combine. Wait 2 weeks after using Phenelzine.
Selegiline	Do not combine. Wait 2 weeks after using Selegiline.
Tranylcypromine	Do not combine. Wait 2 weeks after using Tranylcypromine.

Dulcolax

And:	Action:
Antacids	Wait 1 hour before taking Dulcolax.
Milk	Wait 1 hour before taking Dulcolax.

Duration 12 Hour

No interactions reported.

Ecotrin

And:	Action:
Acarbose	Do not combine without your doctor's approval.
Aluminum Carbonate	This antacid may change the rate of aspirin absorption.
Aluminum Hydroxide	This antacid may change the rate of aspirin absorption.
Aluminum Hydroxide Gel	This antacid may change the rate of aspirin absorption.
Chlorpropamide	Do not combine without your doctor's approval.
Diclofenac	Do not combine without your doctor's approval.
Dicumarol	Do not combine without your doctor's approval.
Etodolac	Do not combine without your doctor's approval.
Fenoprofen	Do not combine without your doctor's approval.
Flurbiprofen	Do not combine without your doctor's approval.
Glimepiride	Do not combine without your doctor's approval.
Glipizide	Do not combine without your doctor's approval.
Glyburide	Do not combine without your doctor's approval.
Ibuprofen	Do not combine without your doctor's approval.
Indomethacin	Do not combine without your doctor's approval.
Ketoprofen	Do not combine without your doctor's approval.
Ketorolac	Do not combine without your doctor's approval.
Magaldrate	This antacid may change the rate of aspirin absorption.
Magnesium Hydroxide	This antacid may change the rate of aspirin absorption.
Magnesium Oxide	This antacid may change the rate of aspirin absorption.
Meclofenamate	Do not combine without your doctor's approval.
Mefenamic Acid	Do not combine without your doctor's approval.
Metformin	Do not combine without your doctor's approval.
Miglitol	Do not combine without your doctor's approval.
Nabumetone	Do not combine without your doctor's approval.
Naproxen	Do not combine without your doctor's approval.
Oxaprozin	Do not combine without your doctor's approval.

Phenylbutazone	Do not combine without your doctor's approval.
Piroxicam	Do not combine without your doctor's approval.
Probenecid	Do not combine without your doctor's approval.
Sulfinpyrazone	Do not combine without your doctor's approval.
Sulindac	Do not combine without your doctor's approval.
Tolazamide	Do not combine without your doctor's approval.
Tolbutamide	Do not combine without your doctor's approval.
Tolmetin	Do not combine without your doctor's approval.
Troglitazone	Do not combine without your doctor's approval.
Warfarin	Do not combine without your doctor's approval.

Ex-Lax

No interactions reported.

Ex-Lax Gentle Nature Laxative Pills

No interactions reported.

Ex-Lax Stool Softener

No interactions reported.

Excedrin

And:	*Action:*
Acarbose	Do not combine without your doctor's approval.
Alcohol	Do not combine without your doctor's approval.
Allopurinol	Do not combine without your doctor's approval.
Chlorpropamide	Do not combine without your doctor's approval.
Dicumarol	Do not combine without your doctor's approval.
Glimepiride	Do not combine without your doctor's approval.
Glipizide	Do not combine without your doctor's approval.
Glyburide	Do not combine without your doctor's approval.
Metformin	Do not combine without your doctor's approval.
Miglitol	Do not combine without your doctor's approval.
Probenecid	Do not combine without your doctor's approval.
Sulfinpyrazone	Do not combine without your doctor's approval.
Tolazamide	Do not combine without your doctor's approval.
Tolbutamide	Do not combine without your doctor's approval.
Troglitazone	Do not combine without your doctor's approval.
Warfarin	Do not combine without your doctor's approval.

Excedrin P.M.

And:	Action:
Alcohol	The acetaminophen in the medication may cause liver damage in heavy drinkers.
Alprazolam	Do not combine without your doctor's approval.
Buspirone	Do not combine without your doctor's approval.
Chlordiazepoxide	Do not combine without your doctor's approval.
Chlorpromazine	Do not combine without your doctor's approval.
Chlorprothixene	Do not combine without your doctor's approval.
Clorazepate	Do not combine without your doctor's approval.
Diazepam	Do not combine without your doctor's approval.
Droperidol	Do not combine without your doctor's approval.
Estazolam	Do not combine without your doctor's approval.
Ethchlorvynol	Do not combine without your doctor's approval.
Ethinamate	Do not combine without your doctor's approval.
Fluphenazine	Do not combine without your doctor's approval.
Flurazepam	Do not combine without your doctor's approval.
Glutethimide	Do not combine without your doctor's approval.
Haloperidol	Do not combine without your doctor's approval.
Hydroxyzine	Do not combine without your doctor's approval.
Lorazepam	Do not combine without your doctor's approval.
Loxapine	Do not combine without your doctor's approval.
Meprobamate	Do not combine without your doctor's approval.
Mesoridazine	Do not combine without your doctor's approval.
Midazolam	Do not combine without your doctor's approval.
Molindone	Do not combine without your doctor's approval.
Oxazepam	Do not combine without your doctor's approval.
Perphenazine	Do not combine without your doctor's approval.
Prazepam	Do not combine without your doctor's approval.
Prochlorperazine	Do not combine without your doctor's approval.
Promethazine	Do not combine without your doctor's approval.
Propofol	Do not combine without your doctor's approval.
Quazepam	Do not combine without your doctor's approval.
Secobarbital	Do not combine without your doctor's approval.
Temazepam	Do not combine without your doctor's approval.
Thioridazine	Do not combine without your doctor's approval.
Thiothixene	Do not combine without your doctor's approval.

Triazolam	Do not combine without your doctor's approval.
Trifluoperazine	Do not combine without your doctor's approval.
Zolpidem	Do not combine without your doctor's approval.

Excedrin, Aspirin Free

And:	Action:
Alcohol	The acetaminophen in the medication may cause liver damage in heavy drinkers.

Extended-Release Bayer 8-Hour Aspirin

See Bayer Aspirin

Extra Strength Bufferin

See Bufferin

Femstat 3

No interactions reported.

FiberCon

And:	Action:
Demeclocycline	Take FiberCon at least 1 hour before or 2 hours after taking this drug.
Doxycycline	Take FiberCon at least 1 hour before or 2 hours after taking this drug.
Methacycline	Take FiberCon at least 1 hour before or 2 hours after taking this drug.
Minocycline	Take FiberCon at least 1 hour before or 2 hours after taking this drug.
Oxytetracycline	Take FiberCon at least 1 hour before or 2 hours after taking this drug.
Tetracycline	Take FiberCon at least 1 hour before or 2 hours after taking this drug.

Fleet Children's Enema

See Fleet Enema

Fleet Enema

And:	Action:
Calcium Channel Blockers	Do not combine.
Water Pills	Do not combine.

Fleet Prep Kits

And:	Action:
Aluminum Carbonate	Do not combine. Wait 1 hour before using Fleet.

Aluminum Hydroxide	Do not combine. Wait 1 hour before using Fleet.
Aluminum Hydroxide Gel	Do not combine. Wait 1 hour before using Fleet.
Dairy products	Do not combine. Wait 1 hour before using Fleet.
Magaldrate	Do not combine. Wait 1 hour before using Fleet.
Magnesium Hydroxide	Do not combine. Wait 1 hour before using Fleet.
Magnesium Oxide	Do not combine. Wait 1 hour before using Fleet.
Sodium Bicarbonate	Do not combine. Wait 1 hour before using Fleet.

Fleet Sof-Lax

And:	Action:
Mineral Oil	Do not combine without your doctor's approval.

Fleet Sof-Lax Overnight

And:	Action:
Mineral Oil	Do not combine without your doctor's approval.

Fletcher's Castoria

No interactions reported.

Fletcher's Cherry Flavor

No interactions reported.

4-Way Fast Acting Nasal Spray

No interactions reported.

4-Way 12 Hour

No interactions reported.

Gas-X

No interactions reported.

Gaviscon

See Maalox

Genuine Bayer Aspirin

See Bayer Aspirin

Goody's Headache Powder

And:	Action:
Alcohol	The acetaminophen in the medication may cause liver damage in heavy drinkers.

Goody's Pain Relief Tablets

And:	Action:
Alcohol	The acetaminophen in the medication may cause liver damage in heavy drinkers.

Halfprin

See Bayer Aspirin

Halls Cough Suppressant

No interactions reported.

Imodium A-D

And:	Action:
Antibiotics	Do not combine without your doctor's approval.

Infants' Mylicon

No interactions reported.

Kaopectate

No interactions reported.

Kondremul

And:	Action:
Stool Softener Laxatives	Do not combine.

Konsyl Fiber Tablets

And:	Action:
Demeclocycline	Take Konsyl at least 1 hour before or 2 hours after taking the antibiotic.
Doxycycline	Take Konsyl at least 1 hour before or 2 hours after taking the antibiotic.
Methacycline	Take Konsyl at least 1 hour before or 2 hours after taking the antibiotic.
Minocycline	Take Konsyl at least 1 hour before or 2 hours after taking the antibiotic.
Oxytetracycline	Take Konsyl at least 1 hour before or 2 hours after taking the antibiotic.
Tetracycline	Take Konsyl at least 1 hour before or 2 hours after taking the antibiotic.

Konsyl Powder

And:	Action:
Prescription Drugs	Allow 2 hours between doses of the drug and the laxative.

Legatrin PM

See Tylenol PM

Maalox

And:	Action:
Alendronate	Allow 2 to 3 hours between doses of the antacid and the drug.
Allopurinol	Allow 2 to 3 hours between doses of the antacid and the drug.

Arthritis Drugs	Allow 2 to 3 hours between doses of the antacid and the drug.
Aspirin	Allow 2 to 3 hours between doses of the antacid and the drug.
Atenolol	Allow 2 to 3 hours between doses of the antacid and the drug.
Captopril	Allow 2 to 3 hours between doses of the antacid and the drug.
Chlordiazepoxide	Allow 2 to 3 hours between doses of the antacid and the drug.
Cimetidine	Allow 2 to 3 hours between doses of the antacid and the drug.
Ciprofloxacin	Allow 2 to 3 hours between doses of the antacid and the drug.
Demeclocycline	Allow 2 to 3 hours between doses of the antacid and the drug.
Digoxin	Allow 2 to 3 hours between doses of the antacid and the drug.
Doxycycline	Allow 2 to 3 hours between doses of the antacid and the drug.
Enoxacin	Allow 2 to 3 hours between doses of the antacid and the drug.
Fosfomycin	Allow 2 to 3 hours between doses of the antacid and the drug.
Gabapentin	Allow 2 to 3 hours between doses of the antacid and the drug.
Glipizide	Allow 2 to 3 hours between doses of the antacid and the drug.
Glyburide	Allow 2 to 3 hours between doses of the antacid and the drug.
Isoniazid	Allow 2 to 3 hours between doses of the antacid and the drug.
Ketoconazole	Allow 2 to 3 hours between doses of the antacid and the drug.
Levothyroxine	Allow 2 to 3 hours between doses of the antacid and the drug.
Lomefloxacin	Allow 2 to 3 hours between doses of the antacid and the drug.
Meat	Antacid action reduced by high-protein foods.
Methacycline	Allow 2 to 3 hours between doses of the antacid and the drug.
Methenamine	Allow 2 to 3 hours between doses of the antacid and the drug.
Metronidazole	Allow 2 to 3 hours between doses of the antacid and the drug.
Minocycline	Allow 2 to 3 hours between doses of the antacid and the drug.
Misoprostol	Allow 2 to 3 hours between doses of the antacid and the drug.
Mycophenolate	Allow 2 to 3 hours between doses of the antacid and the drug.
Norfloxacin	Allow 2 to 3 hours between doses of the antacid and the drug.
Ofloxacin	Allow 2 to 3 hours between doses of the antacid and the drug.
Oxytetracycline	Allow 2 to 3 hours between doses of the antacid and the drug.
Penicillamine	Allow 2 to 3 hours between doses of the antacid and the drug.
Phenytoin	Allow 2 to 3 hours between doses of the antacid and the drug.
Quinidine	Allow 2 to 3 hours between doses of the antacid and the drug.
Sodium Polystyrene Sulfonate	Allow 2 to 3 hours between doses of the antacid and the drug.
Sucralfate	Allow 2 to 3 hours between doses of the antacid and the drug.
Tetracycline	Allow 2 to 3 hours between doses of the antacid and the drug.

| Tilodronate | Allow 2 to 3 hours between doses of the antacid and the drug. |
| Ursodiol | Allow 2 to 3 hours between doses of the antacid and the drug. |

Maalox Antacid/Anti-Gas

See Maalox

Maalox Anti-Gas

No interactions reported.

Maltsupex

No interactions reported.

Maximum Strength Fast-Acting Mylanta Antacid Tablets

See Mylanta Tablets and Gelcaps

Maximum Strength Fast-Acting Mylanta Liquid

See Mylanta Liquid

Maximum Strength Multi-Symptom Formula Midol

See Midol Menstrual Formula

Maximum Strength Nytol

See Nytol

Maximum Strength Unisom

See Unisom

Metamucil

| And: | Action: |
| Prescription Drugs | Allow 2 hours between doses of the drug and the laxative. |

Midol Menstrual Formula

And:	Action:
Alcohol	May cause extra drowsiness. Do not combine.
Alprazolam	May cause extra drowsiness. Check with your doctor.
Buspirone	May cause extra drowsiness. Check with your doctor.
Caffeine-containing food, beverages, and medications	Combined use may cause nervousness, irritability, sleeplessness, and occasionally, rapid heartbeat.
Chlordiazepoxide	May cause extra drowsiness. Check with your doctor.
Chlorpromazine	May cause extra drowsiness. Check with your doctor.
Chlorprothixene	May cause extra drowsiness. Check with your doctor.
Clorazepate	May cause extra drowsiness. Check with your doctor.
Diazepam	May cause extra drowsiness. Check with your doctor.
Droperidol	May cause extra drowsiness. Check with your doctor.

Estazolam	May cause extra drowsiness. Check with your doctor.
Ethchlorvynol	May cause extra drowsiness. Check with your doctor.
Ethinamate	May cause extra drowsiness. Check with your doctor.
Fluphenazine	May cause extra drowsiness. Check with your doctor.
Flurazepam	May cause extra drowsiness. Check with your doctor.
Glutethimide	May cause extra drowsiness. Check with your doctor.
Haloperidol	May cause extra drowsiness. Check with your doctor.
Hydroxyzine	May cause extra drowsiness. Check with your doctor.
Lorazepam	May cause extra drowsiness. Check with your doctor.
Loxapine	May cause extra drowsiness. Check with your doctor.
Meprobamate	May cause extra drowsiness. Check with your doctor.
Mesoridazine	May cause extra drowsiness. Check with your doctor.
Midazolam	May cause extra drowsiness. Check with your doctor.
Molindone	May cause extra drowsiness. Check with your doctor.
Oxazepam	May cause extra drowsiness. Check with your doctor.
Perphenazine	May cause extra drowsiness. Check with your doctor.
Prazepam	May cause extra drowsiness. Check with your doctor.
Prochlorperazine	May cause extra drowsiness. Check with your doctor.
Promethazine	May cause extra drowsiness. Check with your doctor.
Propofol	May cause extra drowsiness. Check with your doctor.
Quazepam	May cause extra drowsiness. Check with your doctor.
Secobarbital	May cause extra drowsiness. Check with your doctor.
Temazepam	May cause extra drowsiness. Check with your doctor.
Thioridazine	May cause extra drowsiness. Check with your doctor.
Thiothixene	May cause extra drowsiness. Check with your doctor.
Triazolam	May cause extra drowsiness. Check with your doctor.
Trifluoperazine	May cause extra drowsiness. Check with your doctor.
Zolpidem	May cause extra drowsiness. Check with your doctor.

Midol PMS Formula

And:	*Action:*
Alcohol	May cause extra drowsiness. Do not combine.
Alprazolam	May cause extra drowsiness. Check with your doctor.
Buspirone	May cause extra drowsiness. Check with your doctor.
Chlordiazepoxide	May cause extra drowsiness. Check with your doctor.
Chlorpromazine	May cause extra drowsiness. Check with your doctor.

Chlorprothixene	May cause extra drowsiness. Check with your doctor.
Clorazepate	May cause extra drowsiness. Check with your doctor.
Diazepam	May cause extra drowsiness. Check with your doctor.
Droperidol	May cause extra drowsiness. Check with your doctor.
Estazolam	May cause extra drowsiness. Check with your doctor.
Ethchlorvynol	May cause extra drowsiness. Check with your doctor.
Ethinamate	May cause extra drowsiness. Check with your doctor.
Fluphenazine	May cause extra drowsiness. Check with your doctor.
Flurazepam	May cause extra drowsiness. Check with your doctor.
Glutethimide	May cause extra drowsiness. Check with your doctor.
Haloperidol	May cause extra drowsiness. Check with your doctor.
Hydroxyzine	May cause extra drowsiness. Check with your doctor.
Lorazepam	May cause extra drowsiness. Check with your doctor.
Loxapine	May cause extra drowsiness. Check with your doctor.
Meprobamate	May cause extra drowsiness. Check with your doctor.
Mesoridazine	May cause extra drowsiness. Check with your doctor.
Midazolam	May cause extra drowsiness. Check with your doctor.
Molindone	May cause extra drowsiness. Check with your doctor.
Oxazepam	May cause extra drowsiness. Check with your doctor.
Perphenazine	May cause extra drowsiness. Check with your doctor.
Prazepam	May cause extra drowsiness. Check with your doctor.
Prochlorperazine	May cause extra drowsiness. Check with your doctor.
Promethazine	May cause extra drowsiness. Check with your doctor.
Propofol	May cause extra drowsiness. Check with your doctor.
Quazepam	May cause extra drowsiness. Check with your doctor.
Secobarbital	May cause extra drowsiness. Check with your doctor.
Temazepam	May cause extra drowsiness. Check with your doctor.
Thioridazine	May cause extra drowsiness. Check with your doctor.
Thiothixene	May cause extra drowsiness. Check with your doctor.
Triazolam	May cause extra drowsiness. Check with your doctor.
Trifluoperazine	May cause extra drowsiness. Check with your doctor.
Zolpidem	May cause extra drowsiness. Check with your doctor.

Midol Teen Menstrual Formula

No interactions reported.

Motrin

And:	Action:
Acetaminophen	Do not combine without your doctor's approval.
Aspirin	Do not combine without your doctor's approval.

Mycelex-7

No interactions reported.

Mylanta AR

No interactions reported.

Mylanta Gas Relief

No interactions reported.

Mylanta Liquid

And:	Action:
Alendronate	Allow 2 to 3 hours between doses of the antacid and the drug.
Allopurinol	Allow 2 to 3 hours between doses of the antacid and the drug.
Arthritis Drugs	Allow 2 to 3 hours between doses of the antacid and the drug.
Aspirin	Allow 2 to 3 hours between doses of the antacid and the drug.
Atenolol	Allow 2 to 3 hours between doses of the antacid and the drug.
Captopril	Allow 2 to 3 hours between doses of the antacid and the drug.
Chlordiazepoxide	Allow 2 to 3 hours between doses of the antacid and the drug.
Cimetidine	Allow 2 to 3 hours between doses of the antacid and the drug.
Ciprofloxacin	Allow 2 to 3 hours between doses of the antacid and the drug.
Demeclocycline	Allow 2 to 3 hours between doses of the antacid and the drug.
Digoxin	Allow 2 to 3 hours between doses of the antacid and the drug.
Doxycycline	Allow 2 to 3 hours between doses of the antacid and the drug.
Enoxacin	Allow 2 to 3 hours between doses of the antacid and the drug.
Fosfomycin	Allow 2 to 3 hours between doses of the antacid and the drug.
Gabapentin	Allow 2 to 3 hours between doses of the antacid and the drug.
Glipizide	Allow 2 to 3 hours between doses of the antacid and the drug.
Glyburide	Allow 2 to 3 hours between doses of the antacid and the drug.
Isoniazid	Allow 2 to 3 hours between doses of the antacid and the drug.
Ketoconazole	Allow 2 to 3 hours between doses of the antacid and the drug.
Levothyroxine	Allow 2 to 3 hours between doses of the antacid and the drug.
Lomefloxacin	Allow 2 to 3 hours between doses of the antacid and the drug.
Meat	Antacid action reduced by high-protein foods.
Methacycline	Allow 2 to 3 hours between doses of the antacid and the drug.

Methenamine	Allow 2 to 3 hours between doses of the antacid and the drug.
Metronidazole	Allow 2 to 3 hours between doses of the antacid and the drug.
Minocycline	Allow 2 to 3 hours between doses of the antacid and the drug.
Misoprostol	Allow 2 to 3 hours between doses of the antacid and the drug.
Mycophenolate	Allow 2 to 3 hours between doses of the antacid and the drug.
Norfloxacin	Allow 2 to 3 hours between doses of the antacid and the drug.
Ofloxacin	Allow 2 to 3 hours between doses of the antacid and the drug.
Oxytetracycline	Allow 2 to 3 hours between doses of the antacid and the drug.
Penicillamine	Allow 2 to 3 hours between doses of the antacid and the drug.
Phenytoin	Allow 2 to 3 hours between doses of the antacid and the drug.
Quinidine	Allow 2 to 3 hours between doses of the antacid and the drug.
Sodium Polystyrene Sulfonate	Allow 2 to 3 hours between doses of the antacid and the drug.
Sucralfate	Allow 2 to 3 hours between doses of the antacid and the drug.
Tetracycline	Allow 2 to 3 hours between doses of the antacid and the drug.
Tilodronate	Allow 2 to 3 hours between doses of the antacid and the drug.
Ursodiol	Allow 2 to 3 hours between doses of the antacid and the drug.

Mylanta Soothing Lozenges

See Tums

Mylanta Tablets and Gelcaps

And:	Action:
Alendronate	Allow 2 to 3 hours between doses of the antacid and the drug.
Allopurinol	Allow 2 to 3 hours between doses of the antacid and the drug.
Arthritis Drugs	Allow 2 to 3 hours between doses of the antacid and the drug.
Aspirin	Allow 2 to 3 hours between doses of the antacid and the drug.
Atenolol	Allow 2 to 3 hours between doses of the antacid and the drug.
Captopril	Allow 2 to 3 hours between doses of the antacid and the drug.
Chlordiazepoxide	Allow 2 to 3 hours between doses of the antacid and the drug.
Cimetidine	Allow 2 to 3 hours between doses of the antacid and the drug.
Ciprofloxacin	Allow 2 to 3 hours between doses of the antacid and the drug.
Demeclocycline	Allow 2 to 3 hours between doses of the antacid and the drug.
Digoxin	Allow 2 to 3 hours between doses of the antacid and the drug.
Doxycycline	Allow 2 to 3 hours between doses of the antacid and the drug.
Enoxacin	Allow 2 to 3 hours between doses of the antacid and the drug.
Fosfomycin	Allow 2 to 3 hours between doses of the antacid and the drug.
Gabapentin	Allow 2 to 3 hours between doses of the antacid and the drug.

Glipizide	Allow 2 to 3 hours between doses of the antacid and the drug.
Glyburide	Allow 2 to 3 hours between doses of the antacid and the drug.
Isoniazid	Allow 2 to 3 hours between doses of the antacid and the drug.
Ketoconazole	Allow 2 to 3 hours between doses of the antacid and the drug.
Levothyroxine	Allow 2 to 3 hours between doses of the antacid and the drug.
Lomefloxacin	Allow 2 to 3 hours between doses of the antacid and the drug.
Methacycline	Allow 2 to 3 hours between doses of the antacid and the drug.
Methenamine	Allow 2 to 3 hours between doses of the antacid and the drug.
Metronidazole	Allow 2 to 3 hours between doses of the antacid and the drug.
Minocycline	Allow 2 to 3 hours between doses of the antacid and the drug.
Misoprostol	Allow 2 to 3 hours between doses of the antacid and the drug.
Mycophenolate	Allow 2 to 3 hours between doses of the antacid and the drug.
Norfloxacin	Allow 2 to 3 hours between doses of the antacid and the drug.
Ofloxacin	Allow 2 to 3 hours between doses of the antacid and the drug.
Oxytetracycline	Allow 2 to 3 hours between doses of the antacid and the drug.
Penicillamine	Allow 2 to 3 hours between doses of the antacid and the drug.
Phenytoin	Allow 2 to 3 hours between doses of the antacid and the drug.
Quinidine	Allow 2 to 3 hours between doses of the antacid and the drug.
Sodium Polystyrene Sulfonate	Allow 2 to 3 hours between doses of the antacid and the drug.
Sucralfate	Allow 2 to 3 hours between doses of the antacid and the drug.
Tetracycline	Allow 2 to 3 hours between doses of the antacid and the drug.
Tilodronate	Allow 2 to 3 hours between doses of the antacid and the drug.
Ursodiol	Allow 2 to 3 hours between doses of the antacid and the drug.

Naphcon A

No interactions reported.

Nasalcrom

No interactions reported.

Neo-Synephrine

No interactions reported.

Neo-Synephrine 12 Hour

No interactions reported.

Nephrox

And:	Action:
Alendronate	Allow 2 to 3 hours between doses of the antacid and the drug.
Allopurinol	Allow 2 to 3 hours between doses of the antacid and the drug.

Arthritis Drugs	Allow 2 to 3 hours between doses of the antacid and the drug.
Aspirin	Allow 2 to 3 hours between doses of the antacid and the drug.
Atenolol	Allow 2 to 3 hours between doses of the antacid and the drug.
Captopril	Allow 2 to 3 hours between doses of the antacid and the drug.
Chlordiazepoxide	Allow 2 to 3 hours between doses of the antacid and the drug.
Cimetidine	Allow 2 to 3 hours between doses of the antacid and the drug.
Ciprofloxacin	Allow 2 to 3 hours between doses of the antacid and the drug.
Demeclocycline	Allow 2 to 3 hours between doses of the antacid and the drug.
Digoxin	Allow 2 to 3 hours between doses of the antacid and the drug.
Doxycycline	Allow 2 to 3 hours between doses of the antacid and the drug.
Enoxacin	Allow 2 to 3 hours between doses of the antacid and the drug.
Fosfomycin	Allow 2 to 3 hours between doses of the antacid and the drug.
Gabapentin	Allow 2 to 3 hours between doses of the antacid and the drug.
Glipizide	Allow 2 to 3 hours between doses of the antacid and the drug.
Glyburide	Allow 2 to 3 hours between doses of the antacid and the drug.
Isoniazid	Allow 2 to 3 hours between doses of the antacid and the drug.
Ketoconazole	Allow 2 to 3 hours between doses of the antacid and the drug.
Levothyroxine	Allow 2 to 3 hours between doses of the antacid and the drug.
Lomefloxacin	Allow 2 to 3 hours between doses of the antacid and the drug.
Meat	Antacid action reduced by high-protein foods.
Methacycline	Allow 2 to 3 hours between doses of the antacid and the drug.
Methenamine	Allow 2 to 3 hours between doses of the antacid and the drug.
Metronidazole	Allow 2 to 3 hours between doses of the antacid and the drug.
Minocycline	Allow 2 to 3 hours between doses of the antacid and the drug.
Misoprostol	Allow 2 to 3 hours between doses of the antacid and the drug.
Mycophenolate	Allow 2 to 3 hours between doses of the antacid and the drug.
Norfloxacin	Allow 2 to 3 hours between doses of the antacid and the drug.
Ofloxacin	Allow 2 to 3 hours between doses of the antacid and the drug.
Oxytetracycline	Allow 2 to 3 hours between doses of the antacid and the drug.
Penicillamine	Allow 2 to 3 hours between doses of the antacid and the drug.
Phenytoin	Allow 2 to 3 hours between doses of the antacid and the drug.
Quinidine	Allow 2 to 3 hours between doses of the antacid and the drug.
Sodium Polystyrene Sulfonate	Allow 2 to 3 hours between doses of the antacid and the drug.
Sucralfate	Allow 2 to 3 hours between doses of the antacid and the drug.
Tetracycline	Allow 2 to 3 hours between doses of the antacid and the drug.

| Tilodronate | Allow 2 to 3 hours between doses of the antacid and the drug. |
| Ursodiol | Allow 2 to 3 hours between doses of the antacid and the drug. |

N'Ice

No interactions reported.

Nicoderm CQ

And:	*Action:*
Asthma medications	Dosage of the asthma medicine may need adjustment. Check with your doctor.
Drugs for depression	Dosage of the antidepressant may need adjustment. Check with your doctor.

Nicorette

See Nicoderm CQ

Nicotrol

See Nicoderm CQ

No Doz

| *And:* | *Action:* |
| Caffeine | Combined use may cause nervousness, irritability, sleeplessness, and occasionally, rapid heartbeat. |

Nolahist

And:	*Action:*
Alcohol	May cause extra drowsiness. Do not combine.
Alprazolam	May cause extra drowsiness. Check with your doctor.
Buspirone	May cause extra drowsiness. Check with your doctor.
Chlordiazepoxide	May cause extra drowsiness. Check with your doctor.
Chlorpromazine	May cause extra drowsiness. Check with your doctor.
Chlorprothixene	May cause extra drowsiness. Check with your doctor.
Clorazepate	May cause extra drowsiness. Check with your doctor.
Diazepam	May cause extra drowsiness. Check with your doctor.
Droperidol	May cause extra drowsiness. Check with your doctor.
Estazolam	May cause extra drowsiness. Check with your doctor.
Ethchlorvynol	May cause extra drowsiness. Check with your doctor.
Ethinamate	May cause extra drowsiness. Check with your doctor.
Fluphenazine	May cause extra drowsiness. Check with your doctor.
Flurazepam	May cause extra drowsiness. Check with your doctor.
Glutethimide	May cause extra drowsiness. Check with your doctor.
Haloperidol	May cause extra drowsiness. Check with your doctor.

Hydroxyzine	May cause extra drowsiness. Check with your doctor.
Lorazepam	May cause extra drowsiness. Check with your doctor.
Loxapine	May cause extra drowsiness. Check with your doctor.
Meprobamate	May cause extra drowsiness. Check with your doctor.
Mesoridazine	May cause extra drowsiness. Check with your doctor.
Midazolam	May cause extra drowsiness. Check with your doctor.
Molindone	May cause extra drowsiness. Check with your doctor.
Oxazepam	May cause extra drowsiness. Check with your doctor.
Perphenazine	May cause extra drowsiness. Check with your doctor.
Prazepam	May cause extra drowsiness. Check with your doctor.
Prochlorperazine	May cause extra drowsiness. Check with your doctor.
Promethazine	May cause extra drowsiness. Check with your doctor.
Propofol	May cause extra drowsiness. Check with your doctor.
Quazepam	May cause extra drowsiness. Check with your doctor.
Secobarbital	May cause extra drowsiness. Check with your doctor.
Temazepam	May cause extra drowsiness. Check with your doctor.
Thioridazine	May cause extra drowsiness. Check with your doctor.
Thiothixene	May cause extra drowsiness. Check with your doctor.
Triazolam	May cause extra drowsiness. Check with your doctor.
Trifluoperazine	May cause extra drowsiness. Check with your doctor.
Zolpidem	May cause extra drowsiness. Check with your doctor.

12 Hour Nostrilla

No interactions reported.

Novahistine

And:	Action:
Alcohol	May cause extra drowsiness. Do not combine.
Alprazolam	May cause extra drowsiness. Check with your doctor.
Buspirone	May cause extra drowsiness. Check with your doctor.
Chlordiazepoxide	May cause extra drowsiness. Check with your doctor.
Chlorpromazine	May cause extra drowsiness. Check with your doctor.
Chlorprothixene	May cause extra drowsiness. Check with your doctor.
Clorazepate	May cause extra drowsiness. Check with your doctor.
Diazepam	May cause extra drowsiness. Check with your doctor.
Droperidol	May cause extra drowsiness. Check with your doctor.
Estazolam	May cause extra drowsiness. Check with your doctor.

Ethchlorvynol	May cause extra drowsiness. Check with your doctor.
Ethinamate	May cause extra drowsiness. Check with your doctor.
Fluphenazine	May cause extra drowsiness. Check with your doctor.
Flurazepam	May cause extra drowsiness. Check with your doctor.
Furazolidone	Do not combine. Wait 2 weeks after using Furazolidone.
Glutethimide	May cause extra drowsiness. Check with your doctor.
Haloperidol	May cause extra drowsiness. Check with your doctor.
Hydroxyzine	May cause extra drowsiness. Check with your doctor.
Isocarboxazid	Do not combine. Wait 2 weeks after using Isocarboxazid.
Lorazepam	May cause extra drowsiness. Check with your doctor.
Loxapine	May cause extra drowsiness. Check with your doctor.
Meprobamate	May cause extra drowsiness. Check with your doctor.
Mesoridazine	May cause extra drowsiness. Check with your doctor.
Midazolam	May cause extra drowsiness. Check with your doctor.
Molindone	May cause extra drowsiness. Check with your doctor.
Oxazepam	May cause extra drowsiness. Check with your doctor.
Perphenazine	May cause extra drowsiness. Check with your doctor.
Phenelzine	Do not combine. Wait 2 weeks after using Phenelzine.
Prazepam	May cause extra drowsiness. Check with your doctor.
Prochlorperazine	May cause extra drowsiness. Check with your doctor.
Promethazine	May cause extra drowsiness. Check with your doctor.
Propofol	May cause extra drowsiness. Check with your doctor.
Quazepam	May cause extra drowsiness. Check with your doctor.
Secobarbital	May cause extra drowsiness. Check with your doctor.
Selegiline	Do not combine. Wait 2 weeks after using Selegiline.
Temazepam	May cause extra drowsiness. Check with your doctor.
Thioridazine	May cause extra drowsiness. Check with your doctor.
Thiothixene	May cause extra drowsiness. Check with your doctor.
Tranylcypromine	Do not combine. Wait 2 weeks after using Tranylcypromine.
Triazolam	May cause extra drowsiness. Check with your doctor.
Trifluoperazine	May cause extra drowsiness. Check with your doctor.
Zolpidem	May cause extra drowsiness. Check with your doctor.

Novahistine DMX

And:	Action:
Furazolidone	Do not combine. Wait 2 weeks after using Furazolidone.
Isocarboxazid	Do not combine. Wait 2 weeks after using Isocarboxazid.

Phenelzine	Do not combine. Wait 2 weeks after using Phenelzine.
Selegiline	Do not combine. Wait 2 weeks after using Selegiline.
Tranylcypromine	Do not combine. Wait 2 weeks after using Tranylcypromine.

Nuprin

And:	Action:
Acetaminophen	Do not combine without your doctor's approval.
Aspirin	Do not combine without your doctor's approval.

Nytol

And:	Action:
Alcohol	Do not combine. Alcohol increases Nytol's effect.
Alprazolam	Increases Nytol's effect.
Aprobarbital	Increases Nytol's effect.
Buprenorphine	Increases Nytol's effect.
Buspirone	Increases Nytol's effect.
Butabarbital	Increases Nytol's effect.
Butalbital	Increases Nytol's effect.
Chlordiazepoxide	Increases Nytol's effect.
Chlorpromazine	Increases Nytol's effect.
Chlorprothixene	Increases Nytol's effect.
Clorazepate	Increases Nytol's effect.
Clozapine	Increases Nytol's effect.
Codeine	Increases Nytol's effect.
Dezocine	Increases Nytol's effect.
Diazepam	Increases Nytol's effect.
Droperidol	Increases Nytol's effect.
Estazolam	Increases Nytol's effect.
Ethchlorvynol	Increases Nytol's effect.
Ethinamate	Increases Nytol's effect.
Fentanyl	Increases Nytol's effect.
Fluphenazine	Increases Nytol's effect.
Flurazepam	Increases Nytol's effect.
Furazolidone	Increases and prolongs Nytol's effect.
Glutethimide	Increases Nytol's effect.
Haloperidol	Increases Nytol's effect.
Hydrocodone	Increases Nytol's effect.

Hydromorphone	Increases Nytol's effect.
Hydroxyzine	Increases Nytol's effect.
Isocarboxazid	Increases and prolongs Nytol's effect.
Ketamine	Increases Nytol's effect.
Levomethadyl	Increases Nytol's effect.
Levorphanol	Increases Nytol's effect.
Lorazepam	Increases Nytol's effect.
Loxapine	Increases Nytol's effect.
Meperidine	Increases Nytol's effect.
Mephobarbital	Increases Nytol's effect.
Meprobamate	Increases Nytol's effect.
Mesoridazine	Increases Nytol's effect.
Methadone	Increases Nytol's effect.
Methohexital	Increases Nytol's effect.
Methotrimeprazine	Increases Nytol's effect.
Midazolam	Increases Nytol's effect.
Molindone	Increases Nytol's effect.
Morphine	Increases Nytol's effect.
Oxazepam	Increases Nytol's effect.
Oxycodone	Increases Nytol's effect.
Pentobarbital	Increases Nytol's effect.
Perphenazine	Increases Nytol's effect.
Phenelzine	Increases and prolongs Nytol's effect.
Phenobarbital	Increases Nytol's effect.
Prazepam	Increases Nytol's effect.
Prochlorperazine	Increases Nytol's effect.
Promethazine	Increases Nytol's effect.
Propofol	Increases Nytol's effect.
Propoxyphene	Increases Nytol's effect.
Quazepam	Increases Nytol's effect.
Risperidone	Increases Nytol's effect.
Secobarbital	Increases Nytol's effect.
Selegiline	Increases and prolongs Nytol's effect.
Temazepam	Increases Nytol's effect.
Thiamylal Sodium	Increases Nytol's effect.
Thioridazine	Increases Nytol's effect.

Thiothixene	Increases Nytol's effect.
Tranylcypromine	Increases and prolongs Nytol's effect.
Triazolam	Increases Nytol's effect.
Trifluoperazine	Increases Nytol's effect.
Zolpidem	Increases Nytol's effect.

OcuHist

No interactions reported.

Orudis KT

And:	Action:
Dicumarol	Do not combine without your doctor's approval.
Diuretics	Do not combine without your doctor's approval.
Lithium	Do not combine without your doctor's approval.
Methotrexate	Do not combine without your doctor's approval.
Other Pain and Fever Reducers	Do not combine with Orudis KT.
Other Ketoprofen-Containing Products	Do not combine with Orudis KT.
Probenecid	Do not combine without your doctor's approval.
Warfarin	Do not combine without your doctor's approval.

Otrivin

No interactions reported.

Pamprin Maximum Pain Relief

And:	Action:
Acarbose	Do not combine without your doctor's approval.
Arthritis Medications	Do not combine without your doctor's approval.
Chlorpropamide	Do not combine without your doctor's approval.
Dicumarol	Do not combine without your doctor's approval.
Glimepiride	Do not combine without your doctor's approval.
Glipizide	Do not combine without your doctor's approval.
Glyburide	Do not combine without your doctor's approval.
Metformin	Do not combine without your doctor's approval.
Miglitol	Do not combine without your doctor's approval.
Probenecid	Do not combine without your doctor's approval.
Sulfinpyrazone	Do not combine without your doctor's approval.
Tolazamide	Do not combine without your doctor's approval.
Tolbutamide	Do not combine without your doctor's approval.

| Troglitazone | Do not combine without your doctor's approval. |
| Warfarin | Do not combine without your doctor's approval. |

Pamprin Multi-Symptom

See Midol PMS Formula

Panadol

See Tylenol

PediaCare Cough-Cold Chewable Tablets and Liquid

See PediaCare NightRest Cough-Cold Liquid

PediaCare Infants' Decongestant Drops

See PediaCare NightRest Cough-Cold Liquid

PediaCare Infants' Drops Decongestant Plus Cough

See PediaCare NightRest Cough-Cold Liquid

PediaCare NightRest Cough-Cold Liquid

And:	*Action:*
Alprazolam	May cause extra drowsiness. Check with your doctor.
Buspirone	May cause extra drowsiness. Check with your doctor.
Chlordiazepoxide	May cause extra drowsiness. Check with your doctor.
Chlorpromazine	May cause extra drowsiness. Check with your doctor.
Chlorprothixene	May cause extra drowsiness. Check with your doctor.
Clorazepate	May cause extra drowsiness. Check with your doctor.
Diazepam	May cause extra drowsiness. Check with your doctor.
Droperidol	May cause extra drowsiness. Check with your doctor.
Estazolam	May cause extra drowsiness. Check with your doctor.
Ethchlorvynol	May cause extra drowsiness. Check with your doctor.
Ethinamate	May cause extra drowsiness. Check with your doctor.
Fluphenazine	May cause extra drowsiness. Check with your doctor.
Flurazepam	May cause extra drowsiness. Check with your doctor.
Furazolidone	Do not combine. Wait 2 weeks after using Furazolidone.
Glutethimide	May cause extra drowsiness. Check with your doctor.
Haloperidol	May cause extra drowsiness. Check with your doctor.
Hydroxyzine	May cause extra drowsiness. Check with your doctor.
Isocarboxazid	Do not combine. Wait 2 weeks after using Isocarboxazid.
Lorazepam	May cause extra drowsiness. Check with your doctor.
Loxapine	May cause extra drowsiness. Check with your doctor.
Meprobamate	May cause extra drowsiness. Check with your doctor.

Mesoridazine	May cause extra drowsiness. Check with your doctor.
Midazolam	May cause extra drowsiness. Check with your doctor.
Molindone	May cause extra drowsiness. Check with your doctor.
Oxazepam	May cause extra drowsiness. Check with your doctor.
Perphenazine	May cause extra drowsiness. Check with your doctor.
Phenelzine	Do not combine. Wait 2 weeks after using Phenelzine.
Prazepam	May cause extra drowsiness. Check with your doctor.
Prochlorperazine	May cause extra drowsiness. Check with your doctor.
Promethazine	May cause extra drowsiness. Check with your doctor.
Propofol	May cause extra drowsiness. Check with your doctor.
Quazepam	May cause extra drowsiness. Check with your doctor.
Secobarbital	May cause extra drowsiness. Check with your doctor.
Selegiline	Do not combine. Wait 2 weeks after using Selegiline.
Temazepam	May cause extra drowsiness. Check with your doctor.
Thioridazine	May cause extra drowsiness. Check with your doctor.
Thiothixene	May cause extra drowsiness. Check with your doctor.
Tranylcypromine	Do not combine. Wait 2 weeks after using Tranylcypromine.
Triazolam	May cause extra drowsiness. Check with your doctor.
Trifluoperazine	May cause extra drowsiness. Check with your doctor.
Zolpidem	May cause extra drowsiness. Check with your doctor.

Pediatric Sudafed Nasal Decongestant Liquid Oral Drops

See Sudafed

Pediatric Vicks 44E

See Vicks 44 Cough Relief

Pediatric Vicks 44M

See Vicks 44M

Pepcid AC

No interactions reported.

Pepto Diarrhea Control

And:	Action:
Antibiotics	Do not combine without your doctor's approval.

Pepto-Bismol

Acarbose	Combine with caution.
Allopurinol	Combine with caution.
Chlorpropamide	Combine with caution.

Dicumarol	Combine with caution.
Glimepiride	Combine with caution.
Glipizide	Combine with caution.
Glyburide	Combine with caution.
Metformin	Combine with caution.
Miglitol	Combine with caution.
Probenecid	Combine with caution.
Sulfinpyrazone	Combine with caution.
Tolazamide	Combine with caution.
Tolbutamide	Combine with caution.
Troglitazone	Combine with caution.
Warfarin	Combine with caution.

Perdiem

No interactions reported.

Peri-Colace

No interactions reported.

Pertussin CS

And:	Action:
Furazolidone	Do not combine. Wait 2 weeks after using Furazolidone.
Isocarboxazid	Do not combine. Wait 2 weeks after using Isocarboxazid.
Phenelzine	Do not combine. Wait 2 weeks after using Phenelzine.
Selegiline	Do not combine. Wait 2 weeks after using Selegiline.
Tranylcypromine	Do not combine. Wait 2 weeks after using Tranylcypromine.

Pertussin DM

See Pertussin CS

Phazyme

No interactions reported.

Phillips' Gelcaps

| And: | Action: |
| Mineral Oil | Do not combine. |

Phillips' Milk of Magnesia

And:	Action:
Alendronate	Allow 2 to 3 hours between doses of the antacid and the drug.
Allopurinol	Allow 2 to 3 hours between doses of the antacid and the drug.
Arthritis Drugs	Allow 2 to 3 hours between doses of the antacid and the drug.
Aspirin	Allow 2 to 3 hours between doses of the antacid and the drug.

Atenolol	Allow 2 to 3 hours between doses of the antacid and the drug.
Captopril	Allow 2 to 3 hours between doses of the antacid and the drug.
Chlordiazepoxide	Allow 2 to 3 hours between doses of the antacid and the drug.
Cimetidine	Allow 2 to 3 hours between doses of the antacid and the drug.
Ciprofloxacin	Allow 2 to 3 hours between doses of the antacid and the drug.
Demeclocycline	Allow 2 to 3 hours between doses of the antacid and the drug.
Digoxin	Allow 2 to 3 hours between doses of the antacid and the drug.
Doxycycline	Allow 2 to 3 hours between doses of the antacid and the drug.
Enoxacin	Allow 2 to 3 hours between doses of the antacid and the drug.
Fosfomycin	Allow 2 to 3 hours between doses of the antacid and the drug.
Gabapentin	Allow 2 to 3 hours between doses of the antacid and the drug.
Glipizide	Allow 2 to 3 hours between doses of the antacid and the drug.
Glyburide	Allow 2 to 3 hours between doses of the antacid and the drug.
Isoniazid	Allow 2 to 3 hours between doses of the antacid and the drug.
Ketoconazole	Allow 2 to 3 hours between doses of the antacid and the drug.
Levothyroxine	Allow 2 to 3 hours between doses of the antacid and the drug.
Lomefloxacin	Allow 2 to 3 hours between doses of the antacid and the drug.
Methacycline	Allow 2 to 3 hours between doses of the antacid and the drug.
Methenamine	Allow 2 to 3 hours between doses of the antacid and the drug.
Metronidazole	Allow 2 to 3 hours between doses of the antacid and the drug.
Minocycline	Allow 2 to 3 hours between doses of the antacid and the drug.
Misoprostol	Allow 2 to 3 hours between doses of the antacid and the drug.
Mycophenolate	Allow 2 to 3 hours between doses of the antacid and the drug.
Norfloxacin	Allow 2 to 3 hours between doses of the antacid and the drug.
Ofloxacin	Allow 2 to 3 hours between doses of the antacid and the drug.
Oxytetracycline	Allow 2 to 3 hours between doses of the antacid and the drug.
Penicillamine	Allow 2 to 3 hours between doses of the antacid and the drug.
Phenytoin	Allow 2 to 3 hours between doses of the antacid and the drug.
Quinidine	Allow 2 to 3 hours between doses of the antacid and the drug.
Sodium Polystyrene Sulfonate	Allow 2 to 3 hours between doses of the antacid and the drug.
Sucralfate	Allow 2 to 3 hours between doses of the antacid and the drug.
Tetracycline	Allow 2 to 3 hours between doses of the antacid and the drug.
Tilodronate	Allow 2 to 3 hours between doses of the antacid and the drug.
Ursodiol	Allow 2 to 3 hours between doses of the antacid and the drug.

Pin-X

No interactions reported.

PMS Multi-Symptom Formula Midol

See Midol PMS Formula

Primatene Mist

Furazolidone	Do not combine. Wait 2 weeks after using Furazolidone.
Isocarboxazid	Do not combine. Wait 2 weeks after using Isocarboxazid.
Phenelzine	Do not combine. Wait 2 weeks after using Phenelzine.
Selegiline	Do not combine. Wait 2 weeks after using Selegiline.
Tranylcypromine	Do not combine. Wait 2 weeks after using Tranylcypromine.

Primatene Tablets

See Primatene Mist

Privine

No interactions reported.

Prodium

No interactions reported.

Propagest

And:	Action:
Acebutolol	Do not combine without your doctor's approval.
Amitriptyline	Do not combine without your doctor's approval.
Amlodipine	Do not combine without your doctor's approval.
Amoxapine	Do not combine without your doctor's approval.
Atenolol	Do not combine without your doctor's approval.
Benazepril	Do not combine without your doctor's approval.
Bendroflumethiazide	Do not combine without your doctor's approval.
Betaxolol	Do not combine without your doctor's approval.
Bisoprolol	Do not combine without your doctor's approval.
Bupropion	Do not combine without your doctor's approval.
Captopril	Do not combine without your doctor's approval.
Carteolol	Do not combine without your doctor's approval.
Chlorothiazide	Do not combine without your doctor's approval.
Chlorthalidone	Do not combine without your doctor's approval.
Clonidine	Do not combine without your doctor's approval.
Deserpidine	Do not combine without your doctor's approval.
Desipramine	Do not combine without your doctor's approval.
Diazoxide	Do not combine without your doctor's approval.
Diltiazem	Do not combine without your doctor's approval.
Doxazosin	Do not combine without your doctor's approval.

Doxepin	Do not combine without your doctor's approval.
Enalapril	Do not combine without your doctor's approval.
Esmolol	Do not combine without your doctor's approval.
Felodipine	Do not combine without your doctor's approval.
Fluoxetine	Do not combine without your doctor's approval.
Fosinopril	Do not combine without your doctor's approval.
Furosemide	Do not combine without your doctor's approval.
Guanabenz	Do not combine without your doctor's approval.
Guanethidine	Do not combine without your doctor's approval.
Hydralazine	Do not combine without your doctor's approval.
Hydrochlorothiazide	Do not combine without your doctor's approval.
Hydroflumethiazide	Do not combine without your doctor's approval.
Imipramine	Do not combine without your doctor's approval.
Indapamide	Do not combine without your doctor's approval.
Isocarboxazid	Do not combine without your doctor's approval.
Isradipine	Do not combine without your doctor's approval.
Labetalol	Do not combine without your doctor's approval.
Lisinopril	Do not combine without your doctor's approval.
Losartan	Do not combine without your doctor's approval.
Maprotiline	Do not combine without your doctor's approval.
Mecamylamine	Do not combine without your doctor's approval.
Methyclothiazide	Do not combine without your doctor's approval.
Methyldopa	Do not combine without your doctor's approval.
Metolazone	Do not combine without your doctor's approval.
Metoprolol	Do not combine without your doctor's approval.
Metyrosine	Do not combine without your doctor's approval.
Minoxidil	Do not combine without your doctor's approval.
Mirtazapine	Do not combine without your doctor's approval.
Moexipril	Do not combine without your doctor's approval.
Nadolol	Do not combine without your doctor's approval.
Nefazodone	Do not combine without your doctor's approval.
Nicardipine	Do not combine without your doctor's approval.
Nifedipine	Do not combine without your doctor's approval.
Nisoldipine	Do not combine without your doctor's approval.
Nitroglycerin	Do not combine without your doctor's approval.
Nortriptyline	Do not combine without your doctor's approval.

Paroxetine	Do not combine without your doctor's approval.
Penbutolol	Do not combine without your doctor's approval.
Phenelzine	Do not combine without your doctor's approval.
Phenoxybenzamine	Do not combine without your doctor's approval.
Phentolamine	Do not combine without your doctor's approval.
Pindolol	Do not combine without your doctor's approval.
Polythiazide	Do not combine without your doctor's approval.
Prazosin	Do not combine without your doctor's approval.
Propranolol	Do not combine without your doctor's approval.
Protriptyline	Do not combine without your doctor's approval.
Quinapril	Do not combine without your doctor's approval.
Ramipril	Do not combine without your doctor's approval.
Rauwolfia Serpentina	Do not combine without your doctor's approval.
Rescinnamine	Do not combine without your doctor's approval.
Reserpine	Do not combine without your doctor's approval.
Sertraline	Do not combine without your doctor's approval.
Sodium Nitroprusside	Do not combine without your doctor's approval.
Sotalol	Do not combine without your doctor's approval.
Spirapril	Do not combine without your doctor's approval.
Terazosin	Do not combine without your doctor's approval.
Timolol	Do not combine without your doctor's approval.
Torsemide	Do not combine without your doctor's approval.
Trandolapril	Do not combine without your doctor's approval.
Tranylcypromine	Do not combine without your doctor's approval.
Trazodone	Do not combine without your doctor's approval.
Trimethaphan	Do not combine without your doctor's approval.
Trimipramine	Do not combine without your doctor's approval.
Valsartan	Do not combine without your doctor's approval.
Venlafaxine	Do not combine without your doctor's approval.
Verapamil	Do not combine without your doctor's approval.

Rheaban

No interactions reported.

Robitussin

No interactions reported.

Robitussin Cold & Cough

And:	Action:
Furazolidone	Do not combine. Wait 2 weeks after using Furazolidone.

Isocarboxazid	Do not combine. Wait 2 weeks after using Isocarboxazid.
Phenelzine	Do not combine. Wait 2 weeks after using Phenelzine.
Selegiline	Do not combine. Wait 2 weeks after using Selegiline.
Tranylcypromine	Do not combine. Wait 2 weeks after using Tranylcypromine.

Robitussin Cold, Cough & Flu

See Robitussin Cold & Cough

Robitussin Cough & Cold

See Robitussin Cold & Cough

Robitussin Cough Suppressant

See Robitussin Cold & Cough

Robitussin Night-Time Cold Formula

And:	*Action:*
Alcohol	May cause extra drowsiness. Do not combine.
Alprazolam	May cause extra drowsiness. Check with your doctor.
Buspirone	May cause extra drowsiness. Check with your doctor.
Chlordiazepoxide	May cause extra drowsiness. Check with your doctor.
Chlorpromazine	May cause extra drowsiness. Check with your doctor.
Chlorprothixene	May cause extra drowsiness. Check with your doctor.
Clorazepate	May cause extra drowsiness. Check with your doctor.
Diazepam	May cause extra drowsiness. Check with your doctor.
Droperidol	May cause extra drowsiness. Check with your doctor.
Estazolam	May cause extra drowsiness. Check with your doctor.
Ethchlorvynol	May cause extra drowsiness. Check with your doctor.
Ethinamate	May cause extra drowsiness. Check with your doctor.
Fluphenazine	May cause extra drowsiness. Check with your doctor.
Flurazepam	May cause extra drowsiness. Check with your doctor.
Furazolidone	Do not combine. Wait 2 weeks after using Furazolidone.
Glutethimide	May cause extra drowsiness. Check with your doctor.
Haloperidol	May cause extra drowsiness. Check with your doctor.
Hydroxyzine	May cause extra drowsiness. Check with your doctor.
Isocarboxazid	Do not combine. Wait 2 weeks after using Isocarboxazid.
Lorazepam	May cause extra drowsiness. Check with your doctor.
Loxapine	May cause extra drowsiness. Check with your doctor.
Meprobamate	May cause extra drowsiness. Check with your doctor.
Mesoridazine	May cause extra drowsiness. Check with your doctor.
Midazolam	May cause extra drowsiness. Check with your doctor.

Molindone	May cause extra drowsiness. Check with your doctor.
Oxazepam	May cause extra drowsiness. Check with your doctor.
Perphenazine	May cause extra drowsiness. Check with your doctor.
Phenelzine	Do not combine. Wait 2 weeks after using Phenelzine.
Prazepam	May cause extra drowsiness. Check with your doctor.
Prochlorperazine	May cause extra drowsiness. Check with your doctor.
Promethazine	May cause extra drowsiness. Check with your doctor.
Propofol	May cause extra drowsiness. Check with your doctor.
Quazepam	May cause extra drowsiness. Check with your doctor.
Secobarbital	May cause extra drowsiness. Check with your doctor.
Selegiline	Do not combine. Wait 2 weeks after using Selegiline.
Temazepam	May cause extra drowsiness. Check with your doctor.
Thioridazine	May cause extra drowsiness. Check with your doctor.
Thiothixene	May cause extra drowsiness. Check with your doctor.
Tranylcypromine	Do not combine. Wait 2 weeks after using Tranylcypromine.
Triazolam	May cause extra drowsiness. Check with your doctor.
Trifluoperazine	May cause extra drowsiness. Check with your doctor.
Zolpidem	May cause extra drowsiness. Check with your doctor.

Robitussin Pediatric Cough & Cold Formula

See Robitussin Cold & Cough

Robitussin Pediatric Cough Suppressant

See Robitussin Cold & Cough

Robitussin Pediatric Drops

See Robitussin Cold & Cough

Robitussin Severe Congestion Liqui-Gels

See Robitussin-CF

Robitussin-CF

And:	Action:
Furazolidone	Do not combine. Wait 2 weeks after using Furazolidone.
Isocarboxazid	Do not combine. Wait 2 weeks after using Isocarboxazid.
Phenelzine	Do not combine. Wait 2 weeks after using Phenelzine.
Selegiline	Do not combine. Wait 2 weeks after using Selegiline.
Tranylcypromine	Do not combine. Wait 2 weeks after using Tranylcypromine.

Robitussin-DM

See Robitussin-CF

Robitussin-PE

See Robitussin-CF

Rogaine

No interactions reported.

Rolaids

And:	Action:
Alendronate	Allow 2 to 3 hours between doses of the antacid and the drug.
Allopurinol	Allow 2 to 3 hours between doses of the antacid and the drug.
Arthritis Drugs	Allow 2 to 3 hours between doses of the antacid and the drug.
Aspirin	Allow 2 to 3 hours between doses of the antacid and the drug.
Atenolol	Allow 2 to 3 hours between doses of the antacid and the drug.
Captopril	Allow 2 to 3 hours between doses of the antacid and the drug.
Chlordiazepoxide	Allow 2 to 3 hours between doses of the antacid and the drug.
Cimetidine	Allow 2 to 3 hours between doses of the antacid and the drug.
Ciprofloxacin	Allow 2 to 3 hours between doses of the antacid and the drug.
Demeclocycline	Allow 2 to 3 hours between doses of the antacid and the drug.
Digoxin	Allow 2 to 3 hours between doses of the antacid and the drug.
Doxycycline	Allow 2 to 3 hours between doses of the antacid and the drug.
Enoxacin	Allow 2 to 3 hours between doses of the antacid and the drug.
Fosfomycin	Allow 2 to 3 hours between doses of the antacid and the drug.
Gabapentin	Allow 2 to 3 hours between doses of the antacid and the drug.
Glipizide	Allow 2 to 3 hours between doses of the antacid and the drug.
Glyburide	Allow 2 to 3 hours between doses of the antacid and the drug.
Isoniazid	Allow 2 to 3 hours between doses of the antacid and the drug.
Ketoconazole	Allow 2 to 3 hours between doses of the antacid and the drug.
Levothyroxine	Allow 2 to 3 hours between doses of the antacid and the drug.
Lomefloxacin	Allow 2 to 3 hours between doses of the antacid and the drug.
Methacycline	Allow 2 to 3 hours between doses of the antacid and the drug.
Methenamine	Allow 2 to 3 hours between doses of the antacid and the drug.
Metronidazole	Allow 2 to 3 hours between doses of the antacid and the drug.
Minocycline	Allow 2 to 3 hours between doses of the antacid and the drug.
Misoprostol	Allow 2 to 3 hours between doses of the antacid and the drug.
Mycophenolate	Allow 2 to 3 hours between doses of the antacid and the drug.
Norfloxacin	Allow 2 to 3 hours between doses of the antacid and the drug.
Ofloxacin	Allow 2 to 3 hours between doses of the antacid and the drug.

Oxytetracycline	Allow 2 to 3 hours between doses of the antacid and the drug.
Penicillamine	Allow 2 to 3 hours between doses of the antacid and the drug.
Phenytoin	Allow 2 to 3 hours between doses of the antacid and the drug.
Quinidine	Allow 2 to 3 hours between doses of the antacid and the drug.
Sodium Polystyrene Sulfonate	Allow 2 to 3 hours between doses of the antacid and the drug.
Sucralfate	Allow 2 to 3 hours between doses of the antacid and the drug.
Tetracycline	Allow 2 to 3 hours between doses of the antacid and the drug.
Tilodronate	Allow 2 to 3 hours between doses of the antacid and the drug.
Ursodiol	Allow 2 to 3 hours between doses of the antacid and the drug.

Ryna Liquid

And:	Action:
Alcohol	May cause extra drowsiness. Check with your doctor.
Alprazolam	May cause extra drowsiness. Check with your doctor.
Buspirone	May cause extra drowsiness. Check with your doctor.
Chlordiazepoxide	May cause extra drowsiness. Check with your doctor.
Chlorpromazine	May cause extra drowsiness. Check with your doctor.
Chlorprothixene	May cause extra drowsiness. Check with your doctor.
Clorazepate	May cause extra drowsiness. Check with your doctor.
Diazepam	May cause extra drowsiness. Check with your doctor.
Droperidol	May cause extra drowsiness. Check with your doctor.
Estazolam	May cause extra drowsiness. Check with your doctor.
Ethchlorvynol	May cause extra drowsiness. Check with your doctor.
Ethinamate	May cause extra drowsiness. Check with your doctor.
Fluphenazine	May cause extra drowsiness. Check with your doctor.
Flurazepam	May cause extra drowsiness. Check with your doctor.
Furazolidone	Do not combine. Wait 2 weeks after using Furazolidone.
Glutethimide	May cause extra drowsiness. Check with your doctor.
Haloperidol	May cause extra drowsiness. Check with your doctor.
Hydroxyzine	May cause extra drowsiness. Check with your doctor.
Isocarboxazid	Do not combine. Wait 2 weeks after using Isocarboxazid.
Lorazepam	May cause extra drowsiness. Check with your doctor.
Loxapine	May cause extra drowsiness. Check with your doctor.
Meprobamate	May cause extra drowsiness. Check with your doctor.
Mesoridazine	May cause extra drowsiness. Check with your doctor.
Midazolam	May cause extra drowsiness. Check with your doctor.

Molindone	May cause extra drowsiness. Check with your doctor.
Oxazepam	May cause extra drowsiness. Check with your doctor.
Perphenazine	May cause extra drowsiness. Check with your doctor.
Phenelzine	Do not combine. Wait 2 weeks after using Phenelzine.
Prazepam	May cause extra drowsiness. Check with your doctor.
Prochlorperazine	May cause extra drowsiness. Check with your doctor.
Promethazine	May cause extra drowsiness. Check with your doctor.
Propofol	May cause extra drowsiness. Check with your doctor.
Quazepam	May cause extra drowsiness. Check with your doctor.
Secobarbital	May cause extra drowsiness. Check with your doctor.
Selegiline	Do not combine. Wait 2 weeks after using Selegiline.
Temazepam	May cause extra drowsiness. Check with your doctor.
Thioridazine	May cause extra drowsiness. Check with your doctor.
Thiothixene	May cause extra drowsiness. Check with your doctor.
Tranylcypromine	Do not combine. Wait 2 weeks after using Tranylcypromine.
Triazolam	May cause extra drowsiness. Check with your doctor.
Trifluoperazine	May cause extra drowsiness. Check with your doctor.
Zolpidem	May cause extra drowsiness. Check with your doctor.

Ryna-C Liquid

See Ryna Liquid

Ryna-CX Liquid

See Ryna Liquid

Safe Tussin 30

And:	*Action:*
Furazolidone	Do not combine. Wait 2 weeks after using Furazolidone.
Isocarboxazid	Do not combine. Wait 2 weeks after using Isocarboxazid.
Phenelzine	Do not combine. Wait 2 weeks after using Phenelzine.
Selegiline	Do not combine. Wait 2 weeks after using Selegiline.
Tranylcypromine	Do not combine. Wait 2 weeks after using Tranylcypromine.

Senokot

No interactions reported.

Sinarest

And:	*Action:*
Alcohol	May cause extra drowsiness. Do not combine.
Alprazolam	May cause extra drowsiness. Check with your doctor.

Buspirone	May cause extra drowsiness. Check with your doctor.
Chlordiazepoxide	May cause extra drowsiness. Check with your doctor.
Chlorpromazine	May cause extra drowsiness. Check with your doctor.
Chlorprothixene	May cause extra drowsiness. Check with your doctor.
Clorazepate	May cause extra drowsiness. Check with your doctor.
Diazepam	May cause extra drowsiness. Check with your doctor.
Droperidol	May cause extra drowsiness. Check with your doctor.
Estazolam	May cause extra drowsiness. Check with your doctor.
Ethchlorvynol	May cause extra drowsiness. Check with your doctor.
Ethinamate	May cause extra drowsiness. Check with your doctor.
Fluphenazine	May cause extra drowsiness. Check with your doctor.
Flurazepam	May cause extra drowsiness. Check with your doctor.
Furazolidone	Do not combine. Wait 2 weeks after using Furazolidone.
Glutethimide	May cause extra drowsiness. Check with your doctor.
Haloperidol	May cause extra drowsiness. Check with your doctor.
Hydroxyzine	May cause extra drowsiness. Check with your doctor.
Isocarboxazid	Do not combine. Wait 2 weeks after using Isocarboxazid.
Lorazepam	May cause extra drowsiness. Check with your doctor.
Loxapine	May cause extra drowsiness. Check with your doctor.
Meprobamate	May cause extra drowsiness. Check with your doctor.
Mesoridazine	May cause extra drowsiness. Check with your doctor.
Midazolam	May cause extra drowsiness. Check with your doctor.
Molindone	May cause extra drowsiness. Check with your doctor.
Oxazepam	May cause extra drowsiness. Check with your doctor.
Perphenazine	May cause extra drowsiness. Check with your doctor.
Phenelzine	Do not combine. Wait 2 weeks after using Phenelzine.
Prazepam	May cause extra drowsiness. Check with your doctor.
Prochlorperazine	May cause extra drowsiness. Check with your doctor.
Promethazine	May cause extra drowsiness. Check with your doctor.
Propofol	May cause extra drowsiness. Check with your doctor.
Quazepam	May cause extra drowsiness. Check with your doctor.
Secobarbital	May cause extra drowsiness. Check with your doctor.
Selegiline	Do not combine. Wait 2 weeks after using Selegiline.
Temazepam	May cause extra drowsiness. Check with your doctor.
Thioridazine	May cause extra drowsiness. Check with your doctor.
Thiothixene	May cause extra drowsiness. Check with your doctor.

Tranylcypromine	Do not combine. Wait 2 weeks after using Tranylcypromine.
Triazolam	May cause extra drowsiness. Check with your doctor.
Trifluoperazine	May cause extra drowsiness. Check with your doctor.
Zolpidem	May cause extra drowsiness. Check with your doctor.

Sine-Aid

And:	Action:
Alcohol	The acetaminophen in the medication may cause liver damage in heavy drinkers.
Furazolidone	Do not combine. Wait 2 weeks after using Furazolidone.
Isocarboxazid	Do not combine. Wait 2 weeks after using Isocarboxazid.
Phenelzine	Do not combine. Wait 2 weeks after using Phenelzine.
Selegiline	Do not combine. Wait 2 weeks after using Selegiline.
Tranylcypromine	Do not combine. Wait 2 weeks after using Tranylcypromine.

Sine-Off No Drowsiness Formula

And:	Action:
Furazolidone	Do not combine. Wait 2 weeks after using Furazolidone.
Isocarboxazid	Do not combine. Wait 2 weeks after using Isocarboxazid.
Phenelzine	Do not combine. Wait 2 weeks after using Phenelzine.
Selegiline	Do not combine. Wait 2 weeks after using Selegiline.
Tranylcypromine	Do not combine. Wait 2 weeks after using Tranylcypromine.

Sine-Off Sinus, Cold & Flu Medicine

See Sine-Off Sinus Medicine

Sine-Off Sinus Medicine

And:	Action:
Alcohol	May cause extra drowsiness. Do not combine.
Alprazolam	May cause extra drowsiness. Check with your doctor.
Buspirone	May cause extra drowsiness. Check with your doctor.
Chlordiazepoxide	May cause extra drowsiness. Check with your doctor.
Chlorpromazine	May cause extra drowsiness. Check with your doctor.
Chlorprothixene	May cause extra drowsiness. Check with your doctor.
Clorazepate	May cause extra drowsiness. Check with your doctor.
Diazepam	May cause extra drowsiness. Check with your doctor.
Droperidol	May cause extra drowsiness. Check with your doctor.
Estazolam	May cause extra drowsiness. Check with your doctor.
Ethchlorvynol	May cause extra drowsiness. Check with your doctor.

Ethinamate	May cause extra drowsiness. Check with your doctor.
Fluphenazine	May cause extra drowsiness. Check with your doctor.
Flurazepam	May cause extra drowsiness. Check with your doctor.
Furazolidone	Do not combine. Wait 2 weeks after using Furazolidone.
Glutethimide	May cause extra drowsiness. Check with your doctor.
Haloperidol	May cause extra drowsiness. Check with your doctor.
Hydroxyzine	May cause extra drowsiness. Check with your doctor.
Isocarboxazid	Do not combine. Wait 2 weeks after using Isocarboxazid.
Lorazepam	May cause extra drowsiness. Check with your doctor.
Loxapine	May cause extra drowsiness. Check with your doctor.
Meprobamate	May cause extra drowsiness. Check with your doctor.
Mesoridazine	May cause extra drowsiness. Check with your doctor.
Midazolam	May cause extra drowsiness. Check with your doctor.
Molindone	May cause extra drowsiness. Check with your doctor.
Oxazepam	May cause extra drowsiness. Check with your doctor.
Perphenazine	May cause extra drowsiness. Check with your doctor.
Phenelzine	Do not combine. Wait 2 weeks after using Phenelzine.
Prazepam	May cause extra drowsiness. Check with your doctor.
Prochlorperazine	May cause extra drowsiness. Check with your doctor.
Promethazine	May cause extra drowsiness. Check with your doctor.
Propofol	May cause extra drowsiness. Check with your doctor.
Quazepam	May cause extra drowsiness. Check with your doctor.
Secobarbital	May cause extra drowsiness. Check with your doctor.
Selegiline	Do not combine. Wait 2 weeks after using Selegiline.
Temazepam	May cause extra drowsiness. Check with your doctor.
Thioridazine	May cause extra drowsiness. Check with your doctor.
Thiothixene	May cause extra drowsiness. Check with your doctor.
Tranylcypromine	Do not combine. Wait 2 weeks after using Tranylcypromine.
Triazolam	May cause extra drowsiness. Check with your doctor.
Trifluoperazine	May cause extra drowsiness. Check with your doctor.
Zolpidem	May cause extra drowsiness. Check with your doctor.

Singlet

And:	Action:
Alcohol	May cause extra drowsiness. Do not combine.
Alprazolam	May cause extra drowsiness. Check with your doctor.

Buspirone	May cause extra drowsiness. Check with your doctor.
Chlordiazepoxide	May cause extra drowsiness. Check with your doctor.
Chlorpromazine	May cause extra drowsiness. Check with your doctor.
Chlorprothixene	May cause extra drowsiness. Check with your doctor.
Clorazepate	May cause extra drowsiness. Check with your doctor.
Diazepam	May cause extra drowsiness. Check with your doctor.
Droperidol	May cause extra drowsiness. Check with your doctor.
Estazolam	May cause extra drowsiness. Check with your doctor.
Ethchlorvynol	May cause extra drowsiness. Check with your doctor.
Ethinamate	May cause extra drowsiness. Check with your doctor.
Fluphenazine	May cause extra drowsiness. Check with your doctor.
Flurazepam	May cause extra drowsiness. Check with your doctor.
Furazolidone	Do not combine. Wait 2 weeks after using Furazolidone.
Glutethimide	May cause extra drowsiness. Check with your doctor.
Haloperidol	May cause extra drowsiness. Check with your doctor.
Hydroxyzine	May cause extra drowsiness. Check with your doctor.
Isocarboxazid	Do not combine. Wait 2 weeks after using Isocarboxazid.
Lorazepam	May cause extra drowsiness. Check with your doctor.
Loxapine	May cause extra drowsiness. Check with your doctor.
Meprobamate	May cause extra drowsiness. Check with your doctor.
Mesoridazine	May cause extra drowsiness. Check with your doctor.
Midazolam	May cause extra drowsiness. Check with your doctor.
Molindone	May cause extra drowsiness. Check with your doctor.
Oxazepam	May cause extra drowsiness. Check with your doctor.
Perphenazine	May cause extra drowsiness. Check with your doctor.
Phenelzine	Do not combine. Wait 2 weeks after using Phenelzine.
Prazepam	May cause extra drowsiness. Check with your doctor.
Prochlorperazine	May cause extra drowsiness. Check with your doctor.
Promethazine	May cause extra drowsiness. Check with your doctor.
Propofol	May cause extra drowsiness. Check with your doctor.
Quazepam	May cause extra drowsiness. Check with your doctor.
Secobarbital	May cause extra drowsiness. Check with your doctor.
Selegiline	Do not combine. Wait 2 weeks after using Selegiline.
Temazepam	May cause extra drowsiness. Check with your doctor.
Thioridazine	May cause extra drowsiness. Check with your doctor.
Thiothixene	May cause extra drowsiness. Check with your doctor.

Tranylcypromine	Do not combine. Wait 2 weeks after using Tranylcypromine.
Triazolam	May cause extra drowsiness. Check with your doctor.
Trifluoperazine	May cause extra drowsiness. Check with your doctor.
Zolpidem	May cause extra drowsiness. Check with your doctor.

Sinulin

And:	Action:
Acebutolol	Do not combine without your doctor's approval.
Alcohol	May cause extra drowsiness. Do not combine.
Alprazolam	May cause extra drowsiness. Check with your doctor.
Amitriptyline	Do not combine without your doctor's approval.
Amlodipine	Do not combine without your doctor's approval.
Amoxapine	Do not combine without your doctor's approval.
Atenolol	Do not combine without your doctor's approval.
Benazepril	Do not combine without your doctor's approval.
Bendroflumethiazide	Do not combine without your doctor's approval.
Betaxolol	Do not combine without your doctor's approval.
Bisoprolol	Do not combine without your doctor's approval.
Bupropion	Do not combine without your doctor's approval.
Buspirone	May cause extra drowsiness. Check with your doctor.
Captopril	Do not combine without your doctor's approval.
Carteolol	Do not combine without your doctor's approval.
Chlordiazepoxide	May cause extra drowsiness. Check with your doctor.
Chlorothiazide	Do not combine without your doctor's approval.
Chlorpromazine	May cause extra drowsiness. Check with your doctor.
Chlorprothixene	May cause extra drowsiness. Check with your doctor.
Chlorthalidone	Do not combine without your doctor's approval.
Clonidine	Do not combine without your doctor's approval.
Clorazepate	May cause extra drowsiness. Check with your doctor.
Deserpidine	Do not combine without your doctor's approval.
Desipramine	Do not combine without your doctor's approval.
Diazepam	May cause extra drowsiness. Check with your doctor.
Diazoxide	Do not combine without your doctor's approval.
Diltiazem	Do not combine without your doctor's approval.
Doxazosin	Do not combine without your doctor's approval.
Doxepin	Do not combine without your doctor's approval.

Droperidol	May cause extra drowsiness. Check with your doctor.
Enalapril	Do not combine without your doctor's approval.
Esmolol	Do not combine without your doctor's approval.
Estazolam	May cause extra drowsiness. Check with your doctor.
Ethchlorvynol	May cause extra drowsiness. Check with your doctor.
Ethinamate	May cause extra drowsiness. Check with your doctor.
Felodipine	Do not combine without your doctor's approval.
Fluoxetine	Do not combine without your doctor's approval.
Fluphenazine	May cause extra drowsiness. Check with your doctor.
Flurazepam	May cause extra drowsiness. Check with your doctor.
Fosinopril	Do not combine without your doctor's approval.
Furosemide	Do not combine without your doctor's approval.
Glutethimide	May cause extra drowsiness. Check with your doctor.
Guanabenz	Do not combine without your doctor's approval.
Guanethidine	Do not combine without your doctor's approval.
Haloperidol	May cause extra drowsiness. Check with your doctor.
Hydralazine	Do not combine without your doctor's approval.
Hydrochlorothiazide	Do not combine without your doctor's approval.
Hydroflumethiazide	Do not combine without your doctor's approval.
Hydroxyzine	May cause extra drowsiness. Check with your doctor.
Imipramine	Do not combine without your doctor's approval.
Indapamide	Do not combine without your doctor's approval.
Isocarboxazid	Do not combine without your doctor's approval.
Isradipine	Do not combine without your doctor's approval.
Labetalol	Do not combine without your doctor's approval.
Lisinopril	Do not combine without your doctor's approval.
Lorazepam	May cause extra drowsiness. Check with your doctor.
Losartan	Do not combine without your doctor's approval.
Loxapine	May cause extra drowsiness. Check with your doctor.
Maprotiline	Do not combine without your doctor's approval.
Mecamylamine	Do not combine without your doctor's approval.
Meprobamate	May cause extra drowsiness. Check with your doctor.
Mesoridazine	May cause extra drowsiness. Check with your doctor.
Methyclothiazide	Do not combine without your doctor's approval.
Methyldopa	Do not combine without your doctor's approval.
Metolazone	Do not combine without your doctor's approval.

Metoprolol	Do not combine without your doctor's approval.
Metyrosine	Do not combine without your doctor's approval.
Midazolam	May cause extra drowsiness. Check with your doctor.
Minoxidil	Do not combine without your doctor's approval.
Mirtazapine	Do not combine without your doctor's approval.
Moexipril	Do not combine without your doctor's approval.
Molindone	May cause extra drowsiness. Check with your doctor.
Nadolol	Do not combine without your doctor's approval.
Nefazodone	Do not combine without your doctor's approval.
Nicardipine	Do not combine without your doctor's approval.
Nifedipine	Do not combine without your doctor's approval.
Nisoldipine	Do not combine without your doctor's approval.
Nitroglycerin	Do not combine without your doctor's approval.
Nortriptyline	Do not combine without your doctor's approval.
Oxazepam	May cause extra drowsiness. Check with your doctor.
Paroxetine	Do not combine without your doctor's approval.
Penbutolol	Do not combine without your doctor's approval.
Perphenazine	May cause extra drowsiness. Check with your doctor.
Phenelzine	Do not combine without your doctor's approval.
Phenoxybenzamine	Do not combine without your doctor's approval.
Phentolamine	Do not combine without your doctor's approval.
Pindolol	Do not combine without your doctor's approval.
Polythiazide	Do not combine without your doctor's approval.
Prazepam	May cause extra drowsiness. Check with your doctor.
Prazosin	Do not combine without your doctor's approval.
Prochlorperazine	May cause extra drowsiness. Check with your doctor.
Promethazine	May cause extra drowsiness. Check with your doctor.
Propofol	May cause extra drowsiness. Check with your doctor.
Propranolol	Do not combine without your doctor's approval.
Protriptyline	Do not combine without your doctor's approval.
Quazepam	May cause extra drowsiness. Check with your doctor.
Quinapril	Do not combine without your doctor's approval.
Ramipril	Do not combine without your doctor's approval.
Rauwolfia Serpentina	Do not combine without your doctor's approval.
Rescinnamine	Do not combine without your doctor's approval.
Reserpine	Do not combine without your doctor's approval.

Secobarbital	May cause extra drowsiness. Check with your doctor.
Sertraline	Do not combine without your doctor's approval.
Sodium Nitroprusside	Do not combine without your doctor's approval.
Sotalol	Do not combine without your doctor's approval.
Spirapril	Do not combine without your doctor's approval.
Temazepam	May cause extra drowsiness. Check with your doctor.
Terazosin	Do not combine without your doctor's approval.
Thioridazine	May cause extra drowsiness. Check with your doctor.
Thiothixene	May cause extra drowsiness. Check with your doctor.
Timolol	Do not combine without your doctor's approval.
Torsemide	Do not combine without your doctor's approval.
Trandolapril	Do not combine without your doctor's approval.
Tranylcypromine	Do not combine without your doctor's approval.
Trazodone	Do not combine without your doctor's approval.
Triazolam	May cause extra drowsiness. Check with your doctor.
Trifluoperazine	May cause extra drowsiness. Check with your doctor.
Trimethaphan	Do not combine without your doctor's approval.
Trimipramine	Do not combine without your doctor's approval.
Valsartan	Do not combine without your doctor's approval.
Venlafaxine	Do not combine without your doctor's approval.
Verapamil	Do not combine without your doctor's approval.
Zolpidem	May cause extra drowsiness. Check with your doctor.

Sinutab

And:	Action:
Furazolidone	Do not combine. Wait 2 weeks after using Furazolidone.
Isocarboxazid	Do not combine. Wait 2 weeks after using Isocarboxazid.
Phenelzine	Do not combine. Wait 2 weeks after using Phenelzine.
Selegiline	Do not combine. Wait 2 weeks after using Selegiline.
Tranylcypromine	Do not combine. Wait 2 weeks after using Tranylcypromine.

Sinutab Sinus Allergy

And:	Action:
Alcohol	May cause extra drowsiness. Do not combine.
Alprazolam	May cause extra drowsiness. Check with your doctor.
Buspirone	May cause extra drowsiness. Check with your doctor.
Chlordiazepoxide	May cause extra drowsiness. Check with your doctor.
Chlorpromazine	May cause extra drowsiness. Check with your doctor.

Chlorprothixene	May cause extra drowsiness. Check with your doctor.
Clorazepate	May cause extra drowsiness. Check with your doctor.
Diazepam	May cause extra drowsiness. Check with your doctor.
Droperidol	May cause extra drowsiness. Check with your doctor.
Estazolam	May cause extra drowsiness. Check with your doctor.
Ethchlorvynol	May cause extra drowsiness. Check with your doctor.
Ethinamate	May cause extra drowsiness. Check with your doctor.
Fluphenazine	May cause extra drowsiness. Check with your doctor.
Flurazepam	May cause extra drowsiness. Check with your doctor.
Furazolidone	Do not combine. Wait 2 weeks after using Furazolidone.
Glutethimide	May cause extra drowsiness. Check with your doctor.
Haloperidol	May cause extra drowsiness. Check with your doctor.
Hydroxyzine	May cause extra drowsiness. Check with your doctor.
Isocarboxazid	Do not combine. Wait 2 weeks after using Isocarboxazid.
Lorazepam	May cause extra drowsiness. Check with your doctor.
Loxapine	May cause extra drowsiness. Check with your doctor.
Meprobamate	May cause extra drowsiness. Check with your doctor.
Mesoridazine	May cause extra drowsiness. Check with your doctor.
Midazolam	May cause extra drowsiness. Check with your doctor.
Molindone	May cause extra drowsiness. Check with your doctor.
Oxazepam	May cause extra drowsiness. Check with your doctor.
Perphenazine	May cause extra drowsiness. Check with your doctor.
Phenelzine	Do not combine. Wait 2 weeks after using Phenelzine.
Prazepam	May cause extra drowsiness. Check with your doctor.
Prochlorperazine	May cause extra drowsiness. Check with your doctor.
Promethazine	May cause extra drowsiness. Check with your doctor.
Propofol	May cause extra drowsiness. Check with your doctor.
Quazepam	May cause extra drowsiness. Check with your doctor.
Secobarbital	May cause extra drowsiness. Check with your doctor.
Selegiline	Do not combine. Wait 2 weeks after using Selegiline.
Temazepam	May cause extra drowsiness. Check with your doctor.
Thioridazine	May cause extra drowsiness. Check with your doctor.
Thiothixene	May cause extra drowsiness. Check with your doctor.
Tranylcypromine	Do not combine. Wait 2 weeks after using Tranylcypromine.
Triazolam	May cause extra drowsiness. Check with your doctor.
Trifluoperazine	May cause extra drowsiness. Check with your doctor.

Zolpidem	May cause extra drowsiness. Check with your doctor.

Sinutab Sinus Medication

And:	Action:
Alcohol	The acetaminophen in the medication may cause liver damage in heavy drinkers.
Furazolidone	Do not combine. Wait 2 weeks after using Furazolidone.
Isocarboxazid	Do not combine. Wait 2 weeks after using Isocarboxazid.
Phenelzine	Do not combine. Wait 2 weeks after using Phenelzine.
Selegiline	Do not combine. Wait 2 weeks after using Selegiline.
Tranylcypromine	Do not combine. Wait 2 weeks after using Tranylcypromine.

Sleepinal

And:	Action:
Alcohol	Do not combine.
Alprazolam	Do not combine without your doctor's approval.
Buspirone	Do not combine without your doctor's approval.
Chlordiazepoxide	Do not combine without your doctor's approval.
Chlorpromazine	Do not combine without your doctor's approval.
Chlorprothixene	Do not combine without your doctor's approval.
Clorazepate	Do not combine without your doctor's approval.
Diazepam	Do not combine without your doctor's approval.
Droperidol	Do not combine without your doctor's approval.
Estazolam	Do not combine without your doctor's approval.
Ethchlorvynol	Do not combine without your doctor's approval.
Ethinamate	Do not combine without your doctor's approval.
Fluphenazine	Do not combine without your doctor's approval.
Flurazepam	Do not combine without your doctor's approval.
Glutethimide	Do not combine without your doctor's approval.
Haloperidol	Do not combine without your doctor's approval.
Hydroxyzine	Do not combine without your doctor's approval.
Lorazepam	Do not combine without your doctor's approval.
Loxapine	Do not combine without your doctor's approval.
Meprobamate	Do not combine without your doctor's approval.
Mesoridazine	Do not combine without your doctor's approval.
Midazolam	Do not combine without your doctor's approval.
Molindone	Do not combine without your doctor's approval.
Oxazepam	Do not combine without your doctor's approval.

Perphenazine	Do not combine without your doctor's approval.
Prazepam	Do not combine without your doctor's approval.
Prochlorperazine	Do not combine without your doctor's approval.
Promethazine	Do not combine without your doctor's approval.
Propofol	Do not combine without your doctor's approval.
Quazepam	Do not combine without your doctor's approval.
Secobarbital	Do not combine without your doctor's approval.
Temazepam	Do not combine without your doctor's approval.
Thioridazine	Do not combine without your doctor's approval.
Thiothixene	Do not combine without your doctor's approval.
Triazolam	Do not combine without your doctor's approval.
Trifluoperazine	Do not combine without your doctor's approval.
Zolpidem	Do not combine without your doctor's approval.

St. Joseph

See Bayer Aspirin

Sucrets

No interactions reported.

Sucrets 4 Hour Cough Suppressant

And:	*Action:*
Furazolidone	Do not combine. Wait 2 weeks after using Furazolidone.
Isocarboxazid	Do not combine. Wait 2 weeks after using Isocarboxazid.
Phenelzine	Do not combine. Wait 2 weeks after using Phenelzine.
Selegiline	Do not combine. Wait 2 weeks after using Selegiline.
Tranylcypromine	Do not combine. Wait 2 weeks after using Tranylcypromine.

Sudafed

And:	*Action:*
Furazolidone	Do not combine. Wait 2 weeks after using Furazolidone.
Isocarboxazid	Do not combine. Wait 2 weeks after using Isocarboxazid.
Phenelzine	Do not combine. Wait 2 weeks after using Phenelzine.
Selegiline	Do not combine. Wait 2 weeks after using Selegiline.
Tranylcypromine	Do not combine. Wait 2 weeks after using Tranylcypromine.

Sudafed Children's Nasal Decongestant Liquid

See Sudafed

Sudafed Cold & Allergy

And:	Action:
Alcohol	May cause extra drowsiness. Do not combine.
Alprazolam	May cause extra drowsiness. Check with your doctor.
Buspirone	May cause extra drowsiness. Check with your doctor.
Chlordiazepoxide	May cause extra drowsiness. Check with your doctor.
Chlorpromazine	May cause extra drowsiness. Check with your doctor.
Chlorprothixene	May cause extra drowsiness. Check with your doctor.
Clorazepate	May cause extra drowsiness. Check with your doctor.
Diazepam	May cause extra drowsiness. Check with your doctor.
Droperidol	May cause extra drowsiness. Check with your doctor.
Estazolam	May cause extra drowsiness. Check with your doctor.
Ethchlorvynol	May cause extra drowsiness. Check with your doctor.
Ethinamate	May cause extra drowsiness. Check with your doctor.
Fluphenazine	May cause extra drowsiness. Check with your doctor.
Flurazepam	May cause extra drowsiness. Check with your doctor.
Furazolidone	Do not combine. Wait 2 weeks after using Furazolidone.
Glutethimide	May cause extra drowsiness. Check with your doctor.
Haloperidol	May cause extra drowsiness. Check with your doctor.
Hydroxyzine	May cause extra drowsiness. Check with your doctor.
Isocarboxazid	Do not combine. Wait 2 weeks after using Isocarboxazid.
Lorazepam	May cause extra drowsiness. Check with your doctor.
Loxapine	May cause extra drowsiness. Check with your doctor.
Meprobamate	May cause extra drowsiness. Check with your doctor.
Mesoridazine	May cause extra drowsiness. Check with your doctor.
Midazolam	May cause extra drowsiness. Check with your doctor.
Molindone	May cause extra drowsiness. Check with your doctor.
Oxazepam	May cause extra drowsiness. Check with your doctor.
Perphenazine	May cause extra drowsiness. Check with your doctor.
Phenelzine	Do not combine. Wait 2 weeks after using Phenelzine.
Prazepam	May cause extra drowsiness. Check with your doctor.
Prochlorperazine	May cause extra drowsiness. Check with your doctor.
Promethazine	May cause extra drowsiness. Check with your doctor.
Propofol	May cause extra drowsiness. Check with your doctor.
Quazepam	May cause extra drowsiness. Check with your doctor.
Secobarbital	May cause extra drowsiness. Check with your doctor.

Selegiline	Do not combine. Wait 2 weeks after using Selegiline.
Temazepam	May cause extra drowsiness. Check with your doctor.
Thioridazine	May cause extra drowsiness. Check with your doctor.
Thiothixene	May cause extra drowsiness. Check with your doctor.
Tranylcypromine	Do not combine. Wait 2 weeks after using Tranylcypromine.
Triazolam	May cause extra drowsiness. Check with your doctor.
Trifluoperazine	May cause extra drowsiness. Check with your doctor.
Zolpidem	May cause extra drowsiness. Check with your doctor.

Sudafed Cold & Cough

And:	Action:
Alcohol	The acetaminophen in the medication may cause liver damage in heavy drinkers.
Furazolidone	Do not combine. Wait 2 weeks after using Furazolidone.
Isocarboxazid	Do not combine. Wait 2 weeks after using Isocarboxazid.
Phenelzine	Do not combine. Wait 2 weeks after using Phenelzine.
Selegiline	Do not combine. Wait 2 weeks after using Selegiline.
Tranylcypromine	Do not combine. Wait 2 weeks after using Tranylcypromine.

Sudafed Cold & Sinus

See Sudafed Cold & Cough

Sudafed Non-Drying Sinus

And:	Action:
Furazolidone	Do not combine. Wait 2 weeks after using Furazolidone.
Isocarboxazid	Do not combine. Wait 2 weeks after using Isocarboxazid.
Phenelzine	Do not combine. Wait 2 weeks after using Phenelzine.
Selegiline	Do not combine. Wait 2 weeks after using Selegiline.
Tranylcypromine	Do not combine. Wait 2 weeks after using Tranylcypromine.

Sudafed Severe Cold Formula

See Sudafed Non-Drying Sinus

Sudafed Sinus

See Sudafed Cold & Cough

Surfak

| And: | Action: |
| Mineral Oil | Do not combine without your doctor's approval. |

Tagamet HB

| And: | Action: |
| Aminophylline | Increases Aminophylline's effect. |

Amlodipine	Interactions have occurred with prescription-strength Tagamet. Check with your doctor.
Dyphylline	Increases Dyphylline's effect.
Felodipine	Interactions have occurred with prescription-strength Tagamet. Check with your doctor.
Isradipine	Interactions have occurred with prescription-strength Tagamet. Check with your doctor.
Nicardipine	Interactions have occurred with prescription-strength Tagamet. Check with your doctor.
Nifedipine	Interactions have occurred with prescription-strength Tagamet. Check with your doctor.
Nimodipine	Interactions have occurred with prescription-strength Tagamet. Check with your doctor.
Phenytoin	Interactions have occurred with prescription-strength Tagamet. Check with your doctor.
Theophylline	Increases Theophylline's effect.
Triazolam	Tagamet may increase the effect of triazolam.
Warfarin	Interactions have occurred with prescription-strength Tagamet. Check with your doctor.

Tavist-1

And:	Action:
Alcohol	May cause extra drowsiness. Do not combine.
Alprazolam	May cause extra drowsiness. Check with your doctor.
Buspirone	May cause extra drowsiness. Check with your doctor.
Chlordiazepoxide	May cause extra drowsiness. Check with your doctor.
Chlorpromazine	May cause extra drowsiness. Check with your doctor.
Chlorprothixene	May cause extra drowsiness. Check with your doctor.
Clorazepate	May cause extra drowsiness. Check with your doctor.
Diazepam	May cause extra drowsiness. Check with your doctor.
Droperidol	May cause extra drowsiness. Check with your doctor.
Estazolam	May cause extra drowsiness. Check with your doctor.
Ethchlorvynol	May cause extra drowsiness. Check with your doctor.
Ethinamate	May cause extra drowsiness. Check with your doctor.
Fluphenazine	May cause extra drowsiness. Check with your doctor.
Flurazepam	May cause extra drowsiness. Check with your doctor.
Furazolidone	Do not combine. Wait 2 weeks after using Furazolidone.
Glutethimide	May cause extra drowsiness. Check with your doctor.
Haloperidol	May cause extra drowsiness. Check with your doctor.

Hydroxyzine	May cause extra drowsiness. Check with your doctor.
Isocarboxazid	Do not combine. Wait 2 weeks after using Isocarboxazid.
Lorazepam	May cause extra drowsiness. Check with your doctor.
Loxapine	May cause extra drowsiness. Check with your doctor.
Meprobamate	May cause extra drowsiness. Check with your doctor.
Mesoridazine	May cause extra drowsiness. Check with your doctor.
Midazolam	May cause extra drowsiness. Check with your doctor.
Molindone	May cause extra drowsiness. Check with your doctor.
Oxazepam	May cause extra drowsiness. Check with your doctor.
Perphenazine	May cause extra drowsiness. Check with your doctor.
Phenelzine	Do not combine. Wait 2 weeks after using Phenelzine.
Prazepam	May cause extra drowsiness. Check with your doctor.
Prochlorperazine	May cause extra drowsiness. Check with your doctor.
Promethazine	May cause extra drowsiness. Check with your doctor.
Propofol	May cause extra drowsiness. Check with your doctor.
Quazepam	May cause extra drowsiness. Check with your doctor.
Secobarbital	May cause extra drowsiness, Check with your doctor.
Seleginine	Do not combine. Wait 2 weeks after using Seleginine.
Temazepam	May cause extra drowsiness. Check with your doctor.
Thioridazine	May cause extra drowsiness. Check with your doctor.
Thiothixene	May cause extra drowsiness. Check with your doctor.
Tranylcypromine	Do not combine. Wait 2 weeks after using Tranylcypromine.
Triazolam	May cause extra drowsiness. Check with your doctor.
Trifluoperazine	May cause extra drowsiness. Check with your doctor.
Zolpidem	May cause extra drowsiness. Check with your doctor.

Tavist-D

See Tavist-1

Teldrin

And:	Action:
Alcohol	May cause extra drowsiness. Do not combine.
Alprazolam	May cause extra drowsiness. Check with your doctor.
Buspirone	May cause extra drowsiness. Check with your doctor.
Chlordiazepoxide	May cause extra drowsiness. Check with your doctor.
Chlorpromazine	May cause extra drowsiness. Check with your doctor.
Chlorprothixene	May cause extra drowsiness. Check with your doctor.
Clorazepate	May cause extra drowsiness. Check with your doctor.

Diazepam	May cause extra drowsiness. Check with your doctor.
Droperidol	May cause extra drowsiness. Check with your doctor.
Estazolam	May cause extra drowsiness. Check with your doctor.
Ethchlorvynol	May cause extra drowsiness. Check with your doctor.
Ethinamate	May cause extra drowsiness. Check with your doctor.
Fluphenazine	May cause extra drowsiness. Check with your doctor.
Flurazepam	May cause extra drowsiness. Check with your doctor.
Furazolidone	Do not combine. Wait 2 weeks after using Furazolidone.
Glutethimide	May cause extra drowsiness. Check with your doctor.
Haloperidol	May cause extra drowsiness. Check with your doctor.
Hydroxyzine	May cause extra drowsiness. Check with your doctor.
Isocarboxazid	Do not combine. Wait 2 weeks after using Isocarboxazid.
Lorazepam	May cause extra drowsiness. Check with your doctor.
Loxapine	May cause extra drowsiness. Check with your doctor.
Meprobamate	May cause extra drowsiness. Check with your doctor.
Mesoridazine	May cause extra drowsiness. Check with your doctor.
Midazolam	May cause extra drowsiness. Check with your doctor.
Molindone	May cause extra drowsiness. Check with your doctor.
Oxazepam	May cause extra drowsiness. Check with your doctor.
Perphenazine	May cause extra drowsiness. Check with your doctor.
Phenelzine	Do not combine. Wait 2 weeks after using Phenelzine.
Prazepam	May cause extra drowsiness. Check with your doctor.
Prochlorperazine	May cause extra drowsiness. Check with your doctor.
Promethazine	May cause extra drowsiness. Check with your doctor.
Propofol	May cause extra drowsiness. Check with your doctor.
Quazepam	May cause extra drowsiness. Check with your doctor.
Secobarbital	May cause extra drowsiness. Check with your doctor.
Selegiline	Do not combine. Wait 2 weeks after using Selegiline.
Temazepam	May cause extra drowsiness. Check with your doctor.
Thioridazine	May cause extra drowsiness. Check with your doctor.
Thiothixene	May cause extra drowsiness. Check with your doctor.
Tranylcypromine	Do not combine. Wait 2 weeks after using Tranylcypromine.
Triazolam	May cause extra drowsiness. Check with your doctor.
Trifluoperazine	May cause extra drowsiness. Check with your doctor.
Zolpidem	May cause extra drowsiness. Check with your doctor.

TheraFlu Flu and Cold Medicine

And:	Action:
Alcohol	May cause extra drowsiness. Do not combine.
Alprazolam	May cause extra drowsiness. Check with your doctor.
Buspirone	May cause extra drowsiness. Check with your doctor.
Chlordiazepoxide	May cause extra drowsiness. Check with your doctor.
Chlorpromazine	May cause extra drowsiness. Check with your doctor.
Chlorprothixene	May cause extra drowsiness. Check with your doctor.
Clorazepate	May cause extra drowsiness. Check with your doctor.
Diazepam	May cause extra drowsiness. Check with your doctor.
Droperidol	May cause extra drowsiness. Check with your doctor.
Estazolam	May cause extra drowsiness. Check with your doctor.
Ethchlorvynol	May cause extra drowsiness. Check with your doctor.
Ethinamate	May cause extra drowsiness. Check with your doctor.
Fluphenazine	May cause extra drowsiness. Check with your doctor.
Flurazepam	May cause extra drowsiness. Check with your doctor.
Furazolidone	Do not combine. Wait 2 weeks after using Furazolidone.
Glutethimide	May cause extra drowsiness. Check with your doctor.
Haloperidol	May cause extra drowsiness. Check with your doctor.
Hydroxyzine	May cause extra drowsiness. Check with your doctor.
Isocarboxazid	Do not combine. Wait 2 weeks after using Isocarboxazid.
Lorazepam	May cause extra drowsiness. Check with your doctor.
Loxapine	May cause extra drowsiness. Check with your doctor.
Meprobamate	May cause extra drowsiness. Check with your doctor.
Mesoridazine	May cause extra drowsiness. Check with your doctor.
Midazolam	May cause extra drowsiness. Check with your doctor.
Molindone	May cause extra drowsiness. Check with your doctor.
Oxazepam	May cause extra drowsiness. Check with your doctor.
Perphenazine	May cause extra drowsiness. Check with your doctor.
Phenelzine	Do not combine. Wait 2 weeks after using Phenelzine.
Prazepam	May cause extra drowsiness. Check with your doctor.
Prochlorperazine	May cause extra drowsiness. Check with your doctor.
Promethazine	May cause extra drowsiness. Check with your doctor.
Propofol	May cause extra drowsiness. Check with your doctor.
Quazepam	May cause extra drowsiness. Check with your doctor.
Secobarbital	May cause extra drowsiness. Check with your doctor.

Selegiline	Do not combine. Wait 2 weeks after using Selegiline.
Temazepam	May cause extra drowsiness. Check with your doctor.
Thioridazine	May cause extra drowsiness. Check with your doctor.
Thiothixene	May cause extra drowsiness. Check with your doctor.
Tranylcypromine	Do not combine. Wait 2 weeks after using Tranylcypromine.
Triazolam	May cause extra drowsiness. Check with your doctor.
Trifluoperazine	May cause extra drowsiness. Check with your doctor.
Zolpidem	May cause extra drowsiness. Check with your doctor.

TheraFlu Flu, Cold & Cough Medicine

See TheraFlu Flu and Cold Medicine

TheraFlu Non-Drowsy Formulas

And:	Action:
Furazolidone	Do not combine. Wait 2 weeks after using Furazolidone.
Isocarboxazid	Do not combine. Wait 2 weeks after using Isocarboxazid.
Phenelzine	Do not combine. Wait 2 weeks after using Phenelzine.
Selegiline	Do not combine. Wait 2 weeks after using Selegiline.
Tranylcypromine	Do not combine. Wait 2 weeks after using Tranylcypromine.

Titralac

See Tums

Titralac Plus

See Tums

Triaminic

And:	Action:
Alcohol	May cause extra drowsiness. Do not combine.
Alprazolam	May cause extra drowsiness. Check with your doctor.
Buspirone	May cause extra drowsiness. Check with your doctor.
Chlordiazepoxide	May cause extra drowsiness. Check with your doctor.
Chlorpromazine	May cause extra drowsiness. Check with your doctor.
Chlorprothixene	May cause extra drowsiness. Check with your doctor.
Clorazepate	May cause extra drowsiness. Check with your doctor.
Diazepam	May cause extra drowsiness. Check with your doctor.
Droperidol	May cause extra drowsiness. Check with your doctor.
Estazolam	May cause extra drowsiness. Check with your doctor.
Ethchlorvynol	May cause extra drowsiness. Check with your doctor.
Ethinamate	May cause extra drowsiness. Check with your doctor.

Fluphenazine	May cause extra drowsiness. Check with your doctor.
Flurazepam	May cause extra drowsiness. Check with your doctor.
Furazolidone	Do not combine. Wait 2 weeks after using Furazolidone.
Glutethimide	May cause extra drowsiness. Check with your doctor.
Haloperidol	May cause extra drowsiness. Check with your doctor.
Hydroxyzine	May cause extra drowsiness. Check with your doctor.
Isocarboxazid	Do not combine. Wait 2 weeks after using Isocarboxazid.
Lorazepam	May cause extra drowsiness. Check with your doctor.
Loxapine	May cause extra drowsiness. Check with your doctor.
Meprobamate	May cause extra drowsiness. Check with your doctor.
Mesoridazine	May cause extra drowsiness. Check with your doctor.
Midazolam	May cause extra drowsiness. Check with your doctor.
Molindone	May cause extra drowsiness. Check with your doctor.
Oxazepam	May cause extra drowsiness. Check with your doctor.
Perphenazine	May cause extra drowsiness. Check with your doctor.
Phenelzine	Do not combine. Wait 2 weeks after using Phenelzine.
Phenylpropanolamine	Do not combine without your doctor's approval.
Prazepam	May cause extra drowsiness. Check with your doctor.
Prochlorperazine	May cause extra drowsiness. Check with your doctor.
Promethazine	May cause extra drowsiness. Check with your doctor.
Propofol	May cause extra drowsiness. Check with your doctor.
Quazepam	May cause extra drowsiness. Check with your doctor.
Secobarbital	May cause extra drowsiness. Check with your doctor.
Selegiline	Do not combine. Wait 2 weeks after using Selegiline.
Temazepam	May cause extra drowsiness. Check with your doctor.
Thioridazine	May cause extra drowsiness. Check with your doctor.
Thiothixene	May cause extra drowsiness. Check with your doctor.
Tranylcypromine	Do not combine. Wait 2 weeks after using Tranylcypromine.
Triazolam	May cause extra drowsiness. Check with your doctor.
Trifluoperazine	May cause extra drowsiness. Check with your doctor.
Zolpidem	May cause extra drowsiness. Check with your doctor.

Triaminic AM Cough and Decongestant Formula

And:	Action:
Furazolidone	Do not combine. Wait 2 weeks after using Furazolidone.
Isocarboxazid	Do not combine. Wait 2 weeks after using Isocarboxazid.

Phenelzine	Do not combine. Wait 2 weeks after using Phenelzine.
Selegiline	Do not combine. Wait 2 weeks after using Selegiline.
Tranylcypromine	Do not combine. Wait 2 weeks after using Tranylcypromine.

Triaminic AM Decongestant Formula

See Triaminic AM Cough and Decongestant Formula

Triaminic DM

And:	Action:
Furazolidone	Do not combine. Wait 2 weeks after using Furazolidone.
Isocarboxazid	Do not combine. Wait 2 weeks after using Isocarboxazid.
Phenelzine	Do not combine. Wait 2 weeks after using Phenelzine.
Phenylpropanolamine	Do not combine without your doctor's approval.
Selegiline	Do not combine. Wait 2 weeks after using Selegiline.
Tranylcypromine	Do not combine. Wait 2 weeks after using Tranylcypromine.

Triaminic Expectorant

See Triaminic DM

Triaminic Infant Oral Decongestant Drops

See Triaminic AM Cough and Decongestant Formula

Triaminic Night Time

See Triaminic

Triaminic Sore Throat Formula

See Triaminic AM Cough and Decongestant Formula

Triaminicin

See Triaminic

Triaminicol

See Triaminic

Tums

And:	Action:
Alendronate	Allow 2 to 3 hours between doses of the antacid and the drug.
Allopurinol	Allow 2 to 3 hours between doses of the antacid and the drug.
Arthritis Drugs	Allow 2 to 3 hours between doses of the antacid and the drug.
Aspirin	Allow 2 to 3 hours between doses of the antacid and the drug.
Atenolol	Allow 2 to 3 hours between doses of the antacid and the drug.
Captopril	Allow 2 to 3 hours between doses of the antacid and the drug.
Chlordiazepoxide	Allow 2 to 3 hours between doses of the antacid and the drug.

Cimetidine	Allow 2 to 3 hours between doses of the antacid and the drug.
Ciprofloxacin	Allow 2 to 3 hours between doses of the antacid and the drug.
Demeclocycline	Allow 2 to 3 hours between doses of the antacid and the drug.
Digoxin	Allow 2 to 3 hours between doses of the antacid and the drug.
Doxycycline	Allow 2 to 3 hours between doses of the antacid and the drug.
Enoxacin	Allow 2 to 3 hours between doses of the antacid and the drug.
Fosfomycin	Allow 2 to 3 hours between doses of the antacid and the drug.
Gabapentin	Allow 2 to 3 hours between doses of the antacid and the drug.
Glipizide	Allow 2 to 3 hours between doses of the antacid and the drug.
Glyburide	Allow 2 to 3 hours between doses of the antacid and the drug.
Isoniazid	Allow 2 to 3 hours between doses of the antacid and the drug.
Ketoconazole	Allow 2 to 3 hours between doses of the antacid and the drug.
Levothyroxine	Allow 2 to 3 hours between doses of the antacid and the drug.
Lomefloxacin	Allow 2 to 3 hours between doses of the antacid and the drug.
Methacycline	Allow 2 to 3 hours between doses of the antacid and the drug.
Methenamine	Allow 2 to 3 hours between doses of the antacid and the drug.
Metronidazole	Allow 2 to 3 hours between doses of the antacid and the drug.
Minocycline	Allow 2 to 3 hours between doses of the antacid and the drug.
Misoprostol	Allow 2 to 3 hours between doses of the antacid and the drug.
Mycophenolate	Allow 2 to 3 hours between doses of the antacid and the drug.
Norfloxacin	Allow 2 to 3 hours between doses of the antacid and the drug.
Ofloxacin	Allow 2 to 3 hours between doses of the antacid and the drug.
Oxytetracycline	Allow 2 to 3 hours between doses of the antacid and the drug.
Penicillamine	Allow 2 to 3 hours between doses of the antacid and the drug.
Phenytoin	Allow 2 to 3 hours between doses of the antacid and the drug.
Quinidine	Allow 2 to 3 hours between doses of the antacid and the drug.
Sodium Polystyrene Sulfonate	Allow 2 to 3 hours between doses of the antacid and the drug.
Sucralfate	Allow 2 to 3 hours between doses of the antacid and the drug.
Tetracycline	Allow 2 to 3 hours between doses of the antacid and the drug.
Tilodronate	Allow 2 to 3 hours between doses of the antacid and the drug.
Ursodiol	Allow 2 to 3 hours between doses of the antacid and the drug.

Tums Antigas/Antacid Formula

See Tums

Tums E-X

See Tums

Tums Ultra

See Tums

Tylenol

And:	Action:
Alcohol	The acetaminophen in the medication may cause liver damage in heavy drinkers.

Tylenol Allergy Sinus

And:	Action:
Alcohol	May cause extra drowsiness, and the acetaminophen in the medication may cause liver damage in heavy drinkers.
Alprazolam	May cause extra drowsiness. Check with your doctor.
Buspirone	May cause extra drowsiness. Check with your doctor.
Chlordiazepoxide	May cause extra drowsiness. Check with your doctor.
Chlorpromazine	May cause extra drowsiness. Check with your doctor.
Chlorprothixene	May cause extra drowsiness. Check with your doctor.
Clorazepate	May cause extra drowsiness. Check with your doctor.
Diazepam	May cause extra drowsiness. Check with your doctor.
Droperidol	May cause extra drowsiness. Check with your doctor.
Estazolam	May cause extra drowsiness. Check with your doctor.
Ethchlorvynol	May cause extra drowsiness. Check with your doctor.
Ethinamate	May cause extra drowsiness. Check with your doctor.
Fluphenazine	May cause extra drowsiness. Check with your doctor.
Flurazepam	May cause extra drowsiness. Check with your doctor.
Furazolidone	Do not combine. Wait 2 weeks after using Furazolidone.
Glutethimide	May cause extra drowsiness. Check with your doctor.
Haloperidol	May cause extra drowsiness. Check with your doctor.
Hydroxyzine	May cause extra drowsiness. Check with your doctor.
Isocarboxazid	Do not combine. Wait 2 weeks after using Isocarboxazid.
Lorazepam	May cause extra drowsiness. Check with your doctor.
Loxapine	May cause extra drowsiness. Check with your doctor.
Meprobamate	May cause extra drowsiness. Check with your doctor.
Mesoridazine	May cause extra drowsiness. Check with your doctor.
Midazolam	May cause extra drowsiness. Check with your doctor.
Molindone	May cause extra drowsiness. Check with your doctor.
Oxazepam	May cause extra drowsiness. Check with your doctor.
Perphenazine	May cause extra drowsiness. Check with your doctor.

Phenelzine	Do not combine. Wait 2 weeks after using Phenelzine.
Prazepam	May cause extra drowsiness. Check with your doctor.
Prochlorperazine	May cause extra drowsiness. Check with your doctor.
Promethazine	May cause extra drowsiness. Check with your doctor.
Propofol	May cause extra drowsiness. Check with your doctor.
Quazepam	May cause extra drowsiness. Check with your doctor.
Secobarbital	May cause extra drowsiness. Check with your doctor.
Selegiline	Do not combine. Wait 2 weeks after using Selegiline.
Temazepam	May cause extra drowsiness. Check with your doctor.
Thioridazine	May cause extra drowsiness. Check with your doctor.
Thiothixene	May cause extra drowsiness. Check with your doctor.
Tranylcypromine	Do not combine. Wait 2 weeks after using Tranylcypromine.
Triazolam	May cause extra drowsiness. Check with your doctor.
Trifluoperazine	May cause extra drowsiness. Check with your doctor.
Zolpidem	May cause extra drowsiness. Check with your doctor.

Tylenol Allergy Sinus NightTime

See Tylenol Allergy Sinus

Tylenol Children's Cold

And:	Action:
Alprazolam	May cause extra drowsiness. Check with your doctor.
Buspirone	May cause extra drowsiness. Check with your doctor.
Chlordiazepoxide	May cause extra drowsiness. Check with your doctor.
Chlorpromazine	May cause extra drowsiness. Check with your doctor.
Chlorprothixene	May cause extra drowsiness. Check with your doctor.
Clorazepate	May cause extra drowsiness. Check with your doctor.
Diazepam	May cause extra drowsiness. Check with your doctor.
Droperidol	May cause extra drowsiness. Check with your doctor.
Estazolam	May cause extra drowsiness. Check with your doctor.
Ethchlorvynol	May cause extra drowsiness. Check with your doctor.
Ethinamate	May cause extra drowsiness. Check with your doctor.
Fluphenazine	May cause extra drowsiness. Check with your doctor.
Flurazepam	May cause extra drowsiness. Check with your doctor.
Furazolidone	Do not combine. Wait 2 weeks after using Furazolidone.
Glutethimide	May cause extra drowsiness. Check with your doctor.
Haloperidol	May cause extra drowsiness. Check with your doctor.

Hydroxyzine	May cause extra drowsiness. Check with your doctor.
Isocarboxazid	Do not combine. Wait 2 weeks after using Isocarboxazid.
Lorazepam	May cause extra drowsiness. Check with your doctor.
Loxapine	May cause extra drowsiness. Check with your doctor.
Meprobamate	May cause extra drowsiness. Check with your doctor.
Mesoridazine	May cause extra drowsiness. Check with your doctor.
Midazolam	May cause extra drowsiness. Check with your doctor.
Molindone	May cause extra drowsiness. Check with your doctor.
Oxazepam	May cause extra drowsiness. Check with your doctor.
Perphenazine	May cause extra drowsiness. Check with your doctor.
Phenelzine	Do not combine. Wait 2 weeks after using Phenelzine.
Prazepam	May cause extra drowsiness. Check with your doctor.
Prochlorperazine	May cause extra drowsiness. Check with your doctor.
Promethazine	May cause extra drowsiness. Check with your doctor.
Propofol	May cause extra drowsiness. Check with your doctor.
Quazepam	May cause extra drowsiness. Check with your doctor.
Secobarbital	May cause extra drowsiness. Check with your doctor.
Selegiline	Do not combine. Wait 2 weeks after using Selegiline.
Temazepam	May cause extra drowsiness. Check with your doctor.
Thioridazine	May cause extra drowsiness. Check with your doctor.
Thiothixene	May cause extra drowsiness. Check with your doctor.
Tranylcypromine	Do not combine. Wait 2 weeks after using Tranylcypromine.
Triazolam	May cause extra drowsiness. Check with your doctor.
Trifluoperazine	May cause extra drowsiness. Check with your doctor.
Zolpidem	May cause extra drowsiness. Check with your doctor.

Tylenol Children's Cold Plus Cough

See Tylenol Children's Cold

Tylenol Children's Flu Liquid

See Tylenol Children's Cold

Tylenol Cold Medication

See Tylenol Allergy Sinus

Tylenol Cold Medication, Hot Liquid Packets

See Tylenol Allergy Sinus

Tylenol Cold Medication, No Drowsiness Formula

See Tylenol Cold Severe Congestion

Tylenol Cold Severe Congestion

And:	Action:
Alcohol	The acetaminophen in the medication may cause liver damage in heavy drinkers.
Furazolidone	Do not combine. Wait 2 weeks after using Furazolidone.
Isocarboxazid	Do not combine. Wait 2 weeks after using Isocarboxazid.
Phenelzine	Do not combine. Wait 2 weeks after using Phenelzine.
Selegiline	Do not combine. Wait 2 weeks after using Selegiline.
Tranylcypromine	Do not combine. Wait 2 weeks after using Tranylcypromine.

Tylenol Cough Medication

See Tylenol Cold Severe Congestion

Tylenol Cough Medication with Decongestant

See Tylenol Cold Severe Congestion

Tylenol Extended Relief Caplets

See Tylenol

Tylenol Extra Strength Adult Liquid Pain Reliever

See Tylenol

Tylenol Extra Strength Gelcaps, Geltabs, Caplets, Tablets

See Tylenol

Tylenol Flu NightTime Gelcaps

See Tylenol Allergy Sinus

Tylenol Flu NightTime, Hot Medication Packets

See Tylenol Allergy Sinus

Tylenol Flu No Drowsiness Formula

See Tylenol Cold Severe Congestion

Tylenol Infants' Cold Drops

And:	Action:
Furazolidone	Do not combine. Wait 2 weeks after using Furazolidone.
Isocarboxazid	Do not combine. Wait 2 weeks after using Isocarboxazid.
Phenelzine	Do not combine. Wait 2 weeks after using Phenelzine.
Selegiline	Do not combine. Wait 2 weeks after using Selegiline.
Tranylcypromine	Do not combine. Wait 2 weeks after using Tranylcypromine.

Tylenol PM

And:	Action:
Alcohol	The acetaminophen in the medication may cause liver damage in heavy drinkers.

Alprazolam	May cause extra drowsiness. Check with your doctor.
Buspirone	May cause extra drowsiness. Check with your doctor.
Chlordiazepoxide	May cause extra drowsiness. Check with your doctor.
Chlorpromazine	May cause extra drowsiness. Check with your doctor.
Chlorprothixene	May cause extra drowsiness. Check with your doctor.
Clorazepate	May cause extra drowsiness. Check with your doctor.
Diazepam	May cause extra drowsiness. Check with your doctor.
Droperidol	May cause extra drowsiness. Check with your doctor.
Estazolam	May cause extra drowsiness. Check with your doctor.
Ethchlorvynol	May cause extra drowsiness. Check with your doctor.
Ethinamate	May cause extra drowsiness. Check with your doctor.
Fluphenazine	May cause extra drowsiness. Check with your doctor.
Flurazepam	May cause extra drowsiness. Check with your doctor.
Glutethimide	May cause extra drowsiness. Check with your doctor.
Haloperidol	May cause extra drowsiness. Check with your doctor.
Hydroxyzine	May cause extra drowsiness. Check with your doctor.
Lorazepam	May cause extra drowsiness. Check with your doctor.
Loxapine	May cause extra drowsiness. Check with your doctor.
Meprobamate	May cause extra drowsiness. Check with your doctor.
Mesoridazine	May cause extra drowsiness. Check with your doctor.
Midazolam	May cause extra drowsiness. Check with your doctor.
Molindone	May cause extra drowsiness. Check with your doctor.
Oxazepam	May cause extra drowsiness. Check with your doctor.
Perphenazine	May cause extra drowsiness. Check with your doctor.
Prazepam	May cause extra drowsiness. Check with your doctor.
Prochlorperazine	May cause extra drowsiness. Check with your doctor.
Promethazine	May cause extra drowsiness. Check with your doctor.
Propofol	May cause extra drowsiness. Check with your doctor.
Quazepam	May cause extra drowsiness. Check with your doctor.
Secobarbital	May cause extra drowsiness. Check with your doctor.
Temazepam	May cause extra drowsiness. Check with your doctor.
Thioridazine	May cause extra drowsiness. Check with your doctor.
Thiothixene	May cause extra drowsiness. Check with your doctor.
Triazolam	May cause extra drowsiness. Check with your doctor.
Trifluoperazine	May cause extra drowsiness. Check with your doctor.
Zolpidem	May cause extra drowsiness. Check with your doctor.

Tylenol Severe Allergy

See Tylenol Allergy Sinus

Tylenol Sinus

See Tylenol Cold Severe Congestion

Unifiber

No interactions reported.

Unisom

And:	Action:
Alcohol	Increases Unisom's effect.
Alprazolam	Increases Unisom's effect.
Aprobarbital	Increases Unisom's effect.
Buprenorphine	Increases Unisom's effect.
Buspirone	Increases Unisom's effect.
Butabarbital	Increases Unisom's effect.
Butalbital	Increases Unisom's effect.
Chlordiazepoxide	Increases Unisom's effect.
Chlorpromazine	Increases Unisom's effect.
Chlorprothixene	Increases Unisom's effect.
Clorazepate	Increases Unisom's effect.
Clozapine	Increases Unisom's effect.
Codeine	Increases Unisom's effect.
Dezocine	Increases Unisom's effect.
Diazepam	Increases Unisom's effect.
Droperidol	Increases Unisom's effect.
Estazolam	Increases Unisom's effect.
Ethchlorvynol	Increases Unisom's effect.
Ethinamate	Increases Unisom's effect.
Fentanyl	Increases Unisom's effect.
Fluphenazine	Increases Unisom's effect.
Flurazepam	Increases Unisom's effect.
Furazolidone	Increases and prolongs the effect of Unisom.
Glutethimide	Increases Unisom's effect.
Haloperidol	Increases Unisom's effect.
Hydrocodone	Increases Unisom's effect.
Hydromorphone	Increases Unisom's effect.

Hydroxyzine	Increases Unisom's effect.
Isocarboxazid	Increases and prolongs the effect of Unisom.
Ketamine	Increases Unisom's effect.
Levomethadyl	Increases Unisom's effect.
Levorphanol	Increases Unisom's effect.
Lorazepam	Increases Unisom's effect.
Loxapine	Increases Unisom's effect.
Meperidine	Increases Unisom's effect.
Mephobarbital	Increases Unisom's effect.
Meprobamate	Increases Unisom's effect.
Mesoridazine	Increases Unisom's effect.
Methadone	Increases Unisom's effect.
Methohexital	Increases Unisom's effect.
Methotrimeprazine	Increases Unisom's effect.
Midazolam	Increases Unisom's effect.
Molindone	Increases Unisom's effect.
Morphine	Increases Unisom's effect.
Oxazepam	Increases Unisom's effect.
Oxycodone	Increases Unisom's effect.
Pentobarbital	Increases Unisom's effect.
Perphenazine	Increases Unisom's effect.
Phenelzine	Increases and prolongs the effect of Unisom.
Phenobarbital	Increases Unisom's effect.
Prazepam	Increases Unisom's effect.
Prochlorperazine	Increases Unisom's effect.
Promethazine	Increases Unisom's effect.
Propofol	Increases Unisom's effect.
Propoxyphene	Increases Unisom's effect.
Quazepam	Increases Unisom's effect.
Risperidone	Increases Unisom's effect.
Secobarbital	Increases Unisom's effect.
Selegiline	Increases and prolongs the effect of Unisom.
Temazepam	Increases Unisom's effect.
Thiamylal Sodium	Increases Unisom's effect.
Thioridazine	Increases Unisom's effect.
Thiothixene	Increases Unisom's effect.

Tranylcypromine	Increases and prolongs the effect of Unisom.
Triazolam	Increases Unisom's effect.
Trifluoperazine	Increases Unisom's effect.
Zolpidem	Increases Unisom's effect.

Unisom With Pain Relief

See Unisom

Vanquish

And:	Action:
Acarbose	Do not combine without your doctor's approval.
Arthritis Medications	Do not combine without your doctor's approval.
Chlorpropamide	Do not combine without your doctor's approval.
Dicumarol	Do not combine without your doctor's approval.
Glimepiride	Do not combine without your doctor's approval.
Glipizide	Do not combine without your doctor's approval.
Glyburide	Do not combine without your doctor's approval.
Metformin	Do not combine without your doctor's approval.
Miglitol	Do not combine without your doctor's approval.
Probenecid	Do not combine without your doctor's approval.
Sulfinpyrazone	Do not combine without your doctor's approval.
Tolazamide	Do not combine without your doctor's approval.
Tolbutamide	Do not combine without your doctor's approval.
Troglitazone	Do not combine without your doctor's approval.
Warfarin	Do not combine without your doctor's approval.

Vasocon-A

No interactions reported.

Vicks 44 Cough Relief

And:	Action:
Furazolidone	Do not combine. Wait 2 weeks after using Furazolidone.
Isocarboxazid	Do not combine. Wait 2 weeks after using Isocarboxazid.
Phenelzine	Do not combine. Wait 2 weeks after using Phenelzine.
Selegiline	Do not combine. Wait 2 weeks after using Selegiline.
Tranylcypromine	Do not combine. Wait 2 weeks after using Tranylcypromine.

Vicks 44D

See Vicks 44 Cough Relief

Vicks 44E

See Vicks 44 Cough Relief

Vicks 44M

And:	Action:
Alcohol	May cause extra drowsiness. Do not combine.
Alprazolam	May cause extra drowsiness. Check with your doctor.
Buspirone	May cause extra drowsiness. Check with your doctor.
Chlordiazepoxide	May cause extra drowsiness. Check with your doctor.
Chlorpromazine	May cause extra drowsiness. Check with your doctor.
Chlorprothixene	May cause extra drowsiness. Check with your doctor.
Clorazepate	May cause extra drowsiness. Check with your doctor.
Diazepam	May cause extra drowsiness. Check with your doctor.
Droperidol	May cause extra drowsiness. Check with your doctor.
Estazolam	May cause extra drowsiness. Check with your doctor.
Ethchlorvynol	May cause extra drowsiness. Check with your doctor.
Ethinamate	May cause extra drowsiness. Check with your doctor.
Fluphenazine	May cause extra drowsiness. Check with your doctor.
Flurazepam	May cause extra drowsiness. Check with your doctor.
Furazolidone	Do not combine. Wait 2 weeks after using Furazolidone.
Glutethimide	May cause extra drowsiness. Check with your doctor.
Haloperidol	May cause extra drowsiness. Check with your doctor.
Hydroxyzine	May cause extra drowsiness. Check with your doctor.
Isocarboxazid	Do not combine. Wait 2 weeks after using Isocarboxazid.
Lorazepam	May cause extra drowsiness. Check with your doctor.
Loxapine	May cause extra drowsiness. Check with your doctor.
Meprobamate	May cause extra drowsiness. Check with your doctor.
Mesoridazine	May cause extra drowsiness. Check with your doctor.
Midazolam	May cause extra drowsiness. Check with your doctor.
Molindone	May cause extra drowsiness. Check with your doctor.
Oxazepam	May cause extra drowsiness. Check with your doctor.
Perphenazine	May cause extra drowsiness. Check with your doctor.
Phenelzine	Do not combine. Wait 2 weeks after using Phenelzine.
Prazepam	May cause extra drowsiness. Check with your doctor.
Prochlorperazine	May cause extra drowsiness. Check with your doctor.
Promethazine	May cause extra drowsiness. Check with your doctor.
Propofol	May cause extra drowsiness. Check with your doctor.

Quazepam	May cause extra drowsiness. Check with your doctor.
Secobarbital	May cause extra drowsiness. Check with your doctor.
Selegiline	Do not combine. Wait 2 weeks after using Selegiline.
Temazepam	May cause extra drowsiness. Check with your doctor.
Thioridazine	May cause extra drowsiness. Check with your doctor.
Thiothixene	May cause extra drowsiness. Check with your doctor.
Tranylcypromine	Do not combine. Wait 2 weeks after using Tranylcypromine.
Triazolam	May cause extra drowsiness. Check with your doctor.
Trifluoperazine	May cause extra drowsiness. Check with your doctor.
Zolpidem	May cause extra drowsiness. Check with your doctor.

Vicks Chloraseptic Cough & Throat Drops

No interactions reported.

Vicks Chloraseptic Sore Throat Lozenges

No interactions reported.

Vicks Chloraseptic Sore Throat Spray

No interactions reported.

Vicks Cough Drops

No interactions reported.

Vicks DayQuil

See Vicks 44 Cough Relief

Vicks DayQuil Allergy

And:	*Action:*
Alcohol	Do not combine.
Furazolidone	Do not combine. Wait 2 weeks after using Furazolidone.
Isocarboxazid	Do not combine. Wait 2 weeks after using Isocarboxazid.
Phenelzine	Do not combine. Wait 2 weeks after using Phenelzine.
Selegiline	Do not combine. Wait 2 weeks after using Selegiline.
Tranylcypromine	Do not combine. Wait 2 weeks after using Tranylcypromine.

Vicks DayQuil, Children's Allergy

See Vicks 44M

Vicks DayQuil Sinus Pressure & Pain Relief

See Vicks 44 Cough Relief

Vicks NyQuil

See Vicks 44M

Vicks NyQuil, Children's

See Vicks 44M

Vicks NyQuil Hot Therapy

See Vicks 44M

Vicks Sinex

No interactions reported.

Vicks Sinex 12-Hour

No interactions reported.

Zantac 75

No interactions reported.

4. Side Effect Guide

If you take several different over-the-counter medicines over a short period of time, then develop an unpleasant reaction, it may be impossible to tell which drug was the culprit. This table will help you track down the source of the problem. It lists the over-the-counter drugs known to cause each type of side effect.

If, for example, you're taking Aleve for pain, Imodium A-D for diarrhea, and Sudafed for head congestion, and you begin having trouble with heartburn, the table will show you that, of the three drugs, only Aleve is prone to cause the problem. Based on this knowledge, you can continue taking the other medications without worry while you find a substitute for Aleve.

The listings include the drugs that specifically note the side effect in the manufacturer's package labeling, as published in *PDR for Nonprescription Drugs*, the doctor's guide to over-the-counter medications. In addition, side effects shared by an entire family of drugs are sometimes listed for each of its members, even if the individual labeling doesn't mention it. The table is restricted to only those side effects likely to occur at recommended dosage levels in a typical person. It does not include symptoms of an overdose. If you suspect that there has been an overdose, don't waste any time; seek medical attention immediately.

Abdominal discomfort

Children's Motrin Oral
   Suspension
Correctol
Dulcolax Tablets and
   Suppositories
Ensure Plus
Fleet Bisacodyl Enema
Fleet Prep Kits
Senna X-Prep Bowel
   Evacuant Liquid
Osmolite HN Liquid Nutrition

Abdominal pain/cramps

Correctol
Ensure Plus
Fleet Bisacodyl Enema
Fleet Prep Kits
Osmolite HN Liquid Nutrition
Peri-Colace

Allergic reactions

Konsyl Powder
Metamucil
Tronolane Anesthetic Cream
   for Hemorrhoids

Blood pressure increase

Bufferin
Ecotrin
Halfprin
Propagest
Sinulin

Blurred vision

Bonine
Donnagel

Bone weakness
(in dialysis patients)

ALternaGEL
Amphojel
Basaljel

Maalox
Maalox Antacid/Anti-Gas
Mylanta Liquid

Burning sensation

Anusol Hemorrhoidal Ointment
Caladryl Cream For Kids
Capzasin-P Topical Analgesic
   Creme
Fleet Babylax
Fleet Bisacodyl Enema
Fleet Prep Kits
Zilactin

Burning, nasal

Afrin 12 Hour
Duration 12 Hour
4-Way 12 Hour Nasal Spray
4-Way Fast Acting Nasal Spray
Neo-Synephrine
Neo-Synephrine 12 Hour
Vicks Sinex

Constipation

Alka-Mints
ALternaGEL
Amphojel
Basaljel
Feosol
Ryna-C Liquid
Ryna-CX Liquid

Contact lens staining

Prodium

Dehydration

Fleet Enema

Delivery complications

Actron
Advil
Advil Cold and Sinus
Aleve
Alka-Seltzer

Alka-Seltzer Plus Cold & Cough
  Medicine Tablets
Alka-Seltzer Plus Cold
  Medicine Tablets
Alka-Seltzer Plus Night-Time
  Cold Medicine Tablets
Alka-Seltzer Plus Sinus
  Medicine Tablets
Aspirin Regimen Bayer
Bayer Arthritis Pain Regimen
  Formula
Bayer Aspirin
Bayer PM
BC Allergy Sinus Cold Powders
BC Powder
BC Sinus Cold Powder
Ecotrin
Goody's Powder and Tablets
Orudis KT
St. Joseph Aspirin
Vanquish

Dementia (in dialysis patients)

ALternaGEL
Amphojel
Basaljel
Maalox
Maalox Antacid/Anti-Gas
Mylanta Liquid

Diarrhea

Ensure Plus
Feosol
Mylanta Liquid
Osmolite HN Liquid Nutrition
Peri-Colace

Dizziness

Actifed Cold & Allergy
Actifed Cold & Sinus
Advil Cold and Sinus
Alka-Seltzer Plus Cold &
  Cough Medicine Tablets

Alka-Seltzer Plus Cold
  Medicine Tablets
Alka-Seltzer Plus Night-Time
  Cold Medicine Tablets
Alka-Seltzer Plus Sinus
  Medicine Tablets
Benadryl Allergy Decongestant
Benadryl Allergy Sinus
  Headache Caplets
Benylin Multisymptom
Bufferin
Cerose DM
Chlor-Trimeton Allergy/
  Decongestant
Comtrex Allergy-Sinus
Contac
Contac Severe Cold and Flu
Coricidin 'D'
Coricidin Cough & Cold Tablets
Dexatrim
Dimetapp
Dimetapp Cold & Allergy
Donnagel
Drixoral Allergy/Sinus
Drixoral Cold & Allergy
Drixoral Cold & Flu
Ecotrin
Novahistine
Novahistine DMX
Pediatric Vicks 44M
Propagest
Robitussin Cold & Cough
Robitussin Cough & Cold
Robitussin Pediatric
  Cough & Cold Formula
Robitussin-CF
Robitussin-PE
Ryna Liquid
Ryna-C Liquid
Ryna-CX Liquid
Sine-Aid
Sinulin
Sinutab
Sudafed

Sudafed Cold & Allergy
Sudafed Sinus
Tylenol Children's Cold
Tylenol Cold Medications
Tylenol Cold Medication,
No Drowsiness Formula
Tylenol Cough Medication
with Decongestant
Tylenol Flu NightTime Gelcaps
and Hot Medication
Tylenol Flu No Drowsiness
Formula
Tylenol Sinus
Vicks 44D
Vicks 44M
Vicks DayQuil
Vicks DayQuil, Children's
Allergy
Vicks Nyquil
Vicks NyQuil, Children's
Cold/Cough

Drowsiness

Actifed Allergy
Daytime/Nighttime Caplets
Actifed Cold & Allergy
Actifed Cold & Sinus
Actifed Sinus Daytime/Nighttime
Alka-Seltzer Plus Cold &
Cough Medicine Liqui-Gels
Alka-Seltzer Plus Cold &
Cough Medicine Tablets
Alka-Seltzer Plus Cold
Medicine Liqui-Gels
Alka-Seltzer Plus Cold
Medicine Tablets
Alka-Seltzer Plus Flu & Body
Aches Tablets
Alka-Seltzer Plus Night-Time
Cold Medicine Liqui-Gels
Alka-Seltzer Plus Night-Time
Cold Medicine Tablets

Alka-Seltzer Plus Sinus
Medicine Tablets
BC Allergy Sinus Cold Powder
Benadryl Allergy
Benadryl Allergy Decongestant
Benadryl Allergy/Cold Tablets
Bonine
Cerose DM
Cheracol Plus
Chlor-Trimeton Allergy
Chlor-Trimeton Allergy/
Decongestant
Comtrex Allergy-Sinus
Comtrex Cold & Flu Reliever
Contac
Contac Day & Night Cold/Flu
Night Caplets
Contac Severe Cold and Flu
Coricidin 'D'
Coricidin Cold & Flu Tablets
Coricidin Cough & Cold Tablets
Dimetapp
Dimetapp Allergy
Dimetapp Allergy Sinus
Dimetapp Cold & Allergy
Dimetapp Cold and Cough
Products
Dimetapp Cold and Fever
Dimetapp DM Elixir
Drixoral Allergy/Sinus
Drixoral Cold & Allergy
Drixoral Cold & Flu
Midol Menstrual Formula
Midol PMS Formula
Nolahist
Novahistine
PediaCare Cough-Cold
PediaCare NightRest Cough-Cold
Pediatric Vicks 44M
Robitussin Night-Time
Cold Formula
Ryna Liquid
Ryna-C Liquid

Sine-Off
Singlet
Sinulin
Sinutab Sinus Allergy
Sudafed Cold & Allergy
Teldrin
Tylenol Allergy Sinus
Tylenol Allergy Sinus NightTime
Tylenol Children's Cold
Tylenol Children's Cold
  Plus Cough
Tylenol Children's Flu Liquid
Tylenol Cold Medications
Tylenol Flu NightTime Gelcaps
  and Hot Medication
Tylenol PM
Tylenol Severe Allergy
Vicks 44M
Vicks DayQuil Allergy
Vicks DayQuil, Children's
  Allergy
Vicks Nyquil
Vicks NyQuil, Children's
  Cold/Cough

Dry mouth

Bonine
Donnagel
Novahistine

Dry skin

Donnagel

Excitability

Actifed Cold & Allergy
Actifed Cold & Sinus
Alka-Seltzer Plus Cold &
  Cough Medicine Liqui-Gels
Alka-Seltzer Plus Cold &
  Cough Medicine Tablets
Alka-Seltzer Plus Cold
  Medicine Liqui-Gels
Alka-Seltzer Plus Cold
  Medicine Tablets

Alka-Seltzer Plus Night-Time
  Cold Medicine Liqui-Gels
Alka-Seltzer Plus Night-Time
  Cold Medicine Tablets
Alka-Seltzer Plus Sinus
  Medicine Tablets
Benadryl Allergy
Benadryl Allergy Decongestant
Cerose DM
Cheracol Plus
Chlor-Trimeton Allergy
Chlor-Trimeton Allergy/
  Decongestant
Comtrex Allergy-Sinus
Contac
Contac Severe Cold & Flu
Coricidin 'D'
Coricidin Cold & Flu Tablets
Dimetapp
Dimetapp Allergy
Dimetapp Allergy Sinus
Dimetapp Cold & Allergy
Dimetapp Cold and Cough
  Products
Dimetapp Cold and Fever
Dimetapp DM Elixir
Drixoral Allergy/Sinus
Drixoral Cold & Allergy
Drixoral Cold & Flu
Nolahist
PediaCare Cough-Cold
PediaCare NightRest Cough-Cold
Pediatric Vicks 44M
Robitussin Night-Time Cold
  Formula
Ryna Liquid
Ryna-C Liquid
Sine-Off
Singlet
Sinulin
Sudafed Cold & Allergy
Teldrin
Tylenol Allergy Sinus
Tylenol Children's Cold

Tylenol Children's Cold
  Plus Cough
Tylenol Cold Medications
Tylenol Flu NightTime Gelcaps
  and Hot Medication
Vicks 44M
Vicks DayQuil Allergy
Vicks DayQuil, Children's
  Allergy
Vicks Nyquil
Vicks NyQuil, Children's
  Cold/Cough

Fainting

Fleet Bisacodyl Enema

Fetal harm

Actron
Advil Cold and Sinus
Aleve
Alka-Seltzer Plus Cold &
  Cough Medicine Tablets
Alka-Seltzer Plus Cold
  Medicine Tablets
Alka-Seltzer Plus Night-Time
  Cold Medicine Tablets
Alka-Seltzer Plus Sinus
  Medicine Tablets
Aspirin Regimen Bayer
Bayer Arthritis Pain Regimen
  Formula
Bayer Aspirin
Bayer PM
BC Allergy Sinus Cold Powder
BC Powder
BC Sinus Cold Powders
Encare Vaginal Contraceptive
  Suppositories
Nuprin
Orudis KT

Flushing

Donnagel

Headache

Dexatrim

Hearing loss

Alka-Seltzer
Aspirin Regimen Bayer
Bayer Arthritis Pain Regimen
  Formula
Bayer Aspirin
Bayer PM
Bufferin
Ecotrin

Heartburn

Aleve
Bufferin
Ecotrin
Halfprin
Novahistine
St. Joseph Aspirin

Insomnia

Actifed Cold & Allergy
Actifed Cold & Sinus
Advil Cold and Sinus
Alka-Seltzer Plus Cold &
  Cough Medicine Tablets
Alka-Seltzer Plus Cold
  Medicine Tablets
Alka-Seltzer Plus Night-Time
  Cold Medicine Tablets
Alka-Seltzer Plus Sinus
  Medicine Tablets
Benadryl Allergy Decongestant
Benadryl Allergy Sinus
  Headache Caplets
Benylin Multisymptom
Cerose DM
Chlor-Trimeton Allergy/
  Decongestant
Comtrex Allergy-Sinus
Contac
Contac Severe Cold and Flu
Coricidin 'D'
Dexatrim
Dimetapp

Dimetapp Cold & Allergy
Drixoral Cold & Allergy
Drixoral Cold & Flu
Nolahist
Novahistine
Novahistine DMX
Pediatric Vicks 44M
Primatene Tablets
Propagest
Robitussin Cold & Cough
Robitussin Cough & Cold
Robitussin Pediatric
   Cough & Cold Formula
Robitussin-CF
Robitussin-PE
Ryna Liquid
Ryna-C Liquid
Ryna-CX Liquid
Sine-Aid
Sinulin
Sinutab
Sudafed
Sudafed Cold & Allergy
Sudafed Sinus
Tylenol Children's Cold
Tylenol Cold Medications
Tylenol Cold Medication,
   No Drowsiness Formula
Tylenol Cough Medication with
   Decongestant
Tylenol Flu NightTime Gelcaps
   and Hot Medication
Tylenol Flu No Drowsiness
   Formula
Tylenol Sinus
Vicks 44D
Vicks 44M
Vicks DayQuil
Vicks DayQuil, Children's
   Allergy
Vicks Nyquil
Vicks NyQuil, Children's
   Cold/Cough

Irritation, anal

Anusol Hemorrhoidal Ointment

Irritation, eyes

Clear Eyes
Eye-Stream Solution
Muro 128
Visine L.R. Eye Drops
Viva-Drops

Irritation, skin

Aspercreme Creme Analgesic Rub
Betadine Solution
Chloresium Ointment and
   Solution
Lotrimin AF
MG 217 Sal-Acid Ointment
Mycelex Cream
Occlusal-HP
Pronto Lice Killing Shampoo
SalAc
Sportscreme

Irritation, vaginal

Encare Vaginal Contraceptive
   Suppositories
Massengill

Itching

Chloresium Ointment and
   Solution

Liver damage

Unisom with Pain Relief

Nausea

Bufferin
Colace
Ecotrin
Ensure Plus
Feosol
Halfprin
Osmolite HN Liquid Nutrition

Peri-Colace
Senna X-Prep Bowel
    Evacuant Liquid
St. Joseph Aspirin

Nervousness

Actifed Cold & Allergy
Actifed Cold & Sinus
Advil Cold and Sinus
Alka-Seltzer Plus Cold & Cough
    Medicine Tablets
Alka-Seltzer Plus Cold Medicine
    Tablets
Alka-Seltzer Plus Night-Time
    Cold Medicine Tablets
Alka-Seltzer Plus Sinus
    Medicine Tablets
Benadryl Allergy Decongestant
Benadryl Allergy Sinus
    Headache Caplets
Benylin Multisymptom
Cerose DM
Chlor-Trimeton Allergy
    Decongestant
Comtrex Allergy-Sinus
Contac
Contac Severe Cold & Flu
Coricidin 'D'
Dexatrim
Dimetapp
Dimetapp Cold & Allergy
Drixoral Allergy/Sinus
Drixoral Cold & Allergy
Drixoral Cold & Flu
Nolahist
Novahistine
Novahistine DMX
Pediatric Vicks 44M
Primatene Tablets
Propagest
Robitussin Cold & Cough
Robitussin Cough & Cold
Robitussin Pediatric Cough &
    Cold Formula

Robitussin-CF
Robitussin-PE
Ryna Liquid
Ryna-C Liquid
Ryna-CX Liquid
Sine-Aid
Sinulin
Sinutab
Sudafed
Sudafed Cold & Allergy
Sudafed Sinus
Tylenol Children's Cold
Tylenol Cold Medications
Tylenol Cold Medication,
    No Drowsiness Formula
Tylenol Cough Medication
    with Decongestant
Tylenol Flu NightTime Gelcaps
    and Hot Medication
Tylenol Flu No Drowsiness
    Formula
Tylenol Sinus
Vicks 44D
Vicks 44M
Vicks DayQuil
Vicks DayQuil, Children's
    Allergy
Vicks Nyquil
Vicks NyQuil, Children's
    Cold/Cough

Pain, eyes

Clear Eyes
Eye-Stream Solution
Visine L.R. Eye Drops
Viva-Drops

Pelvic inflammatory disease

Massengill

Pulse, fast

Propagest
Sinulin

Rash

Colace
Peri-Colace
Phillips' Gelcaps

Redness, eyes

Eye-Stream Solution
Visine L.R. Eye Drops
Viva-Drops

Reye's Syndrome (nausea, vomiting, lethargy)

Alka-Seltzer
Alka-Seltzer Plus Cold & Cough Medicine Tablets
Alka-Seltzer Plus Cold Medicine Tablets
Alka-Seltzer Plus Night-Time Cold Medicine Tablets
Alka-Seltzer Plus Sinus Medicine Tablets
Aspirin Regimen Bayer
Backache Caplets
Bayer Arthritis Pain Regimen Formula
Bayer Aspirin
Bayer PM
BC Allergy Sinus Cold Powders
BC Powder
BC Sinus Cold Powder
Bufferin
Ecotrin
Excedrin
Goody's Powder and Tablets
Pepto-Bismol
St. Joseph Aspirin
Vanquish

Ringing in the ears

Alka-Seltzer
Aspirin Regimen Bayer
Backache Caplets

Bayer Arthritis Pain Regimen Formula
Bayer Aspirin
Bayer PM
BC Allergy Sinus Cold Powders
BC Powder
BC Sinus Cold Powder
Bufferin
Ecotrin
Excedrin
Pepto-Bismol

Runny nose

4-Way 12 Hour Nasal Spray
4-Way Fast Acting Nasal Spray
Neo-Synephrine
Neo-Synephrine 12 Hour
Vicks Sinex

Sensitivity reactions

Anusol Hemorrhoidal Ointment
Betadine Skin Cleanser
Children's Tylenol
Infants' Tylenol
Junior Strength Tylenol
Sine-Aid
Sinulin
Tylenol
Tylenol Allergy Sinus
Tylenol Cold Medication, No Drowsiness Formula
Tylenol Flu NightTime Gelcaps and Hot Medication
Tylenol Severe Allergy
Tylenol Sinus

Sensitivity, sun

Tegrin Dandruff Shampoo
Tegrin for Psoriasis

Sneezing

Afrin 12 Hour
Duration 12 Hour
4-Way 12 Hour Nasal Spray

4-Way Fast Acting Nasal Spray
Neo-Synephrine
Neo-Synephrine 12 Hour
Vicks Sinex

Stinging, nasal

Afrin 12 Hour
Duration 12 Hour
4-Way 12 Hour Nasal Spray
4-Way Fast Acting Nasal Spray
Neo-Synephrine
Neo-Synephrine 12 Hour
Vicks Sinex

Stomach blockage

Ecotrin

Stomach or intestinal bleeding

Bufferin
Ecotrin
Halfprin
St. Joseph Aspirin

Stomach or intestinal disorders

Bufferin
Ecotrin
Halfprin
Novahistine DMX
Prodium
St. Joseph Aspirin

Stomachache

Aleve
Bufferin

Ecotrin
Feosol
Halfprin
St. Joseph Aspirin

Stool color changes

Pepto-Bismol

Throat irritation

Colace

Tongue discoloration

Pepto-Bismol

Urination problems

Donnagel

Urine color change

Prodium

Vaginal dryness

Massengill

Visual disturbances

Clear Eyes
Eye-Stream Solution
Visine L.R. Eye Drops
Viva-Drops

Vomiting

Bufferin
Ecotrin
Halfprin
Novahistine
Senna X-Prep Bowel Evacuant
    Liquid
St. Joseph Aspirin

II. Vitamin/Mineral Supplements

5. Product Selection Tables

If you're shopping for a multivitamin/mineral supplement, this section arms you with a unique comparison grid that will instantly show you which common brands have the highest amounts of any ingredient you're interested in. The grid includes entries for all vitamins and minerals—except sodium—assigned a Recommended Dietary Allowance (Daily Value) by the U.S. Food and Drug Administration.

The amounts listed are drawn from the manufacturer's package labeling, primarily as published in *PDR for Nonprescription Drugs*. For easy comparison, the figures have been converted as necessary from the unit of measure used by the manufacturer to the measurement most frequently employed in the industry. To conserve space, these measurements are not shown in the grid. They are as follows:

Ingredient	Measure
Vitamin A (Retinol, Beta-carotene)	International Units
Vitamin B_1 (Thiamin)	Milligrams
Vitamin B_2 (Riboflavin)	Milligrams
Vitamin B_3 (Niacin)	Milligrams
Vitamin B_5 (Pantothenic Acid)	Milligrams
Vitamin B_6 (Pyridoxine)	Milligrams
Vitamin B_9 (Folic Acid)	Micrograms
Vitamin B_{12} (Cobalamin)	Micrograms
Vitamin C (Ascorbic Acid)	Milligrams
Vitamin D	International Units
Vitamin E	International Units
Biotin	Micrograms
Calcium	Milligrams
Copper	Milligrams
Iodine	Micrograms

Iron	Milligrams
Magnesium	Milligrams
Phosphorus	Milligrams
Potassium	Milligrams
Zinc	Milligrams

The grid is divided into two parts: the first covers general multivitamin/mineral supplements; the second focuses on supplements sold especially for children.

Many of the brands in the grid include other ingredients that have nutritional importance but lack an official Recommended Dietary Allowance from the government. The presence of additional ingredients is noted in the last column of the grid. These ingredients can be found in the pages immediately following the grid, listed alphabetically by brand name.

BRAND	A	B_1	B_2	B_3	B_5	B_6	B_9	B_{12}	C
ACES	5,000	—	—	—	—	—	—	—	500
Caltrate Plus	—	—	—	—	—	—	—	—	—
Centrum	5,000	1.5	1.7	20	10	2	400	6	60
Centrum Silver	5,000	1.5	1.7	20	10	3	400	25	60
Complete for Men	6,666	4.5	5.1	12.3	4.7	4	133	6.5	250
Complete for Women	4,000	2.7	3	7.4	4	2.8	80	3.9	150
DiabeVite	1,250	1.5	1.7	20	10	2	800	6	250
Dical-D Tablets	—	—	—	—	—	—	—	—	—
Dical-D Wafers	—	—	—	—	—	—	—	—	—
Fat Burning Factors	—	3.75	4.25	9.5	10	10	100	20	100
Gerimed	5,000	3	3	25	—	2	—	6	120
Healthy Heart	—	—	—	—	—	50	800	500	600
Hep-Forte	1,200	1	1	10	2	0.5	60	1	10
Heplive	1,200	1	1	10	2	0.5	60	1,000	10
Iberet Filmtab	—	6	6	30	10	5	—	25	150
Iberet-500 Filmtab	—	6	6	30	10	5	—	25	500
Iberet Liquid	—	1.5	1.5	7.5	—	1.25	—	6.25	37.5
Iberet-500 Liquid	—	1.5	1.5	7.5	—	1.25	—	6.25	125
LipoSpray Multi Vitamin	1,500	0.5	0.3	4	3	0.5	100	0.5	15
Mega-B	—	100	100	100	100	100	100	100	—
Megadose	25,000*	80	80	80	80	80	400	80	250
Natural MD Basic Life for Men	5,000	6.75	7.5	19	10	6	200	9	150
Natural MD Basic Life for Women	2,500	3.6	4.1	11.75	7.5	4.5	100	4.9	75

*USP units

D	E	BIOTIN	CALCIUM	COPPER	IODINE	IRON	MAGNESIUM	PHOSPHORUS	POTASSIUM	ZINC	OTHER
—	200	—	—	—	—	—	—	—	—	—	Y
200	—	—	600	1	—	—	40	—	—	7.5	Y
400	30	30	162	2	150	18	100	109	80	15	Y
400	45	30	200	2	150	4	100	48	80	15	Y
133	100	20	67	0.5	50	1.7	33	—	—	10	Y
80	60	12	120	0.3	30	2	40	—	—	6	Y
100	100	300	—	2	—	—	100	—	—	15	Y
133	—	—	117	—	—	—	—	90	—	—	—
200	—	—	232	—	—	—	—	180	—	—	—
—	—	15	—	—	—	—	—	—	—	—	Y
400	30	—	370	—	—	—	—	130	—	15	—
—	400	—	—	—	—	—	—	—	—	—	—
—	10	3.3	—	—	—	—	—	—	—	2	Y
—	10	3,300	—	—	—	—	—	—	—	2	Y
—	—	—	—	—	—	105	—	—	—	—	—
—	—	—	—	—	—	105	—	—	—	—	—
—	—	—	—	—	—	26.25	—	—	—	—	Y
—	—	—	—	—	—	26.25	—	—	—	—	Y
100	3	5	—	—	—	—	—	—	—	—	—
—	—	100	—	—	—	—	—	—	—	—	Y
1,000*	100	80	50	0.5	150	10	7	—	10	25	Y
200	75	15	80	0.75	75	2.5	50	—	—	11.25	Y
100	37.5	7.5	150	0.375	37.5	1.25	50	—	—	6.25	Y

BRAND	A	B_1	B_2	B_3	B_5	B_6	B_9	B_{12}	C
Natural MD Complete Life	3,571	5.7	5.7	5.7	5.7	10.7	85.7	35.7	285.7
Natural MD Essential Life	5,000	7.5	7.5	7.5	7.5	12.5	100	31.25	250
Natural MD Ultimate Life	3,333	5.6	5.6	5.6	5.6	11.1	88.8	44.4	277.7
One-A-Day 50 Plus	5,000	4.5	3.4	20	15	6	400	30	120
One-A-Day Antioxidant Plus	5,000	—	—	—	—	—	—	—	250
One-A-Day Essential	5,000	1.5	1.7	20	10	2	400	6	60
One-A-Day Maximum	5,000	1.5	1.7	20	10	2	400	6	60
One-A-Day Women's	5,000	1.5	1.7	20	10	2	400	6	60
Phyto-Vite	25,000	15	17	100	75	20	400	60	500
Pro-Hepatone	—	2.5	2.5	10	10	2.5	—	32.4	10
Protegra	5,000	—	—	—	—	—	—	—	250
Stress Gum	833.5	0.25	0.28	3.3	0.65	0.33	20	1	30
Stresstabs	—	10	10	100	20	5	400	12	500
Stresstabs + Iron	—	10	10	100	20	5	400	12	500
Stresstabs + Zinc	—	10	10	100	20	5	400	12	500
Theragran	5,000	3	3.4	20	10	3	400	9	90
Theragran-M	5,000	3	3.4	20	10	3	400	9	90
Vitasana	2,000	1.2	1.7	15	—	2	200	1	60

CHILDREN

BRAND	A	B_1	B_2	B_3	B_5	B_6	B_9	B_{12}	C
Bugs Bunny Complete	5,000	1.5	1.7	20	10	2	400	6	60
Bugs Bunny Plus Iron	2,500	1.05	1.2	13.5	—	1.05	300	4.5	60

D	E	BIOTIN	CALCIUM	COPPER	IODINE	IRON	MAGNESIUM	PHOSPHORUS	POTASSIUM	ZINC	OTHER
14.3	85.7	42.9	14.3	0.21	—	—	19.6	—	—	3.2	Y
25	100	75	25	0.25	—	—	17.2	—	—	3.75	Y
11.1	88.8	33.3	11.1	0.22	—	—	21.6	—	—	3.3	Y
400	60	30	120	2	150	—	100	.—	37.5	22.5	Y
—	200	—	—	1	—	—	—	—	—	7.5	Y
400	30	—	—	—	—	—	—	—	—	—	—
400	30	30	130	2	150	18	100	100	37.5	15	Y
400	30	—	450	—	—	27	—	—	—	15	—
400	400	300	500	2	150	4	400	250	70	15	Y
—	10	—	—	—	—	0.32	—	—	—	—	Y
—	200	—	—	1	—	—	—	—	—	7.5	Y
10	15	5	—	—	—	—	—	—	—	—	Y
—	30	45	—	—	—	—	—	—	—	—	—
—	30	45	—	—	—	18	—	—	—	—	—
—	30	45	—	3	—	—	—	—	—	23.9	—
400	30	30	—	—	—	—	—	—	—	—	—
400	30	30	40	2	150	18	100	31	7.5	15	Y
200	15	—	100	1	—	9	10	80	8	1	Y
400	30	40	100	2	150	18	20	100	—	15	—
400	15	—	—	—	—	15	—	—	—	—	—

BRAND	A	B₁	B₂	B₃	B₅	B₆	B₉	B₁₂	C
Bugs Bunny with Extra C	2,500	1.05	1.2	13.5	—	1.05	300	4.5	250
Centrum, Jr. + Extra C	5,000	1.5	1.7	20	10	2	400	6	300
Centrum, Jr. + Extra Calcium	5,000	1.5	1.7	20	10	2	400	6	60
Centrum, Jr. + Iron	5,000	1.5	1.7	20	10	2	400	6	60
Flintstones	2,500	1.05	1.2	13.5	—	1.05	300	4.5	60
Flintstones Complete	5,000	1.5	1.7	20	10	2	400	6	60
Flintstones Plus Calcium	2500	1.05	1.2	13.5	—	1.05	300	4.5	60
Flintstones Plus Extra C	2500	1.05	1.2	13.5	—	1.05	300	4.5	250
Flintstones Plus Iron	2500	1.05	1.2	13.5	—	1.05	300	4.5	60
Sunkist Children's Chewable— Complete	5,000	1.5	1.7	20	10	2	400	6	60
Sunkist Children's Chewable + Extra C	2,500	1.1	1.2	14	—	1	300	5	250

D	E	BIOTIN	CALCIUM	COPPER	IODINE	IRON	MAGNESIUM	PHOSPHORUS	POTASSIUM	ZINC	OTHER
400	15	—	—	—	—	—	—	—	—	—	—
400	30	45	108	2	150	18	40	50	—	15	Y
400	30	45	160	2	150	18	40	50	—	15	Y
400	30	45	108	2	150	18	40	50	—	15	Y
400	15	—	—	—	—	15	—	—	—	—	—
400	30	40	100	2	150	18	20	100	—	15	—
400	15	—	200	—	—	—	—	—	—	—	—
400	15	—	—	—	—	—	—	—	—	—	—
400	15	—	—	—	—	15	—	—	—	—	—
400	30	40	100	2	150	18	20	78	—	10	Y
400	15	—	—	—	—	—	—	—	—	—	Y

Other Ingredients

ACES

Selenium, *100 micrograms*

Caltrate Plus

Boron, *250 micrograms*
Manganese, *1.8 milligrams*

Centrum

Vitamin K, *25 micrograms*
Boron, *150 micrograms*
Chloride, *72 milligrams*
Chromium, *65 micrograms*
Manganese, *3.5 milligrams*
Molybdenum, *160 micrograms*
Nickel, *5 micrograms*
Selenium, *20 micrograms*
Silicon, *2 milligrams*
Tin, *10 micrograms*
Vanadium, *10 micrograms*

Centrum Silver

Vitamin K, *10 micrograms*
Boron, *150 micrograms*
Chloride, *72 milligrams*
Chromium, *130 micrograms*
Manganese, *3.5 milligrams*
Molybdenum, *160 micrograms*
Nickel, *5 micrograms*
Selenium, *20 micrograms*
Silicon, *2 milligrams*
Vanadium, *10 micrograms*

Centrum, Jr. + Extra C

Vitamin K, *10 micrograms*
Chromium, *20 micrograms*
Manganese, *1 milligram*
Molybdenum, *20 micrograms*

Centrum, Jr. + Extra Calcium

Vitamin K, *10 micrograms*
Chromium, *20 micrograms*
Manganese, *1 milligram*
Molybdenum, *20 micrograms*

Centrum, Jr. + Iron

Vitamin K, *10 micrograms*
Chromium, *20 micrograms*
Manganese, *1 milligram*
Molybdenum, *20 micrograms*

Complete for Men

Vitamin K_1, *80 micrograms*
Boron, *200 micrograms*
Chromium, *100 micrograms*
Manganese, *2 milligrams*
Molybdenum, *75 micrograms*
Selenium, *140 micrograms*
Vanadium, *10 micrograms*

Complete for Women

Vitamin K_1, *80 micrograms*
Boron, *800 micrograms*
Chromium, *100 micrograms*
Manganese, *2 milligrams*
Molybdenum, *75 micrograms*
Selenium, *140 micrograms*
Vanadium, *10 micrograms*

DiabeVite

Chromium, *200 micrograms*
Manganese, *2.5 milligrams*
Selenium, *25 micrograms*

Fat Burning Factors

Arginine, *100 milligrams*
Choline bitartrate, *100 milligrams*
Chromium, *200 micrograms*
Inositol, *100 milligrams*
Isoleucine, *25 milligrams*
L-Carnitine, *200 milligrams*
Leucine, *100 milligrams*
Lysine, *200 milligrams*
Valine, *50 milligrams*

Gerimed

Calcium carbonate, *200 milligrams*
Dibasic calcium
    phosphate, *600 milligrams*

Hep-Forte

Choline bitartrate, *21 milligrams*
Desiccated liver, *194.4 milligrams*
dl-Methionine, *10 milligrams*
Inositol, *10 milligrams*
Liver concentrate, *64.8 milligrams*
Liver fraction number 2,
   64.8 milligrams
Yeast (dried), *64.8 milligrams*

Heplive

Choline bitartrate, *21 milligrams*
Desiccated liver, *194.4 milligrams*
dl-Methionine, *10 milligrams*
Inositol, *10 milligrams*
Liver concentrate, *64.8 milligrams*
Liver fraction number 2,
   64.8 milligrams
Yeast (dried), *64.8 milligrams*

Iberet Liquid

Dexpanthenol, *2.5 milligrams*

Iberet-500 Liquid

Dexpanthenol, *2.5 milligrams*

Mega-B

Choline bitartrate, *100 milligrams*
Inositol, *100 milligrams*
Para-Aminobenzoic
   acid (PABA), *100 milligrams*

Megadose

Betaine hydrochloride,
   30 milligrams
Choline bitartrate, *80 milligrams*
Citrus bioflavonoids,
   30 milligrams
Glutamic acid, *30 milligrams*
Hesperidin complex, *5 milligrams*
Inositol, *80 milligrams*
Manganese gluconate,
   6 milligrams

Para-aminobenzoic
   acid (PABA), *80 milligrams*
Rutin, *30 milligrams*

Natural MD Basic Life for Men

Vitamin K_1, *80 micrograms*
Boron, *200 micrograms*
Chromium, *100 micrograms*
Manganese, *2 milligrams*
Molybdenum, *75 micrograms*
Selenium, *105 micrograms*
Vanadium, *10 micrograms*

Natural MD Basic Life for Women

Vitamin K_1, *100 micrograms*
Boron, *1 milligram*
Chromium, *150 micrograms*
Manganese, *2 milligrams*
Molybdenum, *75 micrograms*
Selenium, *105 micrograms*
Vanadium, *10 micrograms*

Natural MD Complete Life

Bilberry extract, *5 milligrams*
Boron, *100 micrograms*
Chondroitin sulfate,
   25 milligrams
Chromium, *150 micrograms*
Citrus bioflavonoids,
   100 milligrams
Co-Enzyme Q-10, *60 milligrams*
Cranberry extract, *20 milligrams*
Garlic concentrate, *400 milligrams*
Glucosamine sulfate,
   25 milligrams
Grape seed extract,
   12.5 milligrams
Green tea extract, *100 milligrams*
L-Carnitine, *50 milligrams*
L-Taurine, *75 milligrams*
Lipoic acid, *50 milligrams*
Lycopene, *1500 micrograms*

Manganese, *1 milligram*
Milk thistle extract, *16 milligrams*
N-Acetylcysteine, *100 milligrams*
Octacosanol, *0.25 milligram*
Pine bark extract, *2.5 milligrams*
Quercetin, *10 milligrams*
Red wine concentrate,
    40 milligrams
Selenium, *150 micrograms*
Shark cartilage, *25 milligrams*

Natural MD Essential Life

Boron, *100 micrograms*
Chromium, *100 micrograms*
Citrus bioflavonoids,
    100 milligrams
Cranberry extract, *20 milligrams*
Garlic concentrate,
    400 milligrams
Green tea extract, *100 milligrams*
Lycopene, *1 gram*
Manganese, *1 milligram*
Red wine concentrate,
    40 milligrams
Selenium, *100 micrograms*

Natural MD Ultimate Life

Bilberry extract, *10 milligrams*
Boron, *100 micrograms*
Chondroitin sulfate,
    50 milligrams
Chromium, *200 micrograms*
Citrus bioflavonoids,
    100 milligrams
Co-Enzyme Q-10, *120 milligrams*
Cranberry extract, *20 milligrams*
Garlic concentrate,
    400 milligrams
Glucosamine sulfate,
    50 milligrams
Grape seed extract, *25 milligrams*
Green tea extract, *100 milligrams*
L-Carnitine, *100 milligrams*
L-Taurine, *150 milligrams*

Lipoic acid, *100 milligrams*
Lycopene, *2 milligrams*
Manganese, *1 milligram*
Milk thistle extract, *32 milligrams*
N-Acetylcysteine, *200 milligrams*
Octacosanol, *0.5 milligram*
Pine bark extract, *5 milligrams*
Quercetin, *20 milligrams*
Red wine concentrate,
    40 milligrams
Selenium, *200 micrograms*
Shark cartilage, *50 milligrams*

One-A-Day 50 Plus

Vitamin K, *20 micrograms*
Chloride, *34 milligrams*
Chromium, *180 micrograms*
Manganese, *4 milligrams*
Molybdenum, *93.75 micrograms*
Selenium, *105 micrograms*

One-A-Day Antioxidant Plus

Manganese, *1.5 milligrams*
Selenium, *15 micrograms*

One-A-Day Maximum

Chloride, *34 milligrams*
Chromium, *10 micrograms*
Manganese, *2.5 milligrams*
Molybdenum, *10 micrograms*
Selenium, *10 micrograms*

Phyto-Vite

Vitamin K, *70 micrograms*
Bilberry standardized
    extract, *10 milligrams*
Boron, *1 milligram*
Catalase and peroxidase
    enzymes, *3,500 Units*
Choline, *50 milligrams*
Chromium, *200 micrograms*
Citrus bioflavonoids with
    Hesperidin, *50 milligrams*

Essential fatty acids,
100 milligrams
Ginkgo biloba standardized
extract, *20 milligrams*
Grape seed proanthocyanidins,
5 milligrams
Inositol, *50 milligrams*
Manganese, *5 milligrams*
PABA, *25 milligrams*
Phytonutrient blend,
800 milligrams
Red grape polyphenols,
5 milligrams
Rutin and Quercetin,
50 milligrams
Selenium, *200 micrograms*

Pro-Hepatone

Choline bitartrate, *100 milligrams*
Desiccated liver, *64.8 milligrams*
Desoxycholic acid, *25 milligrams*
Fructose, *100 milligrams*
Gluthathione, *5 milligrams*
Glycine, *100 milligrams*
Inositol, *100 milligrams*
L-Arginine, *5 milligrams*
L-Aspartic acid, *10 milligrams*
L-Cysteine HCl, *10 milligrams*
L-Glutamine, *10 milligrams*
L-Ornithine, *5 milligrams*
Lecithin, *100 milligrams*
Liver concentrate,
64.8 milligrams

Methionine, *100 milligrams*
Thiotic acid, *5 milligrams*
Unsaturated fatty acid,
640 milligrams

Protegra

Manganese, *1.5 milligrams*
Selenium, *15 micrograms*

Stress Gum

Chromium, *5 micrograms*
Selenium, *5 micrograms*

Sunkist Children's Chewable—Complete

Vitamin K, *10 micrograms*
Manganese, *1 milligram*

Sunkist Children's Chewable + Extra C

Vitamin K, *5 micrograms*

Theragran-M

Vitamin K, *28 micrograms*
Chloride, *7.5 milligrams*
Chromium, *26 micrograms*
Manganese, *3.5 milligrams*
Molybdenum, *32 micrograms*
Selenium, *21 micrograms*

Vitasana

Manganese, *2 milligrams*
Standardized G115 ginseng
extract, *80 milligrams*

6. Vitamin/Mineral Profiles

If you're curious about the precise role played by any of the ingredients in a commercial multivitamin/mineral supplement (or, for that matter, their role in your everyday diet), the profiles in this section will provide you with a brief answer.

More important, they'll also tell you whether you can overdose on the substance, and what problems might result if you do. They'll provide you with the exact recommended allowances for every age group. And they'll tell you how to boost the amount in your diet, in case your chosen vitamin supplement doesn't provide enough.

You'll find that, with most ingredients, it takes sustained megadosing to produce any ill effects. Nevertheless, if you develop any of the symptoms listed in these profiles and suspect a possible overdose, you should check with your doctor immediately. This is especially true if you are also taking prescription drugs.

Alpha-Tocopherol

See Vitamin E

Arginine

See Nonessential Amino Acids

Ascorbic Acid

See Vitamin C

Aspartic Acid

See Nonessential Amino Acids

Beta-Carotene

See Vitamin A

Beta-Tocopherol

See Vitamin E

Biotin

What it is

Biotin, sometimes called vitamin H, is produced naturally within the body by normal intestinal bacteria. This supply is all that a normal, healthy adult needs. Biotin is one of the water-soluble vitamins. There is no synthetic form available.

What it does

Biotin helps the body form fatty acids and process amino acids, starches, and sugars.

Why you need it

Biotin helps maintain the health of the body's sweat glands, nerve tissue, blood cells, bone marrow, skin, hair, and male sex glands.

Can you take too much?

Scientists currently consider natural biotin supplements to be nontoxic. Doses of 50 to 100 times the recommended intake have caused no ill effects.

Recommended daily allowances

The government has not yet established an official recommended dietary allowance (RDA) for biotin.

■ ADULTS

The estimated adequate intake for everyone 11 years of age and older is 100 to 200 micrograms per day.

■ CHILDREN

The following daily amounts are estimated to be adequate for children.

Infants up to 6 months: 35 micrograms
Ages 6 to 12 months: 50 micrograms
Ages 1 to 3 years: 65 micrograms
Ages 4 to 6 years: 85 micrograms
Ages 7 to 10 years: 120 micrograms

Best dietary sources

Biotin is found in dairy products, including butter, cheese, and milk; nuts, including cashews, peanuts, and walnuts; vegetables, including green peas, lentils, soybeans, and split peas; meats; organ meats, especially calves' liver; chicken; eggs; fish, including mackerel and tuna; whole-grain foods, including brown rice, bulgur, wheat, and oats; sunflower seeds; and brewer's yeast.

Branched-Chain Amino Acids

What they are

Three essential amino acids—leucine, isoleucine, and valine—form the so-called branched chain. Amino acids are the building blocks of protein. These three are among those considered essential because they cannot be manufactured in the body and must be obtained through diet.

What they do

Along with the other amino acids, the branched-chain acids are the raw material used by the body to manufacture human proteins. These proteins are a vital component of all the body's cells.

Why you need them

Scientific evidence shows that branched-chain amino acids may help restore muscle mass following surgery, an injury, or trauma. They also help in people who have liver disease. There currently is no evidence that extra branched-chain amino acids are beneficial for healthy individuals. However, a general deficiency of protein in the diet can cause a loss of stamina, lowered resistance to infection, slow healing of wounds, weakness, and depression.

Can you take too much?

Amino acids are rarely toxic, even in large amounts.

Recommended daily allowances

There is no official recommended dietary allowance for the branched-chain amino acids, either separately or as a group. The estimated adult daily requirement for leucine is nearly 9 milligrams per pound of body weight. Infants require almost 5 times that amount; children need approximately twice the adult requirement. For isoleucine, the estimated adult daily requirement is about 6 milligrams per pound of body weight. Infants require more than 3 times that amount; the requirement for children is about twice the adult amount.

The estimated adult daily requirement for valine is also about 6 milligrams per pound of body weight. Infants require more than 4 times that amount, while children need about twice the adult requirement. Your total daily requirement for protein in general is the number of grams equal to half your body weight. For instance, if you weigh 160 pounds, you need 80 grams of protein daily.

Best dietary sources

These and other amino acids are available in most meat and dairy products.

Calcifidol

See Vitamin D

Calcitrol

See Vitamin D

Calcium

What it is

Calcium and phosphorus—the two most abundant minerals in our bodies—work together to keep our bones and teeth healthy. Calcium is found in many foods—most notably dairy products—and is also available as natural and synthetic supplements. You will need a prescription for certain forms of calcium; others can be purchased over the counter.

What it does

Fully 99 percent of our calcium deposits are stored in the bones. In response to the body's needs, calcium moves out of the bones into the bloodstream and then back into the bones for continued storage. Most of the remaining 1 percent of our calcium supply is located in body fluids, where it helps transmit nerve impulses. Calcium also promotes blood coagulation and plays an essential role in enabling muscles, such as the heart, to relax and contract.

Why you need it

Calcium is essential to a child's normal growth and development, and everyone needs an adequate supply to keep bones and teeth strong and healthy. Because of the part it plays in muscle activity, some people take it to prevent muscle cramps; others use it to alleviate their severe muscle spasms that accompany a disorder called tetany. One of calcium's more recently—and widely—publicized benefits is its ability to stave off the brittle-bone disease osteoporosis when used in combination with estrogen.

Can you take too much?

Doses above 2,000 milligrams per day can lead to potentially serious problems, including development of kidney stones. A loss of appetite, constipation, drowsiness, dry mouth or a metallic taste in the mouth, headache, and a feeling of fatigue or weakness could be early warning signs that there is too much calcium in your system. Later signs may include confusion, depression, nausea, vomiting, pain in bones or muscles, high blood pressure, increased thirst or urination, increased sensitivity of the eyes or skin to light, itchy skin or rash, and a slow or irregular heartbeat. If you notice any of these symptoms and you think the amount of calcium you have been taking could be the source of the problem, stop using the supplements and call your doctor. If you think your heartbeat is either irregular or slow, seek medical attention

Recommended daily allowances

■ ADULTS

The basic allowance for everyone 18 years of age and older is 800 milligrams.

Women need an additional 400 milligrams of calcium each day during pregnancy and as long as they breastfeed. Do not take megadoses of calcium during pregnancy or while breastfeeding. Calcium does pass into the breast milk.

Many experts believe that we need more calcium than the official recommendation and suggest the following amounts: 1,000 milligrams of calcium per day for premenopausal women and, due to the risk of osteoporosis, 1,500 milligrams for postmenopausal women and for both elderly men and women past the age of 65.

■ CHILDREN
Infants up to 6 months: 400 milligrams
Ages 6 to 12 months: 600 milligrams
Ages 1 to 10 years: 800 milligrams
Ages 11 to 24 years: 1,200 milligrams

All calcium supplements are not created equal. The body absorbs only part of the calcium it takes in, and different forms of calcium provide varying amounts of this mineral. Calcium citrate may provide a bit more usable calcium than other forms, and is less likely to have side effects. Calcium carbonate is often recommended because it contains the highest percentage of absorbable calcium. It is also the cheapest and has the added advantage of acting as an antacid. Two 1,250- or 1,500-milligram tablets of calcium carbonate per day will provide 1,000 milligrams of what is called "available" calcium to the body.

To get the same 1,000 milligrams from other forms of calcium, you need to take up to 12 tablets a day. Divide the following amounts into more than one dose and take them after meals: two 1,600-milligram tablets of calcium phosphate, five 950-milligram tablets of calcium citrate, eleven 1,000-milligram tablets of calcium gluconate, twelve 650-milligram tablets of calcium lactate, and 12 teaspoons of calcium glubionate. Chelated calcium tablets and combinations of calcium and other vitamins and minerals such as vitamin D and magnesium offer no special advantage. Also avoid bonemeal and dolomite—they may contain toxic lead, mercury, and arsenic.

Whichever supplement you choose, check the information supplied with it to determine the dosage that will supply the amount of calcium you need. Remember too, that smoking and drinking alcohol, coffee, or tea increases the amount of calcium that your body will lose.

Best dietary sources

Calcium is found in dairy products, shrimp, canned salmon and sardines, green leafy vegetables, Brazil nuts and almonds, molasses, soybeans, and tofu.

One cup of yogurt contains up to 415 milligrams of calcium. There are 300 milligrams in 1 cup of skim milk, and 290 milligrams in 1 cup of whole milk. One slice of Swiss cheese provides 270 milligrams; 1 cup of cottage cheese, 230 milligrams; 1 ounce of cheddar cheese, 200 milligrams; 1 stalk of broccoli, cooked, 160 milligrams; and one 4-ounce piece of tofu, 150 milligrams.

Carotene

See Vitamin A

Chloride

What it is

Chloride is a component of hydrochloric (stomach) acid. This mineral is also found in various salt products. Natural and synthetic supplements are available.

What it does

Chloride helps maintain the acid balance in the body's cells and fluids.

Why you need it

Chloride is essential to good health. Without it, the delicate chemical balance in the body will go awry.

Can you take too much?

Too much—or too little—chloride in your system can lead to weakness or confusion. At the extreme, you could go into a coma.

Recommended daily allowances

■ ADULTS

The RDA for everyone 18 years of age and older is 1.75 to 5.1 grams.

■ CHILDREN

Infants up to 6 months: 0.275 to 0.7 gram

Ages 6 to 12 months: 0.4 to 1.2 grams

Ages 1 to 3 years: 0.5 to 1.5 grams

Ages 4 to 6 years: 0.7 to 2.1 grams
Ages 7 to 10 years: 0.925 to 2.775 grams
Ages 11 to 17 years: 1.4 to 4.2 grams

Best dietary sources:
Most of our chloride intake comes from table salt, which contains sodium chloride; salt substitutes, which contain potassium chloride and sea salt.

Cholecalciferol

See Vitamin D

Choline

What it is
Choline, present to some degree in all our food, plays an important role in the nervous system. Natural and synthetic supplements are available. Choline is also a component of lecithin, another nutrient available in supplement form. It is part of the B complex of vitamins.

What it does
The body uses choline to make acetylcholine, a substance essential for transmission of signals in many parts of the nervous system. Choline also aids in the transport of fats into the body's cells, and is vital to the health of the liver and kidneys.

Why you need it
Although choline deficiency is rare, it can lead to internal bleeding in the kidneys, excessively high blood pressure, heart disease, and degeneration of the liver.

If you have high cholesterol and triglyceride levels and are taking nicotinic acid (a form of niacin) as a treatment, you may need choline supplements, since high levels of niacin can deplete the choline in your system.

Can you take too much?
Sustained megadosing (above 6,000 milligrams) can cause dizziness, nausea, and vomiting. If you develop any of these symptoms, stop taking the choline supplement and call your physician.

Recommended daily allowances

The government has not yet established a recommended dietary allowance (RDA) for choline. A typical diet provides 500 to 900 milligrams daily. Taking more than 1 gram of supplementary choline per day is not generally recommended; and healthy women should not take choline supplements at all during pregnancy or while breastfeeding.

Best dietary sources

Foods richest in choline include cabbage, cauliflower, chickpeas, green beans, lentils, soybeans, split peas, calves' liver, eggs, rice, and soy lecithin.

Chromium

What it is

Chromium is one of the minerals that the body needs in only trace amounts. It is found in a variety of meats, seafood, dairy products, eggs, and whole-grain foods.

What it does

Chromium helps the body to convert blood sugar (glucose) into energy. It also makes insulin work more efficiently and effectively.

Why you need it

Because chromium makes it easier for the body to burn glucose, chromium supplements have recently been touted as energy-boosters. In addition, chromium's alliance with insulin makes it especially important for diabetics. It can help some people who develop diabetes as older adults better tolerate glucose, thereby reducing the amount of insulin they need to control their sugar levels.

Can you take too much?

The chromium in food and vitamin/mineral supplements poses no danger. Indeed, Americans are thought to not get enough. However, long-term exposure on the job has reportedly led to skin problems, perforation of the nasal septum, liver or kidney impairment, and lung cancer in some people.

Recommended daily allowances

The government has not yet established the recommended daily amount (RDA) of chromium. The estimated safe and adequate daily intake is as follows:

■ ADULTS

All adults: 50 to 200 micrograms.

■ CHILDREN

Infants up to six months: 1 to 40 micrograms
Ages 6 to 12 months: 20 to 60 micrograms
Ages 1 to 3 years: 20 to 80 micrograms
Ages 4 to 6 years: 30 to 120 micrograms
Age 7 and older: 50 to 200 micrograms

Women should avoid chromium supplements during pregnancy and while they are breastfeeding an infant.

Best dietary sources

You can obtain chromium from meats, including beef, chicken, and calves' liver; fish, oysters, and other seafood; cheese and other dairy products; eggs; fresh fruit; potatoes (with skin); whole-grain products; brewer's yeast; and condiments such as black pepper and thyme.

Cobalamin

See Vitamin B$_{12}$

Cobalt

What it is

Cobalt, one of the minerals we need in just trace amounts, is stored in the liver. This mineral is readily available in a well-balanced diet, and deficiencies are rare.

What it does

Cobalt is closely related to vitamin B$_{12}$, and is therefore essential to the production of the red blood cells that carry oxygen throughout the body.

Why you need it

An inadequate supply of cobalt can lead to the condition called pernicious anemia. Symptoms include digestive problems, weight loss, and a burning feeling in the tongue.

What's too much?

Megadoses of cobalt—in the range of 20 to 30 milligrams per day—can lead to serious problems. Cobalt toxicity can cause the thyroid gland to grow too large in infants or to become enlarged in adults. The heart may also grow too large and, and congestive heart failure could result. In addition, excessive cobalt exposure can lead to an abnormally high level of red blood cells.

Recommended daily allowances

Cobalt deficiencies are extremely rare, and the government has yet to establish a recommended dietary allowance.

Best dietary sources

The small amounts of cobalt in a well-balanced diet will satisfy the cobalt requirements of most people. The richest sources are meats, particularly kidney and liver; clams and oysters; milk; figs; and buckwheat. There is some cobalt available in vegetables such as cabbage, lettuce, and spinach; but strict vegetarians are at greater risk of a deficiency than others.

Copper

What it is

Copper is one of the minerals used by the body in only trace amounts. It is an essential ingredient of proteins and enzymes.

What it does

Copper plays a major role in the body's ability to store and use iron. This important mineral triggers the release of iron, which then forms the hemoglobin in red blood cells. The body also uses this mineral to produce various enzymes it needs to maintain its tissues.

Why you need it

Because of its role in the production of hemoglobin, copper helps to prevent anemia. A deficiency of copper, though rare, can lead to weakness, poor respiration, and skin sores.

Can you take too much?

Nausea, vomiting, stomach pain, and muscle aches may be signs that you have too much copper in your system. Excessive amounts of copper can lead to anemia in some people.

Recommended daily allowances

The government has not yet established a recommended dietary allowance (RDA) for copper. Estimated safe and adequate daily intake is as follows:

■ ADULTS

All adults: 2 to 3 milligrams

Women should not take megadoses of copper during pregnancy or while they are breastfeeding.

■ CHILDREN

Infants up to 6 months: 0.5 to 0.7 milligram
Ages 6 to 12 months: 0.7 to 1 milligram
Ages 1 to 3 years: 1 to 1.5 milligrams
Ages 4 to 6 years: 1.5 to 2 milligrams
Ages 7 to 10 years: 2 to 2.5 milligrams
Age 11 and older: 2 to 3 milligrams

Best dietary sources

You can obtain copper from nuts, including Brazil nuts, cashews, hazelnuts, peanuts, and walnuts; barley and lentils; honey and blackstrap molasses; mussels, oysters, and salmon; mushrooms; oats; and wheat germ.

Cyanocobalamin

See Vitamin B₁₂

Cysteine

See Nonessential Amino Acids

Delta-Tocopherol

See Vitamin E

DHA

See Omega-3 Fatty Acids

Dibasic Calcium Phosphate

See Calcium

Dihydrotachysterol

See Vitamin D

Docosahexaenoic Acid

See Omega-3 Fatty Acids

Eicosapentaenoic Acid

See Omega-3 Fatty Acids

EPA

See Omega-3 Fatty Acids

Ergocalciferol

See Vitamin D

Evening Primrose Oil

See Gamma-Linolenic Acid

Ferrous Fumarate

See Iron

Ferrous Gluconate

See Iron

Ferrous Sulfate

See Iron

Fiber

What it is

Fiber is the material that gives plants their stability and structure. There are two types: soluble fiber, which dissolves within the digestive system, and insoluble fiber, which is unaffected by digestion. Both pass through the body without being absorbed.

Fiber is found to some degree in all vegetables, fruits, nuts, and grains, and is also available as a supplement.

What it does

Fiber acts much like a sponge, and is able to absorb many times its weight in water. Soluble fiber absorbs cholesterol-containing bile from the digestive system and clears it from the body.

Why you need it

Insoluble fiber adds bulk to bowel movements, helping to prevent constipation, hemorrhoids, diverticulosis, and—over the long-term—colorectal cancer. Soluble fiber helps reduce the levels of cholesterol and triglycerides in the blood and works to moderate blood sugar levels as well.

Can you take too much?

A sudden increase in fiber intake can cause bloating and gas. Tremendous amounts could cause a blockage in the large intestine, although this is a rare occurrence. A diet with 25 grams of fiber for each 1,000 calories eaten is considered high in fiber.

Recommended daily allowances

There is no official recommended dietary allowance (RDA) for fiber. Nutrition experts advise intake of at least 20 to 30 grams a day.

Although no problems have surfaced, women who are pregnant or breastfeeding should not use fiber supplements unless prescribed by a physician. Fiber supplements are hazardous to children younger than two years of age.

Best dietary sources

Good sources of fiber include: fruits and vegetables, nuts, seeds, and whole-grain products. Beans and lentils are excellent sources of soluble fiber.

Fish Oils

See Omega-3 Fatty Acids

Fluoride

What it is

Fluoride, one of the minerals we require in only trace amounts, is best known as sodium fluoride, an ingredient in many toothpastes. Fluoride occurs naturally in some foods, and supplements are also available, with a physician's prescription.

What it does

Fluoride helps the body retain the calcium it needs for strong bones and teeth.

Why you need it

Fluoride supplements are prescribed to prevent dental cavities in children living where the fluoride level in the drinking water is inadequate. Children who need extra fluoride generally keep taking supplements until they are 16 years old. Physicians also use fluoride, along with calcium and vitamin D, to treat osteoporosis. It is important to note that this treatment must be supervised by a doctor.

Can you take too much?

A dose of fluoride 2,500 times the standard recommendation can be fatal. Smaller overdoses can eventually lead to stomach cramps or pain, diarrhea, black stools, and vomiting, which could be bloody. A feeling of faintness, shallow breathing, increased saliva, tremors, and an unusual feeling of excitement are also potential warning signs of fluoride toxicity. Stop taking fluoride and call your doctor if you develop any of these symptoms.

Recommended daily allowances

The government has not yet established a recommended dietary allowance (RDA) for fluoride. The estimated safe and adequate daily intake is as follows:

■ ADULTS

All adults: 1.5 to 4 milligrams

The experts disagree about whether it is safe—or beneficial—to take fluoride supplements during pregnancy. At this time experts feel that breastfeeding mothers who take additional fluoride need not anticipate problems with their infants. However, it is best to discuss your specific needs with your physician and to avoid taking megadoses of fluoride while pregnant or breastfeeding.

■ CHILDREN

Infants up to 6 months: 0.1 to 0.5 milligram
Ages 6 to 12 months: 0.2 to 1 milligram
Ages 1 to 3 years: 0.5 to 1.5 milligrams
Ages 4 to 6 years: 1 to 2.5 milligrams
Ages 7 to 10 years: 1.5 to 2.5 milligrams
Age 11 and older: 1.5 to 4 milligrams

Best dietary sources

Fluoride can be found in organ meats, including calves' liver and kidneys; fish and seafood, including cod, canned salmon, and canned sardines; apples; eggs; and tea. Note, however, that the amount of fluoride in these foods can vary greatly. It is much higher in areas where the soil is rich, and the water is fluoridated.

Folacin

See Folic Acid

Folate

See Folic Acid

Folic Acid

What it is

Folic acid is a water-soluble vitamin known by many other names—vitamin B_9, folate, folacin, and tetrahydrofolic acid. It is available in fresh leafy green vegetables and liver. Folic acid is also manufactured synthetically and is included in most multivitamin supplements. An injectable form is available by prescription.

What it does

Folic acid is essential for the formation of the DNA that makes up our genes and the RNA that transmits their instructions. It is particularly important in the body's production of red blood cells. Folic acid deficiency results in megaloblastic anemia, an anemia similar to that caused by vitamin B_{12} deficiency. Symptoms include weight loss, digestive problems, and a burning feeling in the tongue.

Why you need it

Folic acid helps us grow and develop normally. It also regulates nerve cell development in the embryo and the developing baby. Folic acid supplements are used to treat the anemia that may occur with alcoholism, liver disease, pregnancy, breastfeeding, or the use of oral contraceptives.

Can you take too much?

Very high amounts of folic acid have been taken over long periods of time without any adverse effects. However, there is a chance that prolonged use of large amounts might lead to the formation of folacin crystals in the kidneys or cause severe neurologic problems. Symptoms such as loss of appetite, nausea, gas, and abdominal bloating may occur if you take more than 1,500 micrograms of folic acid per day.

Recommended daily allowances

■ ADULTS

For everyone 11 years and older the official recommended dietary allowance is 400 micrograms.

Women need an additional 400 micrograms of folic acid each day during pregnancy. (It is believed that folic acid supplementation during pregnancy may prevent the development of neural tube defects that can lead to mental retardation.) Breastfeeding mothers need an extra 100 micrograms of folic acid per day.

Many others may also require additional folic acid. People who do not eat a well-balanced diet, those over the age of 55, people who abuse alcohol or other drugs, and women who take oral contraceptives should discuss the need for folic acid supplementation with their physicians.

■ CHILDREN
Infants up to 6 months: 30 micrograms
Ages 6 to 12 months: 45 micrograms
Ages 1 to 3 years: 100 micrograms
Ages 4 to 6 years: 200 micrograms
Ages 7 to 10 years: 300 micrograms

Best dietary sources

Folic acid is available in green leafy vegetables such as broccoli, spinach, and romaine lettuce. It is important to note that cooking these vegetables reduces the amount of folic acid the body receives. Other natural sources of folic acid include: fruits—especially oranges and orange juice—calves' liver, brewer's yeast, wheat germ, rice, barley, beans, peas, split peas, chickpeas, lentils, soybeans, and sprouts.

One-half pound of fresh spinach contains 463 micrograms of folic acid; 1 tablespoon of brewer's yeast provides 308 micrograms. One-half cup of dry soybeans has 236 micrograms of folic acid; 1 cup of fresh orange juice provides 164 micrograms.

Gamma-Linolenic Acid

What it is
Gamma-linolenic acid (GLA) is manufactured in the body from linolenic acid, one of the three essential fatty acids required in our diets. It is also found in oil expressed from the seeds of the evening primrose plant, and is available in a supplement called evening primrose oil.

What it does
Gamma-linolenic acid plays a role in the production of prostaglandins, hormone-like substances that, under some conditions, may help the body fight inflammation.

Why you need it
Some researchers believe that anti-inflammatory properties of certain prostaglandins that gamma-linolenic acid helps form may play a role in the body's ability to fight arthritis.

Can you take too much?
There is currently no evidence that gamma-linolenic acid is toxic.

Recommended daily allowances
No recommended allowance has been established for this substance.

Best dietary sources
Gamma-linolenic acid is found in fish.

Gamma-Tocopherol

See Vitamin E

GLA

See Gamma-Linolenic Acid

Glutamic Acid

See Nonessential Amino Acids

Glutamine

See Nonessential Amino Acids

Glycine

See Nonessential Amino Acids

Histidine

See Nonessential Amino Acids

Inositol

What it is

Inositol is part of the vitamin B complex. The body manufactures its own supply of this substance, which it then uses to produce lecithin, a compound that aids in the body's utilization of fats. Inositol is found in many foods and is available both as a separate supplement and as a component of lecithin supplements.

What it does

As a component of lecithin, inositol is responsible for transferring needed fats from the liver to the body's cells.

Why you need it

By assisting in the proper utilization of fat and cholesterol, inositol lowers blood cholesterol levels, thus protecting the arteries and heart from excessive cholesterol buildup.

Can you take too much?

Inositol has not been found toxic at any dosage level.

Recommended daily allowances

The government has not yet established a recommended dietary allowance (RDA) for inositol, but doctors usually order no more than 500 to 1,000 milligrams daily when prescribing a supplement.

Best dietary sources

Inositol is found in dried beans, chickpeas, and lentils; cantaloupe and citrus fruit (other than lemons); calves' liver, pork, and veal; nuts; oats; rice; whole-grain products; lecithin granules, and wheat germ.

Iodine

What it is

Iodine, one of the minerals that we need in only trace amounts, appears in various fish and seafood products and is also available as a natural supplement. A physician's prescription is necessary for the larger dosage strengths.

What it does
Iodine is an important ingredient in the thyroid hormones that regulate many bodily functions.

Why you need it
Iodine is essential for proper functioning of the thyroid gland. Doctors use this mineral to shrink the thyroid prior to surgery and in tests to see how well the gland is working. Iodine is also useful in the treatment of goiter, an enlargement of the thyroid gland that appears as a swelling in the neck area. Iodine helps the cells function normally and keeps skin, hair, and nails healthy.

Can you take too much?
Warning signs that you may have too much iodine in your system include confusion, an irregular heartbeat, and stools that are either bloody or black and tarry. If you develop any of these symptoms of potential iodine toxicity, stop taking the supplement and call your doctor.

Recommended daily allowances
■ ADULTS

All adults: 150 micrograms

Women require an additional 25 micrograms of iodine each day during pregnancy. Women who are breastfeeding an infant need an extra 50 micrograms per day.

Although pregnant women need some additional iodine, too much can have serious consequences. Excessive amounts can give the baby an enlarged thyroid or an underactive thyroid. Cretinism, a form of dwarfism accompanied by mental deficiency, is another possible birth defect related to excessive iodine intake during pregnancy.

Breastfeeding mothers should avoid taking iodine supplements and megadoses while nursing an infant. The iodine that appears in breast milk may cause a skin rash, and can keep the baby's thyroid from functioning properly.

■ CHILDREN
Infants up to 6 months: 40 micrograms
Ages 6 to 12 months: 50 micrograms
Ages 1 to 3 years: 70 micrograms
Ages 4 to 6 years: 90 micrograms
Ages 7 to 10 years: 120 micrograms
Age 11 and older: 150 micrograms

Best dietary sources

Fish and seafood, including cod, haddock, herring, lobster, oysters, shrimp, and canned salmon are the primary sources of iodine. Other natural sources include cod-liver oil, sunflower seeds, iodized table salt, sea salt, and seaweed.

Iron

What it is

Although we've all heard that iron is essential for good blood, it is actually one of the minerals that we need in only trace amounts. Iron is supplied in a wide range of foods and in several different supplement formulations, including ferrous fumarate, ferrous gluconate, ferrous sulfate, and, for deep muscle injections, iron dextran.

What it does

Iron is an essential part of hemoglobin, the red part of red blood cells that carries oxygen throughout the body. Hemoglobin stores approximately 60 to 70 percent of the body's iron supply. Additional iron stored in the muscle tissue helps deliver the oxygen needed to make the muscles contract.

Why you need it

Iron deficiency leads to anemia—failure of the blood to supply sufficient oxygen to the body's cells. Signs of severe anemia include weakness, dizziness, headache, drowsiness, fatigue, and irritability.

Can you take too much?

Damage from a single dose of iron is unlikely. You would need to take more than 1,000 times the RDA for the dose to be fatal. However, iron can build up to toxic levels gradually within the body, especially in older men. Early signs that you may have too much iron in your system are abdominal pain, severe nausea, diarrhea, or vomiting with blood. As iron toxicity intensifies, you may begin to feel weak or even collapse. Your skin may look pale, while your lips, hands, and fingernails begin to take on a bluish tinge. Shallow breathing and a weak, rapid heartbeat are also among the later warning signs of iron overdose. Extreme toxicity can cause convulsions and coma.

When first taking an iron supplement, you may find your stools turning black or gray. This is not a problem. However, if you notice blood in the stool, seek treatment immediately.

Emergency treatment is also essential if you have chest pain, chills, hives, shortness of breath or a skin rash or if you lose consciousness. If you develop these symptoms, discontinue taking the supplement and call your doctor.

Recommended daily allowances

■ ADULTS

Males 11 to 18: 18 milligrams
Males 19 and older: 10 milligrams
Females 11 to 50: 18 milligrams
Females 51 and older: 10 milligrams

Women need an extra 30 to 60 milligrams of iron each day during pregnancy and while breastfeeding. However, pregnant women should not take an iron supplement during the first trimester unless prescribed by their physician. Nursing mothers who are healthy and eat a well-balanced diet may not need an iron supplement. In any event, do not take megadoses during pregnancy or while breastfeeding, and do not give your baby an iron supplement without first checking with the doctor.

■ CHILDREN

Infants up to 6 months: 10 milligrams
Ages 6 months to 3 years: 15 milligrams
Ages 4 to 10 years: 10 milligrams

Best dietary sources

Good sources of iron include enriched bread; prune juice; nuts, including cashews, pistachios, and walnuts; caviar; cheddar cheese, egg yolks; chickpeas; lentils; pumpkin seeds; blackstrap molasses; mussels; wheat germ; whole-grain products; and seaweed.

One cup of prune juice contains 10.5 milligrams of iron, a cup of cooked chickpeas nearly 7 milligrams, and a cup of cooked spinach 4.2 milligrams. Cooking in iron pots and pans greatly increases the amount of iron in your food.

Humans have trouble absorbing iron, even from foods rich in the mineral. A person with normal iron levels will probably absorb only about 10 percent of the iron available in food. A person with an iron deficiency, however, will absorb from 20 to 30 percent of the available iron. Vitamin C increases the body's ability to absorb iron.

Isoleucine

See Branched-Chain Amino Acids

L-Carnitine

What it is

L-carnitine is a product of two of the essential amino acids that the body cannot produce on its own: lysine and methionine. It can be obtained from meat and dairy products and is also available as natural and synthetic supplements.

What it does

Lysine, methionine, and the other essential amino acids must all be on hand before the body can manufacture the proteins needed to repair and maintain its tissues.

Why you need it

Without the essential amino acids, including those in l-carnitine, normal growth and development is impossible. Unless you're a strict vegetarian, however, a deficiency is unlikely. Muscle weakness is the main sign that you may have a deficiency of l-carnitine in your system.

Can you take too much?

Like most amino acids, l-carnitine is rarely toxic, taken in large amounts.

Recommended daily allowances

No allowance has been established.

Best dietary sources

Natural sources of l-carnitine include dairy products, avocados, and lamb, beef, and other red meats. L-carnitine is also found in the soybean product called tempeh.

Lecithin

What it is

Lecithin is a natural compound that includes choline, inositol, phosphorus, and various fatty acids. It is found throughout the body, and is available in a variety of foods, as well as in natural and synthetic supplements.

What it does

The choline and inositol in lecithin both play important roles in the body's handling of fats. Choline is also an ingredient of acetylcholine, an essential chemical messenger in many parts of the nervous system.

Why you need it

By promoting the normal processing of fat and cholesterol, lecithin protects against hardening of the arteries and heart disease. It also helps maintain the health of the liver and kidneys.

If you are taking nicotinic acid (a form of niacin) to lower your cholesterol, you may be advised to take lecithin as a way of boosting your choline intake. High levels of niacin tend to deplete the choline in your system.

Can you take too much?

Excessive dose can cause dizziness, nausea, and vomiting. Follow manufacturers' recommendations, and, if you develop any of these symptoms, stop taking the supplement and call your physician.

Recommended daily allowances

There is no recommended dietary allowance (RDA) for lecithin. Two tablespoons daily is the usual dosage.

Best dietary sources

Good sources of lecithin include cabbage, cauliflower, chickpeas, green beans, lentils, soybeans, corn, split peas, calves' liver and eggs.

Leucine

See Branched-Chain Amino Acids

Lysine

What it is

Lysine is one of the amino acids considered "essential" because they cannot be manufactured in the body and must be obtained through diet. Lysine is available in natural and synthetic supplement form.

What it does

Amino acids are the raw material used by the body to manufacture human proteins. These proteins are a vital component of all the body's cells.

Why you need it

Lysine plays an especially important role in the production of antibodies, hormones, and enzymes. It is also important for the repair of damaged tissue.

Can you take too much?

Amino acids are rarely toxic, even in large amounts.

Recommended daily allowances

There is no official recommended dietary allowance for lysine. The estimated adult daily requirement is approximately 5.5 milligrams per pound of body weight. Infants need 8 times that amount; children, 4 times that amount.

Women who are healthy and eat a well-balanced diet do not require lysine supplementation during pregnancy or while breastfeeding. If you do use a supplement, take it in moderation.

Best dietary sources

Good sources of lysine include red meat, milk, cheese, eggs, fish, lima beans, potatoes, soy products, and yeast.

Magnesium

What it is

Magnesium is one of the minerals that we require in relatively large amounts. It is particularly abundant in green vegetables, and is also available in natural supplements—some of which require a physician's prescription.

What it does

Magnesium plays many roles in the body. It promotes absorption and use of other minerals such as calcium and helps move sodium and potassium across the cell membranes; is involved in the metabolism of proteins, and turns on essential enzymes.

Why you need it

Magnesium helps bones grow and teeth remain strong. It enables nerve impulses to travel through the body, keeps the body's metabolism in balance, and helps the muscles—including the heart—work properly. Small amounts of magnesium work as an antacid; large amounts of magnesium work as a laxative.

Can you take too much?

Although magnesium toxicity is rare, it can lead to serious problems, including severe nausea and vomiting, extreme muscle weakness, and difficulty breathing. The blood pressure can drop to an extremely low level, and the heartbeat may become irregular.

If your heartbeat seems irregular, seek emergency medical treatment immediately. Stop taking magnesium supplements and call your doctor if you notice any of the other signs of potential magnesium toxicity. You should also tell your physician if you lose your appetite, develop diarrhea, abdominal pain, mood changes, fatigue, or weakness; or if you experience discomfort when you urinate.

Recommended daily allowances

■ ADULTS
Males 11 to 14 years: 350 milligrams
Males 15 to 18 years: 400 milligrams
Males 18 and older: 350 milligrams
Females 11 and older: 300 milligrams

Women require an additional 150 milligrams of magnesium each day during pregnancy and while breastfeeding an infant. However, it is best to get the extra amount through your diet. Experts advise *against* taking magnesium supplements during pregnancy—the risk to the developing baby outweighs any benefits of supplementation.

You should also avoid taking large quantities of magnesium while you are breastfeeding. If magnesium supplements are necessary, your physician will recommend that you stop breastfeeding.

■ CHILDREN
Infants up to 6 months: 50 milligrams
Ages 6 to 12 months: 70 milligrams
Ages 1 to 3 years: 150 milligrams
Ages 4 to 6 years: 200 milligrams
Ages 7 to 10 years: 250 milligrams

Best dietary sources

Many foods are rich in magnesium. Good sources include fish and seafood, including bluefish, carp, cod, flounder, halibut, herring, mackerel, ocean perch, shrimp, and swordfish; fruits and fruit juice; leafy green vegetables; dairy products; nuts, including almonds; molasses; soybeans; sunflower seeds; wheat germ; and snails.

One-half cup of dry soybeans contains 278 milligrams of magnesium; 1/2 pound of spinach provides 200 milligrams. One-half of a medium avocado contains 51 milligrams; 1 cup of bottled grape juice has 30 milligrams, a cup of skim milk or buttermilk 34 milligrams, a cup of ice cream 19 milligrams.

Manganese

What it is

Manganese is one of the minerals needed by the body in relatively small (trace) amounts. Found in many beans, nuts, and grains, it is also available by prescription in natural and synthetic supplements.

What It Does

Manganese is concentrated in the pituitary gland, liver, pancreas, kidney, and bones. It is needed for proper utilization of several of the vitamins, including vitamin C; and it plays a role in the body's production of protein, sugar, fat, and cholesterol. It helps nourish the bones and nerves.

Why you need it

Without sufficient manganese, the body's system for processing blood sugar may falter, leading to diabetes. The nervous system may also be affected, resulting in poor coordination and even seizures.

Can you take too much?

Signs of manganese toxicity include depression, trouble sleeping, and impotence. Some people may develop delusions or experience hallucinations following overdoses.

When taking manganese supplements, seek emergency treatment if you have trouble breathing or suffer leg cramps. Your doctor also needs to know if you lose your appetite, have headaches, or feel unusually tired.

Recommended daily allowances

The government has not yet established a recommended dietary allowance (RDA) for manganese. The estimated safe and adequate daily intake is as follows:

■ ADULTS

All adults: 2.5 to 5 milligrams

Women who are pregnant or breastfeeding should not take supplements that contain manganese unless prescribed by their physician and should never take megadoses of this mineral.

■ CHILDREN
Infants up to 6 months: 0.5 to 0.7 milligram
Ages 6 to 12 months: 0.7 to 1 milligram
Ages 1 to 3 years: 1 to 1.5 milligrams
Ages 4 to 6 years: 1.5 to 2 milligrams
Ages 7 to 10 years: 2 to 3 milligrams
Age 11 and older: 2.5 to 5 milligrams

Best dietary sources
You can find manganese in vegetables, including dried beans, peas, and spinach; chestnuts, hazelnuts, peanuts, and pecans; buckwheat, bran, barley, and oatmeal; fruits, including avocados and blackberries; cloves and ginger; coffee; and seaweed.

Menadiol

See Vitamin K

Methionine

What it is
Methionine is one of the amino acids considered essential because they cannot be manufactured in the body and must be obtained through diet. Worse yet for strict vegetarians, this particular amino acid is found only in meat and dairy products. However, natural and synthetic methionine supplements are available.

What it does
Amino acids are the raw material used by the body to manufacture human proteins. These proteins are a vital component of all the body's cells.

Why you need it
Methionine is thought to be necessary for effective use of two other amino acids, cystine and taurine.

Can you take too much?
Amino acids are rarely toxic, even in large amounts.

Recommended daily allowances

There is no official recommended dietary allowance for methionine. The estimated adult daily requirement for methionine and cystine combined is approximately 4.5 milligrams per pound of body weight. Infants need 5 times that amount; children require twice that amount.

Women who are healthy and eat a well-balanced diet do not require methionine supplementation during pregnancy or while breastfeeding. If you do use a supplement, take it in moderation.

Best dietary sources

Methionine is found only in meat, fish, eggs, and milk.

Molybdenum

What it is

Molybdenum is one of the minerals that we need in only trace amounts. It is found in certain vegetables, organ meats, and cereal grains. A molybdenum supplement is available by prescription.

What it does

Molybdenum is part of the bones, teeth, kidney, and liver. It helps the body use its iron reserves, and plays a role in the burning of fat.

Why you need it

Because it is an ingredient of tooth enamel, a shortage of molybdenum can contribute to tooth decay. A deficiency can also lead to anemia (oxygen starvation in the tissues), and even impotence.

Can you take too much?

Regular doses of 10 to 15 milligrams of molybdenum per day—20 to 30 times the estimated safe amount—can cause the painfully swollen joints associated with gout. When people take even slightly more than the estimated safe intake of molybdenum, it can deplete the body of copper. Signs of moderate molybdenum toxicity include diarrhea and a depressed growth rate in children.

Recommended daily allowances

The government has not yet established a recommended dietary allowance (RDA) for molybdenum. The estimated safe and adequate daily intake is as follows:

■ ADULTS

All adults: 150 to 500 micrograms

■ CHILDREN

Infants up to 6 months: 30 to 60 micrograms

Ages 6 to 12 months: 40 to 80 micrograms

Ages 1 to 3 years: 50 to 100 micrograms

Ages 4 to 6 years: 60 to 150 micrograms

Ages 7 to 10 years: 100 to 300 micrograms

Age 11 and older: 150 to 500 micrograms

Best dietary sources

Molybdenum is found in dark green leafy vegetables; organ meats, including liver, kidney, and sweetbreads; beans, peas and other legumes; and cereal grains. The actual amount of molybdenum in grains and vegetables depends on the amount in the soil when the produce was growing.

Myo-Inositol

See Inositol

Niacin

What it is

Niacin, also known as vitamin B_3, is one of the water-soluble vitamins that need constant replenishment.

Niacin supplements are available in two forms, nicotinic acid (the prescription drug Nicolar) and niacinamide, found in over-the-counter supplements. The nicotinic acid form of vitamin B_3 lowers the amount of cholesterol in the blood, thereby reducing the risk of heart disease. Niacinamide does not have this effect.

What it does

Niacin helps release the energy from food and aids the body in synthesizing DNA. It works with other compounds to help the body process fat and produce sugar while aiding the tissues to rid themselves of waste products. The nicotinic acid form of the vitamin lowers the amount of cholesterol and triglycerides in the blood.

Why you need it

Niacin helps the body's skin, nerves, and digestive system stay healthy. It is used to treat dizziness and ringing in the ears and to help prevent premenstrual headaches. Niacin supplements are also given to treat pellagra, a potentially fatal niacin deficiency disease characterized by diarrhea, mental disorders, depression, and skin problems. The nicotinic acid form of niacin is prescribed to reduce the amount of cholesterol and triglycerides in the blood.

Can you take too much?

Too much nicotinic acid—more than 2,000 milligrams a day—over a long period of time may damage the liver or cause a stomach ulcer to flare up. Nausea, vomiting, abdominal cramps or pain, faintness, and a yellowish color to the skin and eyes are warning signs of excessive dosage. The niacinamide form of the vitamin does not have these effects.

Recommended daily allowances

■ ADULTS

Males 11 to 18: 18 milligrams

Males 19 to 22: 19 milligrams

Males 23 to 50: 18 milligrams

Males 50 and older: 16 milligrams

Females 11 to 14: 15 milligrams

Females 15 to 22: 14 milligrams

Females 23 and older: 13 milligrams

Women need an additional 2 milligrams of niacin each day during pregnancy. Breastfeeding mothers need an extra 4 milligrams per day.

■ CHILDREN

Infants up to 6 months: 6 milligrams

Ages 6 to 12 months: 8 milligrams

Ages 1 to 3 years: 9 milligrams

Ages 4 to 6 years: 11 milligrams

Ages 7 to 10 years: 16 milligrams

Best dietary sources

Good sources are lean meats, fish, and poultry, including beef liver, pork, veal, turkey, chicken (white meat), salmon, swordfish, tuna, and halibut. Peanuts, brewer's yeast, and sunflower seeds also provide niacin.

A 4-ounce piece of tofu contains nearly 16 milligrams of niacin. One-half cup of dry soybeans provides 11.5 milligrams. One cup of cottage cheese contains 8 milligrams—about half of the adult RDA.

Niacinamide

See Niacin

Nickel

What it is

Nickel is one of the minerals that we require in only trace amounts. It is available in some types of food, and as a supplement.

What it does

Nickel appears to play only a minor role in human nutrition. It is thought to be involved in the body's use of fats and the blood sugar glucose.

Why you need it

Unlike deficiencies of most other vitamins and minerals, a lack of nickel causes few immediate symptoms. It may aggravate anemia, the condition that results when insufficient oxygen reaches the body's tissues.

Can you take too much?

Although it's difficult to develop a nickel deficiency, too much can definitely be a problem. Symptoms of toxic levels include headache, vertigo, nausea, vomiting, chest pain, and coughing.

Recommended daily allowances

No recommendation has been established. The amount found in a normal diet can range from a few micrograms to hundreds of milligrams, depending on the nickel content of the soil in which the food is grown.

Best dietary sources

Foods that may contain nickel include grains, beans, vegetables, and seafood.

Nicotinamide

See Niacin

Nicotinic Acid

See Niacin

Nonessential Amino Acids

What they are

Amino acids are the raw materials used by the body to manufacture human protein—a vital component of all the body's cells. This group of amino acids is labeled "nonessential" because, when the acids are lacking in the diet, they can be manufactured in the body.

What they do

All the nonessential amino acids must be on hand before the body can synthesize protein; and several have additional, more specialized roles as well.

■ **Arginine** turns on human growth hormone and is considered essential during childhood, when the body's production of this amino acid can't keep up with demand.

■ **Cystine** is an ingredient of the body's major antioxidant, a substance called glutathione. It thereby plays an important role in neutralizing toxic pollutants and by-products within the body.

■ **Glutamic acid** is another component of glutathione. It is related to glutamate, one of the nervous system's chemical messengers. Glutamate appears in our diets as the flavor enhancer MSG.

■ **Glutamine** is a derivative of glutamic acid.

■ **Glycine** is yet another component of the antioxidant glutathione.

■ **Histidine** is needed for growth in children and is deemed essential during the childhood years, when demand outpaces the body's ability to produce this substance.

■ **Taurine** helps regulate the nervous system and the muscles.

■ **Tyrosine**, which is manufactured from the essential amino acid phenylalanine, plays a role in the production of three of the nervous system's messengers: dopamine, epinephrine, and norepinephrine.

Why you need them

Deficiencies of arginine and histidine can stunt growth in small children. Glutamine supplements are prescribed for certain digestive disorders and to treat alcoholism. Taurine is sometimes helpful in the treatment of epilepsy.

Can you take too much?

Large doses of arginine may cause nausea or diarrhea; and excessive amounts of tyrosine can lead to changes in blood pressure and migraine headaches. In general, however, even large amounts of these amino acids in your system are unlikely to cause any severe problems.

Recommended daily allowances

There are no official recommended daily allowances for these nutrients; and it is advisable to take supplements only under a doctor's supervision. Women taking supplements while pregnant or breastfeeding should be especially careful to avoid excessive doses.

Best dietary sources

A complete set of all the amino acids is available in most meat and dairy products. Arginine can also be found in cereals, whole-wheat products, brown rice, chocolate, popcorn, nuts, raisins, and pumpkin and sesame seeds. Other sources of tyrosine include almonds, peanuts, bananas, avocados, lima beans, pickled herring, and pumpkin and sesame seeds.

Oil of Evening Primrose

See Gamma-Linolenic Acid

Omega-3 Fatty Acids

What they are

This group of fatty acids, also known as fish oil, have gained popularity as a protective agent for the heart. Omega-3 supplements contain docosahexaenoic acid (DHA) and eicosapentaenoic acid (EPA).

What they do

The omega-3 fatty acids are believed to lower the levels of triglycerides (fats) and total cholesterol in the blood, while raising the amount of HDL (good) cholesterol. These acids also discourage unwanted clotting that can aggravate plaque buildup.

PABA/613

Why you need them

In people with a cholesterol problem, omega-3 fatty acids can help prevent the buildup of cholesterol-laden plaque that can clog the arteries and lead to heart attack and stroke.

Can you take too much?

Because omega-3 fatty acids discourage clotting, excessive levels can lead to bleeding problems in case of an accident or trauma. Women who menstruate are also in greater danger of developing anemia.

Recommended daily allowances

There is no recommended dietary allowance (RDA) for the omega-3 fatty acids.

To increase your intake of the omega-3 fatty acids, nutritionists generally recommend eating more fish (2 to 3 times a week), rather than taking large amounts of supplements. A 7-ounce serving of certain types of fish easily provides 2 to 4 grams of omega-3 fatty acids.

Best dietary sources

The omega-3 fatty acids are found in cold-water fish. Best sources include cod, tuna, salmon, halibut, shark, and mackerel. Herring, bluefish, shrimp, flounder, and swordfish also provide good amounts of these acids.

A 7-ounce portion of herring contains 3.2 grams of omega-3 acids. The same serving of salmon or bluefish provides 2.4 grams. Seven ounces of tuna has 1 gram.

PABA

What it is

Also known as para-aminobenzoic acid, this water-soluble member of the vitamin B complex is closely associated with folic acid. The body receives a constant supply of PABA from friendly bacteria residing in the intestines.

What it does

PABA plays a role in the breakdown and use of proteins, and in the formation of red blood cells. It also stimulates production of folic acid in the intestines, and helps maintain the health of the skin and hair.

Why you need it

Unless something—such as a sulfa drug—disrupts intestinal production, there appears to be no need for PABA in the diet. If a deficiency does develop, it is signaled by fatigue, depression, nervousness, headache, and digestive disorders. In ointment form, PABA provides burn relief. It is also used as a sunscreen.

Can you take too much?

Sustained megadosing can cause damage to the liver, heart, and kidneys. Symptoms of overdose include nausea and vomiting.

Recommended daily allowances

PABA is normally unneeded; and there is no recommended dietary allowance.

Best dietary sources

PABA can be obtained from liver, yeast, wheat germ, and molasses.

Pantethine

See Pantothenic Acid

Pantothenic Acid

What it is

Pantothenic acid is a water-soluble vitamin also known as vitamin B_5 and pantethine. It is found in a variety of foods and is manufactured synthetically. Your physician can prescribe an injectable form.

What it does

Pantothenic acid helps the body release energy from carbohydrates, protein, and fat.

Why you need it

Pantothenic acid helps the body grow and develop normally. Some people believe that this vitamin also helps wounds heal more quickly by stimulating the cells to grow.

Can you take too much?

Even at doses hundreds of times the usual amount, pantothenic acid causes no problems. However, you may develop diarrhea or retain water if you ingest megadoses of 10 grams or more.

Recommended daily allowances

A recommended dietary allowance (RDA) has not yet been established for pantothenic acid.

■ ADULTS

The estimated adequate intake for males and females 10 years of age and older is 4 to 7 milligrams per day.

Women may need additional pantothenic acid during pregnancy or while breastfeeding.

■ CHILDREN

The estimated adequate daily intake for children is:

Infants up to 6 months: 2 milligrams
Ages 6 months to 3 years: 3 milligrams
Ages 4 to 6 years: 3 to 4 milligrams
Ages 7 to 9 years: 4 to 5 milligrams

Best dietary sources

Pantothenic acid is found in all types of meats, including organ meats and especially liver. It is also available in eggs, lobster, whole-grain cereals, wheat germ, brewer's yeast, corn, peas, lentils, soybeans, peanuts, and sunflower seeds.

One-half cup of dry soybeans contains 1.8 milligrams of pantothenic acid; the same amount of lentils contains 1.3 milligrams. One tablespoon of brewer's yeast or 1 cup of fresh peas provides 1.2 milligrams.

Phenylalanine

What it is

Phenylalanine is one of the amino acids considered "essential" because they cannot be manufactured in the body and must be obtained through diet. Natural and synthetic phenylalanine supplements are also available.

What it does

Amino acids are the raw material used by the body to manufacture human proteins. These proteins are a vital component of all the body's cells.

Why you need it

Phenylalanine has a special role in the production of dopamine, epinephrine, and norepinephrine, three chemical messengers that aid in transmitting signals through the nervous system. However, extra phenylalanine can be both helpful and harmful. Do not take phenylalanine supplements without consulting your physician.

Can you take too much?

Potential side effects of excessive phenylalanine include high or low blood pressure and migraine headaches. If you think you may be having a reaction to phenylalanine, stop taking the supplement and call your doctor right away.

Children born without the ability to process phenylalanine can build up dangerous levels of this amino acid, resulting in mental retardation, seizures, extreme hyperactivity, and psychosis. Tests can uncover this condition, called phenylketonuria, in the newborn; and treatment is available.

Recommended daily allowances

There is no official recommended dietary allowance for phenylalanine. The estimated adult daily requirement for phenylalanine and the related amino acid tyrosine combined is approximately 7 milligrams per pound of body weight. Infants require almost 9 times that amount; children need 10 milligrams per pound.

Women who are healthy and eat a well-balanced diet do not require phenylalanine supplementation during pregnancy or while breastfeeding. If you do use a supplement take it in moderation.

Best dietary sources

Foods rich in phenylalanine include almonds and peanuts; bananas and avocados; cheese and cottage cheese; lima beans; nonfat dried milk; pumpkin and sesame seeds; and pickled herring.

Phosphorus

What it is

Phosphorus is, after calcium, the body's second most plentiful mineral. It is a major component of the bones, and appears in every cell in the body. Supplements are available in the form of various phosphates.

What it does

Phosphorus participates in virtually all the chemical reactions in the body. It helps the body use many of the B vitamins, and plays an important role in the utilization of fats, proteins, and carbohydrates. It stimulates muscle contraction, supports cell division and growth, and participates in transmission of nerve impulses.

Why you need it

As one of the two major ingredients of bones and teeth, phosphorus is essential for normal growth, healing of fractures, and prevention of osteoporosis, the brittle bone disease. It helps the body produce energy and plays an important role in the growth, maintenance, and repair of all of the tissues. A deficiency can lead to ailments ranging from weight loss and fatigue to arthritis, gum disease, and tooth decay.

Can you take too much?

Phosphorus is not toxic. However potassium phosphate supplements often prescribed for kidney stones can cause side effects, including shortness of breath, an irregular heartbeat, or seizures.

When taking potassium phosphate, call your doctor immediately if you notice any of the following potential warning signs: headache; pain in the abdomen, bones or joints; confusion; diarrhea; muscle cramps; swelling in your feet or legs; numbness or tingling in your hands and feet; unusual fatigue or thirst; or a decline in urine output.

Recommended daily allowances

■ ADULTS

All adults: 800 milligrams
Women need an extra 400 milligrams of phosphorus each day during pregnancy and while breastfeeding an infant. See your doctor before taking a supplement. Do not take megadoses of this mineral.

■ CHILDREN

Infants up to 6 months: 240 milligrams
Ages 6 to 12 months: 360 milligrams
Ages 1 to 10 years: 800 milligrams
Ages 11 to 17 years: 1,200 milligrams

Best dietary sources

Potassium phosphate occurs naturally in meats, including red meat and calves' liver; poultry; fish and seafood, including tuna, scallops, and canned sardines; milk and milk products; cheddar, pasteurized and processed cheese; eggs; almonds and peanuts; dried beans, peas, and soybeans; pumpkin and sunflower seeds; and whole-grain products.

Potassium

What it is

Potassium is one of the key minerals required by the body to maintain its normal daily functions. Potassium supplements—often prescribed for people on blood pressure medications—are available in a variety of forms including potassium acetate, potassium bicarbonate, potassium chloride, potassium citrate, and potassium gluconate.

What it does

Along with sodium, potassium regulates the water balance within the body and its cells. It also helps govern the body's acid balance and the electrical charge within the cells. It is essential to the healthy functioning of the brain, heart, muscles, and kidneys.

Why you need it

Potassium keeps the heart beating normally, helps the muscles contract, and feeds the cells by controlling the transfer of nutrients from surrounding fluids. It helps the kidneys remove waste products from the body, works with phosphorus to supply oxygen to the brain, and cooperates with calcium to regulate the nerves.

Can you take too much?

Too much potassium throws off the fluid and electrical balance in the cells and can lead to such serious problems as irregular or rapid heartbeat, a drop in blood pressure, and paralysis of the arms and legs. Convulsions, coma, and even cardiac arrest can follow a severe overdose. Never take more potassium than recommended or prescribed; and call your doctor if you become confused or extremely fatigued, develop nausea or diarrhea, or notice a heaviness in your legs or a numbness and tingling in your hands and feet. Seek emergency medical treatment if your stool is either bloody or black and tarry, if you are having trouble breathing, or if your heartbeat seems to be irregular.

Recommended daily allowances

The amount of salt you use affects your potassium requirements; and there is no standard recommended dietary allowance (RDA) for this mineral. Nutritional experts currently advise cutting back on the amount of table salt you use and increasing the amount of potassium-rich foods you eat. Many experts peg the minimum daily requirement at roughly

2,000 to 2,500 milligrams. Since a normal diet supplies from 2,000 to 6,000 milligrams daily, supplements aren't necessary unless you are taking medications that deplete the body's potassium supply.

Best dietary sources

Potassium is found in fruits, including avocados, bananas, citrus fruits, raisins, and dried peaches; grapefruit, tomato, and orange juice; vegetables, including fresh spinach, parsnips, and potatoes; nuts, including almonds, Brazil nuts, cashews, peanuts, pecans, and walnuts; milk; molasses, dried lentils; canned sardines; and whole-grain cereals.

One cup of cooked spinach contains 1,160 milligrams of potassium. One-half cup of raisins or one-half of a medium avocado provides 650 milligrams. One cooked potato or 1 cup of orange juice contains 500 milligrams.

Pyridoxal Phosphate

See Vitamin B$_6$

Pyridoxine

See Vitamin B$_6$

Retinol

See Vitamin A

Riboflavin

What it is

Riboflavin, also called vitamin B$_2$, is a water-soluble vitamin commonly found in dairy products. It is also produced synthetically.

What it does

Riboflavin plays an important role in the body's production of energy. It helps tissues breathe and get rid of waste. It also helps activate vitamin B$_6$.

Why you need it

Riboflavin helps the body grow and develop. It keeps the mucous membranes healthy and protects the nervous system, skin, and eyes.

Riboflavin is also useful in the treatment of various medical conditions, including infections, stomach and liver disorders, burns, and alcoholism. Researchers also believe that riboflavin helps the body absorb iron more efficiently. It is not uncommon for iron and riboflavin deficiencies to occur simultaneously.

Can you take too much?

Riboflavin appears to be harmless no matter how high the dose. However, too much riboflavin may darken the color of your urine.

Recommended daily allowances

■ ADULTS

Males 11 to 14 years: 1.6 milligrams
Males 15 to 22 years: 1.7 milligrams
Males 23 to 50 years: 1.6 milligrams
Males 51 and older: 1.4 milligrams
Females 11 to 22 years: 1.3 milligrams
Females 23 and older: 1.2 milligrams

Women require an additional 0.3 milligram of riboflavin each day during pregnancy. Breastfeeding mothers need an extra 0.5 milligram of riboflavin per day.

People who exercise a lot—especially women—probably need extra riboflavin as well.

■ CHILDREN

Infants up to 6 months: 0.4 milligram
Ages 6 to 12 months: 0.6 milligram
Ages 1 to 3 years: 0.8 milligram
Ages 4 to 6 years: 1.0 milligram
Ages 7 to 10 years: 1.4 milligrams

Best dietary sources

The body is not able to store riboflavin, so this vitamin must constantly be replenished to prevent a deficiency.

Milk is probably the single best source of riboflavin. One quart of milk contains 1.7 milligrams of riboflavin—enough riboflavin for almost any adult or child. Other good sources of riboflavin include cheese, yogurt, chicken, organ meats, leafy green vegetables, cereal, bread, wheat germ, brewer's yeast, and almonds.

Salt

See Sodium

Selenium

What it is

Selenium is one of the minerals required by the body in only trace amounts. It is a potent antioxidant. Supplements are available in several formulations.

What it does

Working with vitamin E, selenium helps fend off the damage that oxidation can cause to the cells.

Why you need it

Because selenium maintains tissue elasticity by preventing excessive cell damage, a deficiency can cause premature aging. A lack of selenium can also lead to male infertility.

Can you take too much?

Sustained dosages greater than 700 to 1,100 micrograms are not recommended. Toxic levels of selenium can lead to loss of hair, teeth, and nails, a decline in energy, and even paralysis.

Recommended daily allowances

The government has not yet established a recommended dietary allowance (RDA) for selenium. The estimated safe and adequate daily intake is as follows:

■ ADULTS

All adults: 50 to 200 micrograms

Women should not take megadoses of selenium during pregnancy or while breastfeeding.

■ CHILDREN
Infants up to 6 months: 10 to 40 micrograms
Ages 6 to 12 months: 20 to 60 micrograms
Ages 1 to 3 years: 20 to 80 micrograms
Ages 4 to 6 years: 30 to 120 micrograms
Ages 7 and older: 50 to 200 micrograms

Best dietary sources

The amount of selenium in the following foods varies according to the amount in the soil in which they grew. Selenium is found in: vegetables, including broccoli, cabbage, celery, cucumbers, garlic, mushrooms, and onions; kidney, liver, and chicken; whole-grain products, bran, and wheat germ; egg yolks; tuna and seafood; and milk.

Sodium

What it is

Sodium pervades our food supply. As sodium chloride, it is known as salt.

What it does

Sodium maintains the balance of water inside and outside of the body's cells. Together with potassium, it also regulates the body's acid balance and plays a role in governing the electrical charge in the nerves and muscles.

Why you need it

Sodium prevents dehydration and is essential for proper functioning of nerves and muscles. Deficiencies are almost unheard of, but could result in digestive problems, weight loss, and arthritis.

Can you take too much?

Excessive sodium levels can cause body tissue to retain water and swell. Extremely high levels of sodium can lead to dizziness, stupor, and even a coma.

For people with high blood pressure, the extra water retention caused by sodium can make the pressure worse. Blood pressure patients are therefore advised to keep their salt intake below average.

Recommended daily allowances

With other vitamins and minerals, the concern is a possible deficiency. With sodium, the problem is excess. The typical American diet contains as much as 12 grams of sodium per day, while we only need about 3. There is no official recommended dietary allowance (RDA) for sodium. Estimates of the minimum requirements are as follows:

■ ADULTS

All adults: 1.1 to 3.3 grams

According to current guidelines, healthy women need not restrict the amount of sodium in their diets during pregnancy or while breast-feeding.

■ CHILDREN

Infants up to 6 months: 0.11 to 0.35 gram
Ages 6 to 12 months: 0.25 to 0.75 gram
Ages 1 to 3 years: 0.32 to 1 gram
Ages 4 to 6 years: 0.45 to 1.35 grams
Ages 7 to 10 years: 0.6 to 1.8 grams
Ages 11 to 17 years: 0.9 to 2.3 grams

Best dietary sources

Table salt is the primary source. Other foods containing sodium include: bacon, dried and fresh beef, ham, and other meats; milk, butter, and margarine; clams and canned sardines; bread; green beans; and canned tomatoes.

Manufacturers typically add salt to improve the taste of canned vegetables and processed foods. Bouillon, soups, pickles, potato chips and many "snack" foods are especially high in salt.

One teaspoon of salt contains 2 grams of sodium. One cup of cottage cheese provides slightly more than 1/2 gram. One cup of canned corn, 1 cup of canned tomato juice, or 1 slice of pizza (1/6 of a 12-inch pie) each provide about 1/2 gram of sodium.

Sodium Fluoride

See Fluoride

Sulfur

What it is

Sulfur is a component of several amino acids found naturally in protein. Our requirements are met fully through our normal diet. The only people at risk of a deficiency are strict vegetarians.

What it does

Sulfur is one of the raw materials used by the liver to manufacture the bile required by the digestive system. It is also a component of the keratin in skin, nails, and hair.

Why you need it
Sulfur maintains a good complexion and glossy hair.

Can you take too much?
Sulfur is unlikely to cause any problems, even if your body has more than it needs.

Recommended daily allowances
There is no recommended dietary allowance (RDA) for sulfur and no reports of deficiency.

Best dietary sources
Eggs are the richest source of sulfur. It is also available in meat, fish, dried beans, cabbage, milk, and wheat germ.

Taurine

See Nonessential Amino acids

Tetrahydrofolic Acid

See Folic Acid

Thiamin

What it is
Thiamin, one of the water-soluble vitamins, is also called vitamin B_1. Thiamin is widely available in foods and is also produced synthetically. An injectable form is available by prescription.

A well-balanced diet should generally provide enough thiamin for healthy people. However, more adults are deficient in thiamin than in almost any other vitamin. One of the reasons this deficiency has become so common is the high rate of alcoholism. Alcohol impairs the absorption of many nutrients and is especially detrimental to the body's ability to process thiamin.

Very young children and elderly people who do not eat a well-balanced diet are also in danger of developing a serious thiamin deficiency. Although rare, an uncorrected thiamin deficiency can lead to symptoms of beriberi, a disorder that affects the nervous system and may involve the heart and circulatory systems.

What it does

Thiamin plays an important role in converting blood sugar (glucose) into the energy needed to fuel the body. It also helps release energy from fat, and together with adenosine triphosphate, it forms a compound needed to convert carbohydrates into energy.

Why you need it

Thiamin is important for normal growth and development. It keeps the mucous membranes healthy and helps keep the nervous system, heart, and muscles working properly. Physicians prescribe thiamin supplements to treat beriberi. Thiamin supplements are also important for alcoholics. The mental confusion, vision disturbances, and staggering gait typically associated with alcoholism are also symptoms of beriberi.

Can you take too much?

Oral overdoses are extremely rare. People who take several hundred milligrams of thiamin daily—literally hundreds of times the recommended daily amount—may become drowsy. Large injections of thiamin occasionally cause an allergic reaction similar to anaphylactic shock.

Recommended daily allowances

■ ADULTS

Males 11 to 18: 1.4 milligrams
Males 19 to 50: 1.5 milligrams
Males 51 and older: 1.2 milligrams

The RDA for females is:

Females 11 to 22: 1.1 milligrams
Females 23 and older: 1.0 milligram

Women require an additional 0.4 milligram of thiamin each day during pregnancy. Breastfeeding mothers need an extra 0.5 milligram of thiamin per day.

■ CHILDREN

Infants up to 6 months: 0.3 milligram
Ages 6 to 12 months: 0.5 milligram
Ages 1 to 3 years: 0.7 milligram
Ages 4 to 6 years: 0.9 milligram
Ages 7 to 10 years: 1.2 milligrams

Best dietary sources

The body is not able to store thiamin very well, so it is important to constantly replenish your thiamin supply. The best sources are whole-grain cereals, rye and whole-wheat flour, wheat germ, rice bran, dried sunflower seeds, soybeans, navy and kidney beans, meat, pork, and salmon steak.

A tablespoonful of brewer's yeast provides 1.2 milligrams of thiamin; one cup of cooked kidney beans contains 0.51 milligram; two slices of whole-wheat bread have 0.15 milligram.

Threonine

What it is

Threonine is one of the amino acids considered essential because they cannot be manufactured in the body and must be obtained through diet.

What it does

The body must have supplies of all the amino acids, including threonine, on hand in order to manufacture human proteins. These proteins are a vital component of all the body's cells and its many hormones and enzymes.

Why you need it

The body requires a continuing supply of fresh proteins to support normal functions and maintain the tissues in good repair. Without the amino acids, production of these proteins would slow to a halt.

Can you take too much?

Amino acids are rarely toxic, even in large amounts.

Recommended daily allowances

There is no official recommended allowance for threonine. The estimated adult daily requirement is approximately 3.5 milligrams per pound of body weight. Infants require 8 times that amount; children need about 3 times the adult requirement.

Best dietary sources

A complete set of all the amino acids is available in most meat and dairy products.

Tribasic Calcium Phosphate

See Calcium

Tryptophan

What it is

Tryptophan is one of the amino acids considered essential because they cannot be manufactured in the body and must be obtained through diet. Natural and synthetic tryptophan supplements are also available, despite a recent incident in which contaminated supplements caused illness.

What it does

Tryptophan is the raw material for serotonin, one of the chemicals that regulate the transmission of nerve impulses in the brain.

Why you need it

The serotonin manufactured from tryptophan is one of the major chemicals governing mood and behavior. The well-known antidepressant drug Prozac, for instance, works by boosting serotonin levels in the brain. Serotonin also has a calming affect; and a lack of serotonin may spark a headache.

Can you take too much?

When correctly manufactured, tryptophan supplements pose no danger.

Recommended daily allowances

There is no official recommended dietary allowance for tryptophan. The estimated adult daily requirement is less than 1.5 milligrams per pound of body weight. Infants require 7 times that amount; children need less than 2 milligrams per pound.

Best dietary sources

Tryptophan is particularly plentiful in bananas, dried dates, milk, cottage cheese, meat, fish, turkey, and peanuts.

Tyrosine

See Nonessential Amino Acids

Valine

See Branched-Chain Amino Acids

Vanadium

What it is

Vanadium, one of the minerals needed in only trace amounts, can be obtained from fish, meat, whole grain, oils, and vitamin supplements.

What it does

We do not yet know exactly how vanadium works in the body, but we do know that it's present in most body tissues.

Why you need it

Vanadium is needed for proper development of bones, cartilage, and teeth.

Can you take too much?

Megadoses can lead to anemia, eye irritation, and respiratory problems.

Recommended daily allowances

The government has not yet established a recommended dietary allowance (RDA) for vanadium. Adults probably need 100 to 300 micrograms of vanadium per day. Most people get more than 10 times that amount in their daily diet.

Best dietary sources

Vanadium is found in meat, seafood, grains, and vegetable oil.

Vitamin A

What it is

Vitamin A, also known as retinol, is one of the fat-soluble vitamins that can be stored by the body. There are two ways of getting this vitamin from your diet: either as vitamin A itself (especially plentiful in liver) or as beta-carotene, a plant-based substance that the body can convert into vitamin A. Megadoses of vitamin A itself can be toxic. Megadoses of beta-carotene are not, since the body converts only as much as needed into Vitamin A.

What it does

Vitamin A helps regulate cell development, promotes bone growth and tooth development, and boosts the body's immune system and resistance to respiratory infections. By helping to form rhodopsin, a substance the eyes need to function in partial darkness, vitamin A enables us to see at night.

Why you need it

Vitamin A is essential for good vision, especially night vision. It helps keep the skin, hair, and mucous membranes healthy. It also promotes reproduction by helping testicles and ovaries to function properly and aiding in the development of the embryo.

Can you take too much?

A large overdose of vitamin A—500,000 IU or more—can cause headache, vomiting, bone pain, weakness, blurred vision, irritability, and flaking of the skin. Long-term intake of 100,000 IU or more per day can also lead to toxicity. Symptoms include hair loss, headache, bone thickening, an enlarged liver and spleen, anemia, menstrual problems, stiffness, joint pain, weakness, and dry skin. High doses of beta-carotene, on the other hand, have no toxic effects.

Authorities recommend that pregnant women take no more than 5,000 IU of vitamin A per day. The same is true for women taking birth control pills, which tend to increase the amount of retinol in the blood.

Regular doses of 25,000 to 50,000 IU or more per day may cause birth defects.

Recommended daily allowances

The recommended dietary allowance (RDA) for vitamin A is expressed in International Units (IU). One IU contains approximately 5 micrograms of retinol or 30 micrograms of beta-carotene.

■ ADULTS
Males 11 years and older: 5,000 IU.
Females 11 years and older: 4,000 IU.

Women need an additional 1,000 IU each day during pregnancy. Breastfeeding mothers need an extra 2,000 IU per day.

It is important to note that a daily intake of 5,000 IU may not be enough for many people. For example, people who smoke, eat a lot of junk food, or have diabetes or an infection may need more.

■ CHILDREN
Infants up to 12 months: 1,875 IU
Ages 1 to 3 years: 2,000 IU
Ages 4 to 6 years: 2,500 IU
Ages 7 to 10 years: 3,300 IU

Best dietary sources

The average person has up to a two-year supply of vitamin A stored in the liver. However, you need to constantly replenish this supply to prevent a deficiency—and thus night blindness—from developing.

Beta-carotene, the vitamin A precursor, is available in many fruits and vegetables. Good sources include carrots, sweet potatoes, broccoli, spinach, tomatoes, lettuce, winter squash, apricots, cantaloupe, and watermelon.

One sweet potato provides almost 10,000 IU. A single carrot contains almost 5,000 IU, a cup of cooked carrots provides 15,000 IU. Liver is an excellent source of vitamin A itself. One-half pound of calves' liver provides almost 75,000 IU.

Vitamin B_1

See Thiamin

Vitamin B_2

See Riboflavin

Vitamin B_3

See Niacin

Vitamin B_5

See Pantothenic Acid

Vitamin B_6

What it is

Vitamin B_6, also known as pyridoxine and pyridoxal phosphate, is one of the water-soluble vitamins that the body can't store. You need a continued daily supply from food or supplements. A synthetic form is available.

What it does

Vitamin B_6 helps the body process the protein, fat, and carbohydrates in our diet. It works with other vitamins and minerals to supply the energy used in our muscles, and plays a role in cell growth, including the body's production of red blood cells and cells of the immune system.

Why you need it

Vitamin B_6 plays a crucial role in maintaining the body's immune system. It helps the brain work properly and assists in maintaining the proper chemical balance in the body's fluids. It also helps the body resist stress. Physicians prescribe this vitamin to treat certain types of anemia and to counteract poisoning from the prescription drugs cycloserine and isoniazid.

Can you take too much?

There is currently little evidence that more than 50 milligrams of vitamin B_6 per day will do the body any extra good. However, a total daily intake of more than 500 milligrams can lead to serious nerve damage. Clumsiness and numbness in the hands and feet are signs that you may be getting too much vitamin B_6. To be on the safe side, experts recommend that you avoid taking supplements of more than 200 milligrams per day.

Recommended daily allowances

■ ADULTS
Males 11 years and older: 2.2 milligrams
Females 11 years and older: 2.0 milligrams

Women need an additional 0.6 milligram of vitamin B_6 each day during pregnancy. Breastfeeding mothers need an extra 0.5 milligram per day.

■ CHILDREN
Infants up to 6 months: 0.3 milligram
Ages 6 to 12 months: 0.6 milligram
Ages 1 to 3 years: 0.9 milligram
Ages 4 to 6 years: 1.3 milligrams
Ages 7 to 10 years: 1.8 milligrams

Best dietary sources

Vitamin B_6 is available in meats; fish, including salmon, shrimp, and tuna; whole grains, including bran, whole-wheat flour, wheat germ, and rice; bananas; vegetables, including avocados and carrots; and brewer's yeast, hazelnuts, lentils, soybeans, and sunflower seeds.

One-half cup of soybeans provides 0.85 milligram of vitamin B_6; a medium banana has 0.61 milligram; one-half of a medium avocado has 0.46 milligram; and one-quarter cup of wheat germ provides 0.3 milligram.

Vitamin B₉

See Folic Acid

Vitamin B₁₂

What it is

Vitamin B_{12}, a water-soluble vitamin, is also called cobalamin and cyanocobalamin. It is found in meat, fish, dairy products, and eggs—but cannot be obtained from plant-based foods. People who follow a strict vegetarian or macrobiotic diet are at serious risk of developing a vitamin B_{12} deficiency. This is of particular concern for children. A synthetic form of vitamin B_{12} is available, but a prescription is necessary if your physician decides you need high doses or must take it by injection.

What it does

Vitamin B_{12} helps the body process and burn fats and carbohydrates. It also helps the nervous system work properly and aids in growth and cell development—especially blood cells. It is also necessary for production of the protective sheath that covers nerve cells, and helps the body process DNA.

Why you need it

Vitamin B_{12} is essential to the body's growth and development. This vitamin is also useful in the treatment of some types of nerve damage and pernicious anemia. Supplements can help prevent a deficiency in strict vegetarians. Vitamin B_{12} supplementation is particularly important to assure normal growth and development in children who follow a vegetarian diet.

Can you take too much?

Very few problems have been reported with vitamin B_{12}—even when people take as much as 1,000 milligrams per day. However, if you take vitamin B_{12} along with large amounts of vitamin C, you may develop a nosebleed, bleeding from the ears, or a dry mouth.

Recommended daily allowances

■ ADULTS

The RDA for everyone 11 years and older is 3 micrograms. Women need an extra 1 microgram of vitamin B_{12} each day during pregnancy and while they are breastfeeding an infant.

■ CHILDREN

Infants up to 6 months: 0.5 microgram
Ages 6 to 12 months: 1.5 micrograms
Ages 1 to 3 years: 2 micrograms
Ages 4 to 6 years: 2.5 micrograms
Ages 7 to 10 years: 3 micrograms

Best dietary sources

The best sources of vitamin B_{12} are fish, including clams, flounder, herring, mackerel, sardines, and snapper; dairy foods, including milk and milk products, blue cheese, and Swiss cheese; organ meats, especially kidney and liver; other meats, such as beef, pork, and liverwurst; and eggs.

One-half cup of cottage cheese, packed, provides 1 microgram of vitamin B_{12}. One cup of whole or skim milk or one large egg contains 1 microgram. One ounce of cheddar, brick, or mozzarella cheese has 0.28 microgram.

Vitamin C

What it is

Vitamin C, one of the water-soluble vitamins, is also called ascorbic acid.

Some nutritionists have extolled vitamin C as a "cure" for the common cold. While there is no proof for this claim, some studies have indicated that vitamin C can help prevent colds from developing and also ease the symptoms if you do get one.

Researchers may not be convinced, but a great many people believe in vitamin C—it is estimated that more than half of all adults take vitamin C supplements. Taking large doses once a day could, however, be a waste of money, since the body tends to get rid of supplemental vitamin C very quickly. Taking smaller doses several times a day could prove to be more effective.

What it does

Vitamin C plays an essential role in the manufacture of collagen, a substance in connective tissue that essentially holds the bones together. Vitamin C also helps repair damaged tissue and has antioxidant properties.

Why you need it

Vitamin C may or may not cure the common cold, but it is definitely valuable in many other ways. This vitamin helps the body absorb more iron and is therefore useful in the treatment of iron-deficiency and other types of anemia. Vitamin C plays a role in the production of hemoglobin and red blood cells, works to keep the gums and teeth healthy, helps heal broken bones and wounds, and is one of the substances physicians choose to treat urinary tract infections.

Vitamin C continues to be used to treat the deficiency disease scurvy. Although scurvy was much more common in the nineteenth century, it has not disappeared. Symptoms include muscle weakness or wasting, bleeding or swollen gums, loss of teeth, rough skin, delayed wound healing, fatigue, and depression.

Can you take too much?

The body rids itself of extra vitamin C very quickly. Daily doses of as much as 5,000 to 10,000 milligrams taken for several years have failed to produce any serious side effects. However, if too much vitamin C accumulates in the body, facial flushing, headaches, stomach cramps, nausea, or vomiting are possibilities. At a dose of more than 1,000 milligrams per day, you may also notice that you have to urinate more frequently or start having mild diarrhea. Dizziness and faintness may occur following a vitamin C injection.

Recommended daily allowances

■ ADULTS

The RDA for everyone 15 years of age and older is 60 milligrams.

Women need an additional 20 milligrams of vitamin C each day during pregnancy—a developing baby needs the vitamin to support the growth and formation of its bones, teeth and connective tissue. Breastfeeding mothers need an extra 40 milligrams of vitamin C per day to pass on to their rapidly growing babies. If you are pregnant or breastfeeding, your physician will determine the exact amount of vitamin C that you need to take.

People over the age of 55 and smokers may also need a vitamin C supplement.

■ CHILDREN
Infants up to 12 months: 35 milligrams
Ages 1 to 10 years: 45 milligrams
Ages 11 to 14 years: 50 milligrams

Best dietary sources

Most people know that oranges and orange juice contain vitamin C, but the vitamin is also available in many other fruits, and even in vegetables. Sources of vitamin C include broccoli, Brussels sprouts, cabbage, grapefruit, green peppers, lemons, potatoes, spinach, strawberries, sweet and hot peppers, tangerines, and tomatoes.

One cup of orange juice provides 120 milligrams of vitamin C; a medium orange contains 66 milligrams. One stalk of raw broccoli has 160 milligrams of vitamin C; a medium green pepper, raw, provides 70 milligrams.

Vitamin D

What it is

There are two forms of vitamin D: ergocalciferol, which is found in a relatively small selection of foods; and cholecalciferol, which the body manufactures when exposed to the sun. Vitamin D is fat-soluble, can build up inside the body, and therefore is highly toxic when taken in large doses for a long time. Milk fortified with vitamin D is our major dietary source.

What it does

Vitamin D helps to control the formation of bone tissue. It increases the amount of calcium and phosphorus the body absorbs from the small intestine and thus helps regulate the growth, hardening, and repair of the bones.

Why you need it

Vitamin D is essential for the normal growth and development of the teeth, bones, and cartilage in children. It's also needed to keep adult teeth and bones in good repair. Vitamin D prevents rickets, a deficiency disease characterized by malformations of bones and teeth in children and by brittle, easily broken bones in adults.

Can you take too much?

For adults, doses of 50,000 IU per day can prove toxic; and doses of 25,000 IU daily are risky. For a small child, as little as 1,800 IU per day can cause harm. Long-term overdose of vitamin D can cause *irreversible* damage to the kidneys and cardiovascular system, and can retard growth in children. Excessive amounts of the vitamin may lead to high blood pressure and premature hardening of the arteries. Nausea, abdominal pain, loss of appetite, weight loss, seizures, and an irregular heartbeat may be signs that you are taking too much. If you have any concerns, stop taking the vitamin right away and consult your physician.

Vitamin D produced by sunlight is not a concern. Overexposure to the sun does not cause vitamin D toxicity among healthy people.

Recommended daily allowances
■ ADULTS
Ages 19 to 22 years: 600 IU
Ages 23 years and older: 400 IU

Women need an extra 400 IU each day during pregnancy and while they are breastfeeding an infant. The additional vitamin D is important for the baby's normal growth. Do not increase dosage beyond this point, however. Too much vitamin D during pregnancy may cause abnormalities.

People over the age of 55 may also need to take a vitamin D supplement—especially women who have completed menopause.

The increasing use of sunscreens protects against the harmful ultraviolet rays that cause skin cancer; unfortunately, this sensible practice also limits the body's production of vitamin D. If you live in an area that does not typically have a lot of sunshine, you may want to check with your doctor about the possible need for extra vitamin D. This is especially important for children, whose bones and teeth need vitamin D to grow properly.

■ CHILDREN
Through age 18: 800 IU

Best dietary sources
Sunlight is the best source of vitamin D, but you can also boost your body's supply by drinking fortified milk. Other sources include herring, mackerel, salmon, sardines and cod- and halibut-liver oils.

Vitamin E

What it is

Vitamin E, also known as alpha-tocopherol, is a leading antioxidant. Although it is one of the fat soluble vitamins that can build up in the body, it has proven safe in much larger than standard doses. A synthetic form of vitamin E is available, and your doctor can also prescribe vitamin E injections.

What it does

Vitamin E protects the fats found in cell membranes throughout the body from oxidation, or spoilage. Because of this ability to inhibit the natural cell destruction that occurs with age, vitamin E is being tested as a treatment for many of the chronic diseases of the elderly.

Why you need it

In addition to preventing the oxidation of cells and tissue, vitamin E helps to prevent blood clots, thereby reducing the risk of heart disease. It may also discourage development of some types of cancer; and it is needed for production of normal red blood cells. It helps children grow and develop normally and is used to treat vitamin E deficiency in premature or low-birthweight babies.

Can you take too much?

Even at doses of 1,500 IU per day (50 times the RDA), vitamin E has no harmful effects. However, at doses of 2,400 IU per day, it may cause bleeding problems due to its clot-preventing ability. Too much vitamin E may also reduce your body's supply of vitamin A, alter the immune system, and impair sexual function.

Because they can impede formation of blood clots, vitamin E supplements should be avoided for 2 weeks before and after surgery. You should also forgo large doses when taking anticoagulant medications.

Recommended daily allowances

■ ADULTS

Males 18 or older: 30 IU
Females 18 or older: 24 IU

Women need an additional 6 IU each day during pregnancy. Breastfeeding mothers need an extra 9 IU per day.

People over the age of 55, smokers, and people who abuse alcohol may need to take vitamin E supplements.

■ CHILDREN
Infants up to 12 months: 9 to 12 IU
Ages 1 to 7 years: 15 to 21 IU
Ages 11 to 18 years: 24 IU

Best dietary sources
Vegetable oils, including corn, cottonseed, and peanut oils, are the best source of vitamin E. Almonds, hazelnuts, safflower nuts, sunflower seeds, walnuts, wheat germ, whole-wheat flour, and margarine are also rich in vitamin E. Various fruits and vegetables—spinach, lettuce, onions, blackberries, apples, and pears—also contain this vitamin.

Vitamin H

See Biotin

Vitamin K

What it is
There are two forms of vitamin K: phylloquinone, which is found in green leafy vegetables; and menaquinone, which is produced within the body by "friendly" bacteria that reside in the intestinal tract. A deficiency may result if antibiotics or an intestinal disease destroy these bacteria.

What it does
Vitamin K is an essential element in the blood's normal clotting process. It promotes production of the clotting factors, such as pro-thrombin, that stop us from bleeding.

Why you need it
Vitamin K helps prevent abnormal bleeding, and is given to newborns as a precaution against hemorrhagic (bleeding) disease. It is also prescribed to correct deficiencies that result in bleeding disorders.

Can you take too much?
Doses as high as 500 times the usual recommendation have failed to cause any ill effect. However, allergic-type reactions have been reported; and the vitamin could interfere with the liver's ability to function,

although liver problems are not very common. Infants who receive an excessive amount may suffer brain damage.

Recommended daily allowances

The government has not yet established the recommended dietary allowance (RDA) for vitamin K.

■ ADULTS

The estimated adequate daily intake for everyone 18 years of age and older is 70 to 140 micrograms.

There is currently no information on the safety and effectiveness of vitamin K supplements during pregnancy. If you are pregnant or are breastfeeding, do not take vitamin K without consulting your physician.

■ CHILDREN

The estimated adequate daily intake of vitamin K for children is as follows:

Infants up to 6 months: 12 micrograms
Ages 6 to 12 months: 10 to 20 micrograms
Ages 1 to 3 years: 15 to 30 micrograms
Ages 4 to 6 years: 20 to 40 micrograms
Ages 7 to 10 years: 30 to 60 micrograms
Ages 11 to 17 years: 50 to 100 micrograms

Best dietary sources

Vitamin K is found in brussels sprouts, cabbage, cauliflower, oats, soybeans, spinach, cheddar cheese, egg yolks, and green tea.

Zinc

What it is

Zinc is one of the minerals that we require in just trace amounts. It is found in a variety of meat and grain products. Supplements are available as well.

What it does

Zinc is part of the molecular structure of more than 80 enzymes, and works with the red blood cells to transport waste carbon dioxide from body tissue to the lungs for exhalation. It is essential for the production of the RNA and DNA that governs the division, growth, and repair of the body's cells.

Why you need it

Zinc is an extremely important mineral: It helps the body grow and develop, and also promotes normal fetal growth. It preserves our sense of taste and smell, helps wounds heal, and keeps the right amount of vitamin A in our blood. It is also a component of the insulin that regulates our energy supply.

Can you take too much?

Doses of more than 40 times the RDA cause few, if any, problems.

Nausea, vomiting, and diarrhea may follow sustained overdosage. Other consequences include drowsiness, sluggishness, light-headedness, and restlessness. Difficulty writing or walking can also be warning signs of zinc toxicity.

Recommended daily allowances

■ ADULTS

All adults: 15 milligrams

Women need an additional 5 milligrams of zinc each day during pregnancy. Women who are breastfeeding an infant should take an extra 10 milligrams per day. Since women may not get all the zinc they need from their diet, it is important that they discuss the possibility of supplementation with a physician.

■ CHILDREN

Infants up to 6 months: 3 milligrams
Ages 6 to 12 months: 5 milligrams
Ages 1 to 10 years: 10 milligrams
Age 11 and older: 15 milligrams

Best dietary sources

Zinc can be obtained from meat, including beef, lamb, and pork; poultry; seafood, including herring and oysters; egg yolk; milk; maple syrup and blackstrap molasses; sesame and sunflower seeds; soybeans; whole-grain products; wheat bran; wheat germ; and yeast.

III. Appendices

A. Poison Control Centers

If there is one phone number that no home should be without, it is the nearest poison control center. In this section, you'll find a national directory of these centers listed alphabetically by state and city. Many of the centers are certified by the American Association of Poison Control Centers. To be certified, they must serve a large geographic area, be open 24 hours a day, provide direct-dial or toll-free phone service, be supervised by a medical director, and have registered pharmacists or nurses available to answer questions from the public. Certified centers are marked by an asterisk after the name.

In the listings below, telephone numbers designated "TTY" are teletype lines for the hearing-impaired. "TDD" numbers reach a telecommunication device for the deaf.

ALABAMA

BIRMINGHAM

**Regional Poison
Control Center
Children's Hospital of
Alabama (*)**
1600 7th Ave. South
Birmingham, AL 35233-1711
Business: 205-939-9720
Emergency: 205-933-4050
                205-939-9201
                800-292-6678 (AL)
Fax: 205-939-9245

TUSCALOOSA

**Alabama Poison Control
Systems, Inc. (*)**
408 A. Paul Bryant Dr. E.
Tuscaloosa, AL 35401
Business: 205-345-0600
Emergency: 205-345-0600
                800-462-0800 (AL)
Fax: 205-759-7994

ALASKA

ANCHORAGE

**Anchorage Poison Center
Providence Hospital**
P.O. Box 196604
3200 Providence Dr.
Anchorage, AK 99519-6604
Business: 907-562-2211
                ext. 3633
Emergency: 907-261-3193
                800-478-3193 (AK)
Fax: 907-261-3645

FAIRBANKS

**Fairbanks Poison
Control Center**
1650 Cowles St.
Fairbanks, AK 99701
Business: 907-456-7182
Emergency: 907-456-7182
Fax: 907-458-5553

ARIZONA

PHOENIX

**Samaritan Regional
Poison Center (*)
Good Samaritan
Medical Center**
1111 East McDowell Rd.
Phoenix, AZ 85006
Business: 602-495-4884
Emergency: 602-253-3334
Fax: 602-256-7579

TUCSON

**Arizona Poison & Drug
Information Center (*)
University of Arizona
Arizona Health
Sciences Center**
1501 North Campbell Ave.
#1156
Tucson, AZ 85724
Emergency: 520-626-6016
                800-362-0101 (AZ)
Fax: 520-626-2720

ARKANSAS

LITTLE ROCK

**Arkansas Poison and
Drug Information Center
College of Pharmacy -
UAMS**
4301 West Markham St.
Slot 522-2
Little Rock, AR 72205
Business: 501-661-6161
Emergency: 800-376-4766 (AR)

CALIFORNIA

FRESNO

**Central California Regional
Poison Control Center (*)
Valley Children's Hospital**
3151 North Millbrook
Fresno, CA 93703
Business: 209-241-6040
Emergency: 209-445-1222
800-346-5922
(Central CA)
Fax: 209-241-6050

LOS ANGELES

**Los Angeles County
Regional Drug & Poison
Information Center (*)
LAC & USC Medical Center**
1200 North State St.
Los Angeles, CA 90033
Business: 213-226-7741
Emergency: 213-222-3212
800-777-6476
Fax: 213-226-4194

SACRAMENTO

**UC Davis Medical Center
Regional Poison
Control Center (*)**
2315 Stockton Blvd.
Sacramento, CA 95817
Business: 916-734-3415
Emergency: 916-734-3692
800-342-9293
(N. CA only)
Fax: 916-734-7796

SAN DIEGO

**San Diego Regional
Poison Center (*)
UCSD Medical Center**
200 West Arbor Dr.
San Diego, CA 92103-8925
Business: 619-543-3666
Emergency: 619-543-6000
800-876-4766
(San Diego
and Imperial
counties only)
Fax: 619-692-1867

SAN FRANCISCO

**San Francisco Bay Area
Regional Poison
Control Center (*)
SF General Hospital**
1001 Potrero Ave.
Bldg. 80
San Francisco, CA 94110
Business: 415-206-5524
Emergency: 800-523-2222
Fax: 415-821-8513

COLORADO

DENVER

Rocky Mountain Poison and Drug Center (*)
8802 East 9th Ave.
Bldg. 752
Denver, CO 80220
Business: 303-739-1100
Emergency: 303-629-1123
TTY: 303-739-1127
Fax: 303-739-1119

CONNECTICUT

FARMINGTON

Connecticut Poison Control Center (*)
University of Connecticut Health Center
263 Farmington Ave.
Farmington, CT 06032
Business: 203-679-3473
Emergency: 800-343-2722 (CT)
TTY: 203-679-4346
Fax: 203-679-1623

DISTRICT OF COLUMBIA

WASHINGTON, DC

National Capital Poison Center (*)
3201 New Mexico Ave., NW
Suite 310
Washington, DC 20016
Business: 202-362-3867
Emergency: 202-625-3333
TTY: 202-362-8563
Fax: 202-362-8377

FLORIDA

JACKSONVILLE

Florida Poison Information Center of Jacksonville
655 W. 8th St.
Jacksonville, FL 32209
Emergency: 904-549-4480
Fax: 904-549-4063

MIAMI

Florida Poison Information Center of Miami
P.O. Box 016960, R-131
Miami, FL 33101
Emergency: 305-585-5253
Fax: 305-242-9762

TAMPA

Florida Poison Information and Toxicology Resource Center (*)
Tampa General Hospital
P.O. Box 1289
Tampa, FL 33601
Emergency: 813-253-4444
                  800-282-3171 (FL)
Fax: 813-253-4443

GEORGIA

ATLANTA

Georgia Poison Center (*)
Grady Health System
80 Butler St. SE
P.O. Box 26066
Atlanta, GA 30335-3801
Emergency: 404-616-9000
                  800-282-5846 (GA)
Fax: 404-616-6657

MACON

**Regional Poison
Control Center
Medical Center of
Central Georgia**
777 Hemlock St.
Macon, GA 31201
Poison Ctr: 912-633-1427
Fax: 912-633-5082

ILLINOIS

CHICAGO

**Chicago & NE Illinois
Regional Poison
Control Center
Rush-Presbyterian-
St. Luke's Medical Center**
1653 West Congress Pkwy.
Chicago, IL 60612
Business: 312-942-7064
Emergency: 312-942-5969
800-942-5969 (IL)
Fax: 312-942-4260

URBANA

**ASPCA/National Animal
Poison Control Center (*)**
1717 Philo Rd., Suite 36
Urbana, IL 61801
Business: 217-333-2053
800-548-2423
(24-hour
subscribers)
Fax: 217-244-1580

INDIANA

INDIANAPOLIS

**Indiana Poison Center (*)
Methodist Hospital
of Indiana**
1701 North Senate Blvd.
P.O. Box 1367
Indianapolis, IN 46206-1367
Emergency: 317-929-2323
800-382-9097 (IN)
TTY: 317-929-2336
Fax: 317-929-2337

IOWA

DES MOINES

**Variety Club Poison and
Drug Information Center
Iowa Methodist
Medical Center**
1200 Pleasant St.
Des Moines, IA 50309
Business: 515-241-6254
Emergency: 800-362-2327 (IA)
Fax: 515-241-5085

IOWA CITY

**Poison Control Center (*)
University of Iowa Hospitals
and Clinics**
200 Hawkins Dr.
Iowa City, IA 52242
Business: 319-356-2577
Emergency: 800-272-6477
(IA only)

KANSAS

KANSAS CITY

Mid-America Poison
Control Center
University of Kansas
Medical Center
3901 Rainbow Blvd.
Room B-400
Kansas City, KS 66160-7231
Business & 913-588-6633
Emergency: 800-332-6633 (KS)
Fax: 913-588-2350

TOPEKA

Stormont-Vail Regional
Medical Center
Emergency Department
1500 West 10th
Topeka, KS 66604
Business: 913-354-6000
Emergency: 913-354-6100
Fax: 913-354-5004

KENTUCKY

LOUISVILLE

Kentucky Regional Poison
Center (*)
Kosair Children's Hospital
Medical Towers S.
Suite 572
P.O. Box 35070
Louisville, KY 40232-5070
Business: 502-629-7264
Emergency: 502-629-7275
502-589-8222
800-722-5725
(KY)
Fax: 502-629-7277

LOUISIANA

MONROE

Louisiana Drug and Poison
Information Center (*)
Northeast Louisiana
University School
of Pharmacy
Monroe, LA 71209-6430
Business: 318-342-1710
Emergency: 800-256-9822
(LA)
Fax: 318-342-1744

MAINE

PORTLAND

Maine Poison Center (*)
Maine Medical Center
22 Bramhall St.
Portland, ME 04102
Business: 207-871-2950
Emergency: 800-442-6305
(ME)
Fax: 207-871-6226

MARYLAND

BALTIMORE

Maryland Poison Center (*)
University of Maryland
School of Pharmacy
20 North Pine St.
Baltimore, MD 21201
Business: 410-706-7604
Emergency: 410-706-7701
800-492-2414
(MD only)
TTY: 410-706-1858
Fax: 410-706-7184

MASSACHUSETTS

BOSTON

**Massachusetts Poison
Control System (*)**
300 Longwood Ave.
Boston, MA 02115
Emergency: 617-232-2120
          800-682-9211
TTY: 617-355-6089
Fax: 617-738-0032

MICHIGAN

DETROIT

**Poison Control Center (*)
Children's Hospital of
Michigan**
Harper Professional
Office Bldg., Suite 425
Detroit, MI 48201
Business: 313-745-5335
Emergency: 313-745-5711
Fax: 313-745-5493

GRAND RAPIDS

**Blodgett Regional Poison
Center (*)
Blodgett Memorial
Medical Center**
1840 Wealthy St. SE
Grand Rapids, MI 49506
Business: 616-774-5329
Emergency: 800-764-7661 (MI)
Fax: 616-774-7204

MINNESOTA

MINNEAPOLIS

**Hennepin Regional Poison
Center (*) Hennepin County
Medical Center**
701 Park Ave.
Minneapolis, MN 55415
Business: 612-347-3144
Emergency: 612-347-3141
TTY: 612-904-4691
Fax: 612-904-4289

**Minnesota Regional
Poison Center (*)**
8100 34th Ave. South
Box 1309
Minneapolis, MN 55440
Business: 612-851-8100
Emergency: 612-221-2113
Fax: 612-851-8166

MISSISSIPPI

HATTIESBURG

**Poison Center
Forrest General Hospital**
400 South 28th Ave.
Hattiesburg, MS 39401
Business: 601-288-4221
Emergency: 601-288-4235

JACKSON

**Mississippi Regional
Poison Control (*)
University of Mississippi
Medical Center**
2500 North State St.
Jackson, MS 39216
Business: 601-984-1675
Emergency: 601-354-7660
Fax: 601-984-1676

MISSOURI

KANSAS CITY

Poison Control Center (*)
Children's Mercy Hospital
2401 Gillham Rd.
Kansas City, MO 64108
Business: 816-234-3053
Emergency: 816-234-3430
Fax: 816-234-3421

ST. LOUIS

Cardinal Glennon
Children's Hospital
Regional Poison Center (*)
1465 South Grand Blvd.
St. Louis, MO 63104
Emergency: 314-772-5200
            800-366-8888
Fax: 314-577-5355

MONTANA

DENVER, CO

Rocky Mountain Poison and
Drug Center (*)
8802 E. 9th Ave.
Denver, CO 80220
Emergency: 303-629-1123
            800-525-5042 (MT)
Fax: 303-739-1119

NEBRASKA

OMAHA

The Poison Center (*)
Children's Memorial
Hospital
8301 Dodge St.
Omaha, NE 68114
Emergency: 402-390-5555
            (Omaha)
            800-955-9119
            (NE, WY)
Fax: 404-354-3049

NEVADA

LAS VEGAS

Poison Center
Humana Medical Center
3186 Maryland Pkwy.
Las Vegas, NV 89109
Emergency: 800-446-6179 (NV)

RENO

Poison Center
Washoe Medical Center
77 Pringle Way
Reno, NV 89520
Business: 702-328-4129
Emergency: 702-328-4100
Fax: 702-328-5555

NEW HAMPSHIRE

LEBANON

**New Hampshire Poison
Information Center (*)
Dartmouth-Hitchcock
Medical Center**
1 Medical Center Dr.
Lebanon, NH 03756
Emergency: 603-650-5000
          (ask for
          Poison Center)
          800-562-8236
          (NH only)
Fax: 603-650-8986

NEW JERSEY

NEWARK

**New Jersey Poison
Information and
Education System
Newark Beth Israel
Medical Center**
201 Lyons Ave.
Newark, NJ 07112
Emergency: POISON-1
          (800-764-7661)
TTY: POISON-1
          (800-764-7661)
Fax: 201-705-8098

PHILLIPSBURG

**Warren Hospital
Poison Control Center**
185 Roseberry St.
Phillipsburg, NJ 08865
Business: 908-859-6768
Emergency: 908-859-6767
          800-962-1253 (NJ)
Fax: 908-859-6812

NEW MEXICO

ALBUQUERQUE

**New Mexico Poison &
Drug Information Center
University of New Mexico**
Albuquerque, NM 87131-1076
Emergency: 505-843-2551
          800-432-6866 (NM)
Fax: 505-277-5892

NEW YORK

BUFFALO

**Western New York Regional
Poison Control Center
Children's Hospital of
Buffalo**
219 Bryant St.
Buffalo, NY 14222
Business: 716-878-7657
Emergency: 716-878-7654
          800-888-7655
          (NY & W. PA only)

MINEOLA

**L.I. Regional Poison
Control Center (*)
Winthrop University
Hospital**
259 First St.
Mineola, NY 11501
Emergency: 516-542-2323
TTY: 516-747-3323
Fax: 516-739-2070

NEW YORK

New York City Poison
Control Center (*)
NYC Dept. of Health
455 First Ave., Room 123
New York, NY 10016
Business: 212-447-8154
Emergency: 212-340-4494
212-POISONS
(212-764-7667)
TDD: 212-689-9014
Fax: 212-447-8223

NORTH TARRYTOWN

Hudson Valley Poison
Center
Phelps Memorial Hospital
701 N. Broadway
N. Tarrytown, NY 10591
Emergency: 914-353-1000
800-336-6997
Fax: 914-353-1050

ROCHESTER

Finger Lakes Regional
Poison Control Center (*)
University of Rochester
Medical Center
601 Elmwood Ave.
Rochester, NY 14642
Business: 716-273-4155
Emergency: 716-275-3232
800-333-0542 (NY)
Fax: 716-244-1677

SYRACUSE

Central NY Poison
Control Center
SUNY Health Science Center
750 East Adams St.
Syracuse, NY 13210
Business: 315-464-7073
Emergency: 315-476-4766
800-252-5655 (NY)
Fax: 315-464-7077

NORTH CAROLINA

ASHEVILLE

Western North Carolina
Poison Control Center (*)
Memorial Mission Hospital
509 Biltmore Ave.
Asheville, NC 28801
Emergency: 704-255-4490
800-542-4225 (NC)
Fax: 704-255-4467

CHARLOTTE

Carolinas Poison Center (*)
P.O. Box 32861
Charlotte, NC 28232-2861
Business: 704-355-3054
Emergency: 704-355-4000
(Charlotte area)
800-848-6946

NORTH DAKOTA

FARGO

North Dakota Poison Information Center (*) Meritcare Medical Center
720 North 4th St.
Fargo, ND 58122
Business: 701-234-6062
Emergency: 701-234-5575
                    800-732-2200 (ND)
Fax: 701-234-5090

OHIO

AKRON

Akron Regional Poison Control Center Children's Hospital Medical Center
1 Perkins Square
Akron, OH 44308
Business: 330-258-3066
Emergency: 330-379-8562
                    800-362-9922 (OH)
TTY: 330-379-8446
Fax: 330-379-8447

CINCINNATI

Regional Poison Control System Cincinnati Drug and Poison Information Center (*) University of Cincinnati College of Medicine
P.O. Box 670144
Cincinnati, OH 45267-0144
Emergency: 513-558-5111
                    800-872-5111 (OH)
Fax: 513-558-5301

CLEVELAND

Greater Cleveland Poison Control Center (*)
11100 Euclid Ave.
Cleveland, OH 44106
Emergency: 216-231-4455
                    888-231-4455
Fax: 216-844-3242

COLUMBUS

Central Ohio Poison Center (*)
700 Children's Dr.
Columbus, OH 43205-2696
Business: 614-722-2635
Emergency: 614-228-1323
                    800-682-7625
TTY: 614-228-2272
Fax: 614-221-2672

Greater Dayton Area Hospital Association (*) at Central Ohio Poison Center
700 Children's Dr.
Columbus, OH 43205
Business: 614-722-2635
Emergency: 513-222-2227
                    800-762-0727 (OH)

TOLEDO

Poison Information Center of NW Ohio (*) Medical College of Ohio Hospital
3000 Arlington Ave.
Toledo, OH 43614
Business: 419-381-3898
Emergency: 419-381-3897
                    800-589-3897 (OH)
Fax: 419-381-2818

ZANESVILLE

**Drug Information/Poison
Control Center (*)
Bethesda Hospital**
2951 Maple Ave.
Zanesville, OH 43701
Business: 614-454-4246
Emergency: 614-454-4221
614-454-4000
800-686-4221 (OH)
Fax: 614-454-4059

OKLAHOMA

OKLAHOMA CITY

**Oklahoma Poison Control
Center (*) University of
Oklahoma and Children's
Hospital of Oklahoma**
940 Northeast 13th St.
Oklahoma City, OK 73104
Emergency: 405-271-5454 (Bus.)
800-522-4611
(Bus.) (OK)
TDD: 405-271-1122
Fax: 405-271-1816

OREGON

PORTLAND

**Oregon Poison Center (*)
Oregon Health Sciences
University**
3181 SW Sam Jackson Park Rd.
Portland, OR 97201
Emergency: 503-494-8968
800-452-7165 (OR)
Fax: 503-494-4980

PENNSYLVANIA

HERSHEY

**Central Pennsylvania
Poison Center (*)
University Hospital
Milton S. Hershey
Medical Center**
P.O. Box 850
Hershey, PA 17033
Emergency: 800-521-6110
Fax: 717-531-6932

LANCASTER

**Poison Control Center (*)
St. Joseph Hospital and
Health Care Center**
250 College Ave.
Lancaster, PA 17604
Business: 717-299-4546
Emergency: 717-291-8111
Fax: 717-291-8346

PHILADELPHIA

The Poison Control Center (*)
3600 Market St.
Room 220
Philadelphia, PA 19104-2641
Business: 215-590-2003
Emergency: 215-386-2100
800-722-7112
Fax: 215-590-4419

PITTSBURGH

Pittsburgh Poison Center (*)
Children's Hospital
of Pittsburgh
3705 Fifth Ave.
Pittsburgh, PA 15213
Business: 412-692-5600
Emergency: 412-681-6669
Fax: 412-692-7497

RHODE ISLAND

PROVIDENCE

Rhode Island
Poison Center (*)
Rhode Island Hospital
593 Eddy St.
Providence, RI 02903
Emergency: 401-444-5727
Fax: 401-444-8062

SOUTH CAROLINA

COLUMBIA

Palmetto Poison Center (*)
College of Pharmacy
University of South Carolina
Columbia, SC 29208
Business: 803-777-7909
Emergency: 803-777-1117
                 800-922-1117 (SC)
Fax: 803-777-6127

SOUTH DAKOTA

ABERDEEN

Poison Control Center
St. Luke's Midland Regional
Medical Center
305 South State St.
Aberdeen, SD 57401
Business: 605-622-5000
Emergency: 605-622-5100
                 800-592-1889
                 (SD, MN, ND, WY)

RAPID CITY

Rapid City Regional Poison
Center
835 Fairmont Blvd.
P.O. Box 6000
Rapid City, SD 57709
Business &
Emergency: 605-341-3333

SIOUX FALLS

McKennan Poison Center
McKennan Hospital
800 East 21st St.
P.O. Box 5045
Sioux Falls, SD 57117-5045
Business: 605-322-8305
Emergency: 605-322-3894
                 800-843-0505
                  (IA, MN, NE, ND)
                 800-952-0123 (SD)
Fax: 605-322-8378

TENNESSEE

MEMPHIS

Southern Poison Center (*)
847 Monroe Ave.
Suite 230
Memphis, TN 38163
Business: 901-448-6800
Emergency: 901-528-6048
              800-288-9999
              (TN only)
Fax: 901-448-5419

NASHVILLE

Middle Tennessee Poison Center (*)
501 Oxford House
1161 21st Ave. S.
Nashville, TN 37232
Business: 615-936-0760
Emergency: 615-936-2034
              800-288-9999 (TN)
TDD: 615-936-2047
Fax: 615-936-2046

TEXAS

DALLAS

**North Texas Poison Center
Texas Poison Center
Network (*)
Parkland Memorial Hospital**
5201 Harry Hines Blvd.
P.O. Box 35926
Dallas, TX 75235
Business: 214-590-6625
Emergency: 800-POISON-1
              (800-764-7661)
Fax: 214-590-5008

EL PASO

**West Texas Regional
Poison Center (*)**
4815 Alameda Ave.
El Paso, TX 79905
Business: 915-521-7661
Emergency: 800-764-7661
              (800-POISON-1)
Fax: 915-521-7978

GALVESTON

**Southeast Texas
Poison Center (*)
University of Texas
Medical Branch
Trauma Center**
Room 3-112
Galveston, TX 77555-1175
Emergency: 409-765-1420
              800-764-7661
              (TX only)
Fax: 409-772-3917

TEMPLE

**Drug Information Center
Scott and White Memorial
Hospital**
2401 South 31st St.
Temple, TX 76508
Business: 817-724-4636
Fax: 817-724-1731

UTAH

SALT LAKE CITY

**Utah Poison
Control Center (*)**
410 Chipeta Way
Suite 230
Salt Lake City, UT 84108
Emergency: 801-581-2151
801-456-7707
(UT)
Fax: 801-581-4199

VERMONT

BURLINGTON

**Vermont Poison Center (*)
Fletcher Allen Health Care**
111 Colchester Ave.
Burlington, VT 05401
Business: 802-656-2721
Emergency: 802-658-3456
Fax: 802-656-4802

VIRGINIA

CHARLOTTESVILLE

**Blue Ridge Poison Center
Blue Ridge Hospital**
P.O. Box 67
Charlottesville, VA 22901
Emergency: 804-924-5543
800-451-1428
Fax: 804-971-8657

RICHMOND

**Virginia Poison Center
Virginia Commonwealth
University**
P.O. Box 980522
Richmond, VA 23298-0522
Emergency: 804-828-9123
Fax: 804-828-5291

WASHINGTON

SEATTLE

**Washington Poison
Center (*)**
155 NE 100th St.
Suite 400
Seattle, WA 98125-8012
Business: 206-517-2351
Emergency: 206-526-2121
800-732-6985 (WA)
TTY: 206-517-2394
800-572-0638 (WA)
Fax: 206-526-8490

WEST VIRGINIA

CHARLESTON

**West Virginia
Poison Center (*)
West Virginia University**
3110 MacCorkle Ave. SE
Charleston, WV 25304
Business: 304-347-1212
Emergency: 304-348-4211
800-642-3625 (WV)
Fax: 304-348-9560

PARKERSBURG

Poison Center
St. Joseph's Hospital Center
19th St. and Murdoch Ave.
Parkersburg, WV 26101
Emergency: 304-424-4222
Fax: 304-424-4766

WISCONSIN

MADISON

Poison Control Center (*)
University of Wisconsin
Hospital and Clinics
600 Highland Ave.
E5/238
Madison, WI 53792
Business: 608-262-7537
Emergency: 608-262-3702
            800-815-8855 (WI)

MILWAUKEE

Children's Hospital
Poison Center
Children's Hospital of
Wisconsin
9000 W. Wisconsin Ave.
P.O. Box 1997
Milwaukee, WI 53201
Business: 414-266-2000
Emergency: 414-266-2222
            800-815-8855 (WI)
Fax: 414-266-2820

B. Drugs That Should Not Be Crushed

Many common drugs come in pills that should be swallowed whole—never broken, chewed, or crushed. Some of these pills have a special coating that keeps them from dissolving as they pass through the stomach, where digestive acids could neutralize their active ingredients. Others are specially formulated to release the drug slowly, and must remain intact to stay on schedule. (Such products are usually labeled "controlled-release," "extended-release," "timed-release," or "long-acting.")

Listed in this section are many of the products—both prescription and over-the-counter—that are best swallowed whole. If the product is a solid tablet or caplet and you can't swallow pills, you'll need to ask the pharmacist for a liquid form of the drug or look for some other equivalent. If the product comes in capsule form, it's usually safe to empty the contents onto a spoonful of soft food and swallow it that way (without chewing the food). This list is not all-inclusive, so if you have any doubts about a medication you don't see here, double-check with your doctor or pharmacist.

Accutane
Acutrim tablets
Adalat CC
Adipost capsules
Aerolate III
Aerolate JR
Aerolate SR
Allerest tablets
Arthritis Foundation Aspirin
 tablets
Asacol tablets
Atrohist Plus tablets
Atrohist Pediatric capsules
Azulfidine EN-tab tablets
Bayer 8-Hour tablets
Bellergal-S tablets
Bisacodyl tablets
Bontril Slow-Release capsules
Brexin LA
Bromfed capsules
Bromfed-PD capsules
Calan SR
Carbiset-TR
Cardene SR capsules
Cardizem CD
Cardizem SR capsules
Ceclor CD tablets
Charcoal Plus DS
Choledyl SA tablets
ChlorTrimeton Allergy tablets
Claritin-D tablets
Codimal LA capsules
Codimal LA Half capsules
Colestid tablets
Comhist LA capsules
Compazine Spansule capsules
Congess JR capsules
Congess SR capsules
Contac 12 Hour capsules

Contac Maximum Strength
 12 Hour caplets
Cotazym-S capsules
Covera-HS tablets
Creon 5, 10, 20
Cystospaz-M capsules
Dallergy-Jr capsules
Deconamine SR capsules
Deconsal II
Deconsal LA
Depakote tablets
Desoxyn Gradumet tablets
Dexatrim capsules
Dexedrine Spansule
Diamox Sequel capsules
Dilacor XR capsules
Dilatrate-SR capsules
Dimetane Extentab tablets
Dimetapp Extentab tablets
Disobrom tablets
Disophrol Chronotab tablets
Donnatal Extentab tablets
Donnazyme tablets
Doryx capsules
Drixoral tablets
Drize capsules
Dulcolax tablets
Duratuss tablets
Dynabac tablets
Easprin tablets
EC-Naprosyn tablets
Ecotrin tablets
Ecotrin Maximum Strength
Endal tablets
Entex-LA tablets
Entex PSE tablets
ERYC capsules
Ery-Tab tablets
Erythromycin capsules

Erythromycin tablets
Eskalith-CR tablets
Eudal SR tablets
Exgest LA tablets
Extendryl JR capsules
Extendryl SR capsules
Fedahist Gyrocaps capsules
Fedahist Timecaps
Feosol capsules
Fero-Folic 500
Fero-Grad-500 tablets
Fero-Gradumet tablets
Ferro-Sequels capsules
Fumatinic capsules
Glucotrol XL tablets
Guaifed capsules
Guaifed-PD capsules
GuaiMAX-D
Halfprin tablets
Hemaspan caplet
Histafed-LA capsules
Humibid DM tablets
Humibid LA tablets
Humibid Pediatric
Iberet-500 tablets
Iberet-Folic-500 tablets
Imdur
Inderal LA capsules
Inderide LA capsules
Indocin-SR capsules
Ionamin
Isoclor Timesule
Isoptin SR
Isordil Tembid capsules
Isordil Tembid tablets
Isosorbide Dinitrate SR
Kadian capsules
Kaon-CL tablets
Kaon-CL-10 tablets

K-Dur 10 tablets
K-Dur 20 tablets
K-Tab tablets
Klor-Con 8/Klor-Con 10 tablets
Klotrix tablets
Levsinex capsules
Lithobid tablets
Lodine XL tablets
Mag-Tab SR
Mestinon 180 mg tablets
Minocin capsules
Micro-K Extencap capsules
MS Contin tablets
Naldecon tablets
Naprelan tablets
Nasatab LA
Nicobid Tempule capsules
Nitroglyn ER capsules
Nitrong tablets
Norflex tablets
Norpace-CR capsules
Novafed-A capsules
Optilets 500 filmtab
Optilets M 500 filmtab
Oramorph SR
Ornade Spansule capsules
Oruvail capsules
Oxycontin tablets
Pancrease capsules
Pancrease MT 10, 16, 20
  capsules
Papaverine capsules
Pavabid Plateau Cap capsules
PBZ-SR tablets
PCE Dispertabs
Pentasa
Plendil
Pneumomist
Polaramine Repetab tablets

Poly-Histine-D capsules
Poly-Histine-D Ped Caps
Prelu-2 capsules
Prevacid capsules
Prilosec
Procainamide HCl
Procanbid tablets
Procardia XL tablets
Pronestyl-SR tablets
Proventil Repetabs
Quibron-T/SR tablets
Quinaglute Dura-Tab tablets
Quinidex Extentab tablets
Respbid tablets
Ritalin-SR tablets
Rondec-TR tablets
Seldane-D tablets
Sinemet CR
Slo-bid Gyrocaps capsules
Slo-Niacin
Slow-Fe tablets
Slow-K tablets
SLOW-Mag
Sudafed 12-Hour tablets
Sular tablets
SYN-RX tablets
Tavist-D tablets
Tegretol-XR tablets
Teldrin Spansules capsules
Tenuate Dospan tablets

Tessalon Perles
Theo-24 capsules
Theobid capsules
Theoclear-LA capsules
Theochron tablets
Theo-Dur tablets
Theolair-SR tablets
Theo-Time capsules
Thorazine capsules
Tiazac capsules
Toprol XL tablets
Touro A&H capsules
Touro EX tablets
T-Phyl tablets
Tranxene-SD tablets
Trental tablets
Trinalin Repetabs tablets
Tylenol Extended Relief caplets
Uni-Dur tablets
Uniphyl tablets
Ultrase
Vanex Forte caplets
Verelan capsules
Volmax tablets
Voltaren tablets
Wellbutrin SR tablets
Zephrex-LA tablets
Zorprin tablets
Zymase capsules

C. Drugs That May Make You Sensitive to Light

Some drugs in some people can cause what's known as a photosensitivity reaction. Effects can range from itching, scaling, rash, and swelling to skin cancer, premature skin aging, skin and eye burns, cataracts, reduced immunity, damaged blood vessels, and allergic reactions.

Listed in this section are many of the more common drugs—both prescription and over-the-counter—that have been linked with photosensitivity reactions. It's difficult to predict whether any given drug will have this effect on you, but to be on the safe side, you may want to use sunscreens and protective clothing while taking a product on this list. The drugs are organized alphabetically by brand name, with generic names shown in the second column.

Brand	Generic Name
Accupril	Quinapril
Accutane	Isotretinoin
Actifed	Triprolidine/pseudoephedrine
Actifed with codeine	Triprolidine/pseudoephedrine/codeine
Adrucil, Efudex	Fluorouracil
Advil, Motrin, Nuprin	Ibuprofen
Aldactazide	Spironolactone/hydrochlorothiazide
Aldoclor	Methyldopa/chlorothiazide
Aldoril	Methyldopa/hydrochlorothiazide
Aleve, Anaprox, Anaprox DS, Naprelan, Naprosyn, EC-Naprosyn	Naproxen
Alferon N	Interferon ALFA-N3
Altace	Ramipril
Amaryl	Glimepiride
Ambenyl	Bromodiphenhydramine/codeine
Ambien	Zolpidem
Anafranil	Clomipramine
Ancobon	Flucytosine
Ansaid	Flurbiprofen
Apresazide	Hydralazine/hydrochlorothiazide
Aquatensen, Enduron	Methyclothiazide
Asendin	Amoxapine
Avonex	Interferon BETA-1a
Azo Gantanol	Sulfamethoxazole/phenazopyridine
Azo Gantrisin	Sulfasoxazole/phenazopyridine
Azulfidine	Sulfasalazine
Bactrim, Septra	Sulfamethoxazole/trimethoprim
Benadryl	Diphenhydramine
Betapace	Sotalol
Betaseron	Interferon BETA-1B
Bromfed-DM Cough Syrup	Brompheniramine/dextromethorphan/ pseudoephedrine
Capoten	Captopril
Capozide	Captopril/hydrochlorothiazide

Brand	Generic Name
Cardizem, Tiazac	Diltiazem
Chlor-Trimeton Allergy	Chlorpheniramine
Cinobac	Cinoxacin
Cipro	Ciprofloxacin
Claritin	Loratadine
Clinoril	Sulindac
Combipres	Clonidine/chlorthalidone
Compazine	Prochlorperazine
Cordarone	Amiodarone
Corzide	Nadolol/bendroflumethiazide
Cozaar	Losartan potassium
Cytovene	Ganciclovir sodium
Dantrium	Dantrolene sodium
Dapsone	Dapsone, USP
Daypro	Oxaprozin
Declomycin	Demeclocycline
Deconamine	Chlorpheniramine/D-pseudoephedrine
Demi-Regroton	Chlorthalidone/reserpine
Depakene	Valproic acid
Depakote	Divalproex sodium
DiaBeta, Micronase	Glyburide
Diabinese	Chlorpropamide
Diamox	Acetazolamide
Dimetane-DC	Brompheniramine/ phenylpropanolamine/codeine
Dimetane-DX	Brompheniramine/ pseudoephedrine/dextromethorphan
Dipentum	Olsalazine
Diucardin, Saluron	Hydroflumethiazide
Diupres	Reserpine/chlorothiazide
Diuril	Chlorothiazide
Diutensen-R	Methyclothiazide/reserpine
Dolobid	Diflunisal NSAID
DTIC-Dome	Dacarbazine
Dyazide, Maxzide	Hydrochlorothiazide/triamterene

Brand	Generic Name
Dyrenium	Triamterene
Effexor	Venlafaxine
Elavil, Endep	Amitriptyline
Eldepryl	Selegiline
Enduronyl	Methyclothiazide/deserpidine
Ergamisol	Levamisole
Esidrix, HydroDIURIL, Oretic	Hydrochlorothiazide
Esimil	Guanethidine/hydrochlorothiazide
Estar Gel, PsoriGel	Coal tar
Etrafon, Triavil	Perphenazine/amitriptyline
Eulexin	Flutamide
Fansidar	Sulfadoxine/pyrimethamine
Felbatol	Felbamate
Feldene	Piroxicam
Flexeril	Cyclobenzaprine
Floxin	Ofloxacin
Flumezide	Rauwolfia serpentina/ bendroflumethiazide
FUDR Injectable	Floxuridine
Fulvicin, Gris-PEG	Griseofulvin
Gantanol	Sulfamethoxazole
Gantrisin	Sulfasoxazole
Glucotrol	Glipizide
Haldol	Haloperidol
Helidac	Bismuth subsalicylate/ metronidazole/tetracycline HCl
Hibistat	Chlorhexidine gluconate
Hismanal	Astemizole
Hydropres	Reserpine/hydrochlorothiazide
Hygroton, Thalitone	Chlorthalidone
Hyzaar	Losartan potassium/hydrochlorothiazide
Imitrex	Sumatriptan succinate
Inderide	Propranolol/hydrochlorothiazide
Intal	Cromolyn sodium

Brand	Generic Name
Intron A	Interferon ALFA-2B
Invirase	Saquinavir
Lamictal	Lamotrigine
Lamprene	Clofazime
Lasix	Furosemide
Lescol	Fluvastatin
Levoprome	Methotrimeprazine
Limbitrol	Chlordiazepoxide/amitriptyline
Lodine	Etodolac
Lopressor HCT	Metoprolol/hydrochlorothiazide
Lotensin	Benazepril
Lotensin HCT	Benazepril/hydrochlorothiazide
Lozol	Indapamide
Ludiomil	Maprotiline
Maxaquin	Lomefloxacin
Mellaril	Thioridazine
Mepergan	Meperidine/promethazine
Mevacor	Lovastatin
Minizide	Prazosin/polythiazide
Minocin	Minocycline
Moduretic	Amiloride/hydrochlorothiazide
Monopril	Fosinopril
Mykrox, Zaroxolyn	Metolazone
Myochrysine	Gold sodium thiomalate
Naqua	Trichlormethiazide
Nardil	Phenelzine
Naturetin	Bendroflumethiazide
Navane	Thiothixene
NegGram	Nalidixic acid
Neptazane	Methazolamide
Nipent	Pentostatin
Noroxin, Chibroxin	Norfloxacin
Norpramin	Desipramine
Optimine	Azatadine

Brand	Generic Name
Orinase	Tolbutamide
Ornade	Chlorpheniramine/ phenylpropanolamine
Ortho-Novum, Ovral	Estrogen/progestin
Orudis, Oruvail	Ketoprofen
Pamelor	Nortriptyline
Parnate	Tranylcypromine
Paxil	Paroxetine
PBZ	Tripelennamine
Pediazole	Erythromycin ethylsuccinate/ sulfisoxazole
Penetrex	Enoxacin
Pentasa	Mesalamine
Periactin	Cyproheptadine
Phenergan	Promethazine
pHisoHex	Hexachlorophene
Polaramine	Dexchlorpheniramine
Polytrim	Trimethoprim sulfate/ polymyxin B sulfate
Pravachol	Pravastatin
Premarin	Estrogen
Prinivil, Zestril	Lisinopril
Prinzide, Zestoretic	Lisinopril/hydrochlorothiazide
Prograf	Tacrolimus
Prolixin, Permitil	Fluphenazine
ProSom	Estazolam
Pyrazinamide	Pyrazinamide
Quinaglute Dura-Tabs	Quinidine gluconate
Quinidex Extentabs	Quinidine sulfate
Relafen	Nabumetone
Renese	Polythiazide
Retin-A	Tretinoin
Rheumatrex	Methotrexate
Ridaura	Auranofin
Rilutek	Riluzole

Brand	Generic Name
Risperdal	Risperidone
Salutensin	Hydroflumethiazide/reserpine
Seldane	Terfenadine
Seldane-D	Terfenadine/pseudoephedrine
Ser-Ap-Es	Reserpine/hydralazine/ hydrochlorothiazide
Serentil	Mesoridazine
Sinequan	Doxepin
Solganal	Gold glynase compounds
Stelazine	Trifluoperazine
Sumycin	Tetracycline
Surmontil	Trimipramine
Symmetrel	Amantadine
Tavist	Clemastine
Tavist-D	Clemastine/phenylpropanolamine
Tegison	Etretinate
Tegretol	Carbamazepine
Tenoretic	Atenolol/chlorthalidone
Terramycin	Oxytetracycline
Thorazine	Chlorpromazine
Timolide	Timolol/hydrochlorothiazide
Tofranil	Imipramine
Tolinase	Tolazamide
Trecator-SC	Ethionamide
Trilafon	Perphenazine
Trimpex	Trimethoprim
Trinalin Repetabs	Azatadine/pseudoephedrine
Univasc	Moexipril
Urobiotic-250	Oxytetracycline/ sulfamethizole/phenazopyridine
Vaseretic	Enalapril/hydrochlorothiazide
Vasosulf	Sulfacetamide sodium/phenylephrine
Vasotec	Enalapril
Velban	Vinblastine
Vesprin	Triflupromazine

Brand	Generic Name
Vibramycin, Doryx	Doxycycline
Vivactil	Protriptyline
Voltaren, Cataflam	Diclofenac
Ziac	Bisoprolol/hydrochlorothiazide
Zithromax	Azithromycin
Zocor	Simvastatin
Zoloft	Sertraline
Zyrtec	Cetirizine

D. Sulfite-Containing Drugs

If you have asthma, there's a 1-in-20 chance that you'll have a reaction to the sulfites used as preservatives in many common drugs. (Even if you don't have asthma, the chemical might make you feel unwell.) Symptoms of a reaction range from flushing, faintness, weakness, cough, breathing problems, and a blue tinge on the skin to loss of consciousness.

Listed in this section are many of the common drugs—both prescription and over-the-counter—that contain sulfite preservatives. The products are organized alphabetically by brand name, with the generic name included. The list is not all-inclusive; so if you're especially sensitive to sulfites, your best course is to check the ingredients in every drug you take.

Brand	Generic Name
Actinex Cream, 10%	Masoprocol
Adrenalin Inhalation Solution 1:100; Injectable 1:1000	Epinephrine hydrochloride
Aldomet Injection	Methyldopate hydrochloride
Aldomet Oral Suspension	Methyldopa
Amikacin Sulfate Injection, USP. (Elkins-Sinn)	Amikacin sulfate
Amikin Injectable	Amikacin sulfate
Ana-Kit Anaphylaxis Emergency Treatment Kit	Chlorpheniramine maleate/ epinephrine hydrochloride
Antilirium Injectable	Physostigmine salicylate
Aramine Injection	Metaraminol bitartrate
AsthmaNefrin	Epinephrine
Bactrim I.V. Infusion	Trimethoprim/sulfamethoxazole
Betagan Liquifilm	Levobunolol hydrochloride
Bronkosol Solution	Isoetharine hydrochloride
Carmol HC Cream	Hydrocortisone acetate
Cortisporin Otic Solution Sterile	Hydrocortisone/neomycin sulfate/polymyxin B sulfate
Dalalone D.P. Injectable	Dexamethasone acetate
Dalgan Injection	Dezocine
Decadron-LA Sterile Suspension	Dexamethasone acetate
Decadron Ophthalmic Solution	Dexamethasone sodium phosphate
Decadron Phosphate Injection	Dexamethasone sodium phosphate
Decadron Phosphate with Xylocaine Injection, Sterile	Dexamethasone sodium phosphate/lidocaine hydrochloride
Dilaudid-5 Oral Liquid; Dilaudid Tablets—8 mg	Hydromorphone hydrochloride
Dobutrex Solution	Dobutamine hydrochloride
Duranest Injections	Etidocaine hydrochloride
Eldopaque Forte 4% Cream	Hydroquinone
Eldoquin Forte 4% Cream	Hydroquinone

Brand	Generic Name
Epifrin	Epinephrine
EpiPen Auto-Injector	Epinephrine
EpiPen Jr.	Epinephrine
Garamycin Injectable	Gentamicin sulfate
Glaucon Ophthalmic Solution	Epinephrine hydrochloride
Hydeltrasol Injection	Prednisolone sodium phosphate
Hydrocortone Phosphate Injection, Sterile	Hydrocortisone sodium phosphate
Inocor Lactate Injection	Amrinone lactate
Intropin Injection	Dopamine hydrochloride
Isuprel Hydrochloride Injection 1:5000; Inhalation Solution 1:200 & 1:100	Isoproterenol hydrochloride
Levophed Bitartrate Injection	Norepinephrine bitartrate
Levoprome	Methotrimeprazine
Marcaine Hydrochloride/ Epinephrine 1:200,000	Bupivacaine hydrochloride/ epinephrine bitartrate
Mepergan Injection	Meperidine hydrochloride/ promethazine hydrochloride
Minocin Oral Suspension	Minocycline hydrochloride
Moban Concentrate	Molindone hydrochloride
Mydfrin 2.5% Ophthalmic Solution	Phenylephrine hydrochloride
Nebcin Injection	Tobramycin sulfate
Neo-Decadron Ophthalmic Solution, Topical Cream	Neomycin sulfate/ dexamethasone sodium phosphate
NeoStrata AHA Gel	Hydroquinone
Neo-Synephrine Hydrochloride 1% Carpuject; 1% Injection	Phenylephrine hydrochloride
Nephramine Injection	Amino acids
Netromycin Injection	Netilmicin sulfate
Nizoral 2% Cream	Ketoconazole
Norflex Injection	Orphenadrine citrate
Novocain Hydrochloride for Spinal Anesthesia	Procaine hydrochloride

Brand	Generic Name
Nubain Injection	Nalbuphine hydrochloride
Numorphan Injection	Oxymorphone hydrochloride
P1E1, P2E1, P3E1, P4E1, P6E1	Pilocarpine hydrochloride/ epinephrine bitartrate
Phenergan Ampules	Promethazine hydrochloride
Pontocaine Hydrochloride for Spinal Anesthesia	Tetracaine hydrochloride/ dextrose
Pred Forte	Prednisolone acetate
Pred Mild	Prednisolone acetate
Quadrinal Tablets	Ephedrine hydrochloride/ phenobarbital/theophylline calcium salicylate/potassium iodide
Rowasa Suspension Enema	Mesalamine
S-2 Inhalant	Epinephrine
Sensorcaine-MPF with Epinephrine Injection	Bupivacaine hydrochloride
Septra I.V. Infusion and ADD-Vantage Vials	Trimethoprim/sulfamethoxazole
Solaquin Forte 4% Cream; 4% Gel	Hydroquinone
Soma Compound with Codeine	Carisoprodol/aspirin/codeine phosphate
Stelazine Concentrate	Trifluoperazine hydrochloride
Streptomycin Sulfate Injection (Roerig)	Streptomycin sulfate
Sulfacet-R Acne Lotion	Sodium sulfacetamide/sulfur
Sulfamylon Cream	Mafenide acetate
T.R.U.E. Test	Skin test antigens, multiple
Talacen	Pentazocine
Talwin Lactate Carpuject; Multi-Dose Vials	Pentazocine lactate
Tensilon Injectable	Edrophonium chloride
Terramycin Intramuscular Injection	Oxytetracycline
Thorazine Ampules/Multi-Dose Vials	Chlorpromazine
Tobramycin Sulfate Injection (Elkins-Sinn)	Tobramycin sulfate
Tofranil Ampules	Imipramine hydrochloride

Brand	Generic Name
Topicycline for Topical Solution	Tetracycline hydrochloride
Torecan Injection	Triethylperazine maleate
Trilafon Injection	Perphenazine
Tylenol with Codeine Tablets	Acetaminophen/codeine phosphate
Tylox Capsules	Acetaminophen/oxycodone hydrochloride
Tympagesic Otic Solution	Antipyrine/benzocaine/ phenylephrine hydrochloride
Vasoxyl Injection	Methoxamine hydrochloride
Vibramycin Calcium Syrup	Doxycycline calcium
Xylocaine MPF with Epinephrine Injection	Lidocaine hydrochloride/ epinephrine
Yutopar Injection	Ritodrine hydrochloride

E. Lactose- and Galactose-Free Drugs

If dairy products give you gas, bloating, and diarrhea, chances are you suffer from the condition known as lactose intolerance—an inability to digest the natural milk sugar, lactose.

Surprisingly, lactose—or one of its components, galactose—can be found in a number of common over-the-counter medications. If lactose gives you a problem, you'll probably want to look for a medication that's free of the substance. This section provides you with a handy alphabetical list of some leading lactose-free brands. To find other lactose-free remedies, check the Product Selection tables in Section 1.

Actifed capsules

Advil tablets, caplets

Allerest, all tablets

Anacin tablets, caplets

Antiminth suspension

Benadryl tablets, elixirs

Bufferin tablets, caplets

Chlor-Trimeton syrup

Colace capsules, syrup

Comtrex tablets, caplets, liquid

Congespirin tablets

Dimetane Extentabs

Dimetapp tablets, Extentabs, caplets, elixir

Donnagel liquid

Dramamine tablets, liquid

Drixoral SR tablets

Ecotrin tablets, caplets

Empirin tablets

Ex-Lax, all tablets

Feosol capsules, tablets, elixir

Fergon capsules, tablets, elixir

Fer-In-Sol syrup, drops

Geritol tablets, liquid

Imodium A-D liquid

Kaopectate tablets, liquid

Maalox, all liquids, all tablets

Mylanta, all liquids, all tablets

Nuprin tablets, caplets

Parepectolin liquid

Peri-Colace capsules, syrup

Primatene tablets

Riopan tablets, liquids

Robitussin, all syrups

Rolaids tablets

Sinarest tablets

Sine-Aid tablets, caplets

Sudafed caplets, syrups, and all tablets except Sudafed Plus

Teldrin capsules

Tempra tablets, syrup, drops

Theragran liquid

Triaminic, all syrups and drops

Triaminicol syrup

Tums tablets

Tylenol tablets, caplets, elixir, drops, Gelcaps

ViDaylin tablets, liquid